MDCT and MR Imaging of Acute Abdomen

Michael Patlas • Douglas S. Katz
Mariano Scaglione
Editors

MDCT and MR Imaging of Acute Abdomen

New Technologies and Emerging Issues

Springer

Editors
Michael Patlas
Hamilton General Hospital
Department of Radiology
McMaster University
Hamilton
Ontario
Canada

Douglas S. Katz
Department of Radiology
Winthrop-University Hospital
Mineola
New York
USA

Mariano Scaglione
Department of Imaging
Pineta Grande Medical Center
Castel Volturno
Caserta
Italy

ISBN 978-3-030-09991-6 ISBN 978-3-319-70778-5 (eBook)
https://doi.org/10.1007/978-3-319-70778-5

Library of Congress Control Number: 2018935193

Softcover re-print of the Hardcover 1st edition 2018

Printed on acid-free paper

This Springer imprint is published by the registered company Springer International Publishing AG part of Springer Nature.
The registered company address is: Gewerbestrasse 11, 6330 Cham, Switzerland

To my parents, Dr. Natan and Ludmila Patlas, to my wife Nataly, and my children Michal and Jessica.
Michael Patlas

To Darienne, my mate, my friend, my love, and my inspiration.
Douglas Katz

To Pietro and Ruben, my sons, the reason of my life.
Mariano Scaglione

Contents

Evidence-Based Imaging of the Acute Abdomen: Where Is the Evidence?

1

Ania Z. Kielar, Cynthia B. Walsh, and Matthew D. F. McInnes

Abstract

Emergency radiology is still considered an emerging subspecialty compared to more established areas such as neuroradiology and abdominal-pelvic imaging. Although this suggests that less time has passed to allow dedicated research in imaging associated with emergency medicine, it also implies that there are opportunities for study in this field in the future.

In this introductory chapter, we emphasize the importance of evidence-based medicine in radiology and then specifically in the setting of an acute abdomen. Tools available for designing and reporting research are introduced: This includes QUADAS-2 (Quality Assessment of Diagnostic Accuracy Studies), STARD (Standards for Reporting of Diagnostic Accuracy), and PRISMA (Preferred Reporting Items for Systematic Reviews and Meta-Analyses) [1, 2]. We also expand on commonly accessed information currently used to help guide radiologists in diagnosis and decision making with regard to acute abdominal and pelvic conditions.

Perceived barriers to research in emergency radiology are reviewed. Tips and specific tools to implement when designing an emergency radiology research study are provided; this information may also be useful when critically appraising published literature. Finally, an overview of emerging research opportunities and innovative areas in emergency radiology research is introduced, with focus on acute abdominal conditions, all of which will be covered in more detail in subsequent chapters of this textbook.

Keywords

Evidence-based medicine · Levels of evidence Cross-sectional imaging · Abdominal imaging Emergency radiology

A. Z. Kielar, M.D., F.R.C.P.C. (✉)
Department of Medical Imaging, The Ottawa Hospital, Ottawa, Canada

Department of Radiology Ottawa, University of Ottawa, Ottawa, Canada

Ottawa Hospital Research Institute, Ottawa, Canada

Department of Imaging, University of Toronto, Toronto, Canada

C. B. Walsh, M.D., F.R.C.P.C.
Department of Medical Imaging, The Ottawa Hospital, Ottawa, Canada

Department of Radiology Ottawa, University of Ottawa, Ottawa, Canada

M. D. F. McInnes, M.D., F.R.C.P.C.
Department of Medical Imaging, The Ottawa Hospital, Ottawa, Canada

Department of Radiology Ottawa, University of Ottawa, Ottawa, Canada

Ottawa Hospital Research Institute, Ottawa, Canada

M. Patlas et al. (eds.), *MDCT and MR Imaging of Acute Abdomen*,
https://doi.org/10.1007/978-3-319-70778-5_1

Abbreviations

ACR	American College of Radiology
ALARA	As low as reasonably achievable
CT	Computed tomography
ED	Emergency department
EPs	Emergency physicians
LLQ	Left lower quadrant
LUQ	Left upper quadrant
MRI	Magnetic resonance imaging
NPV	Negative predictive value
PICO	Patient, intervention, comparison, outcome
PPV	Positive predictive value
PRISMA	Preferred reporting items for systematic reviews and meta-analyses
QUADAS 2	Quality assessment of diagnostic accuracy studies
RLQ	Right lower quadrant
RUQ	Right upper quadrant
SAR	Specific absorption rate
STARD	Standards for reporting of diagnostic accuracy
US	Ultrasound

1.1 Background: Goals of Imaging Patients in the ED with Abdominal and Pelvic Symptoms

Imaging of patients presenting to the emergency department with abdominal symptoms has key goals of providing safe, accurate, and timely diagnoses of clinically significant abdominal and pelvic disorders. Patients with acute abdominal symptoms can have a wide range of underlying etiologies, including acute on chronic conditions. With an aging population, concomitant comorbidities may affect the emergency physician's ability to make a confident diagnosis based on physical examination alone. Increasing rates of obesity in North America and elsewhere also affect the accuracy of physical examination and lead to greater reliance on imaging. However, obesity can also negatively affect the quality of imaging, and may modify the type or modality of imaging chosen for evaluation by the radiologist [3].

Although establishing a final diagnosis is of primary concern in an emergent setting, the concept of ALARA (as low as reasonably achievable) principle should still be followed when considering imaging of patients presenting to the ED, especially those patients under 30 years of age. Radiology-initiated campaigns of "Image Wisely" in adults and "Image Gently" in children have a substantial role in emergency radiology, although imaging algorithms for assessing this patient population vary depending on the acuity of symptoms and patients' underlying level of hemodynamic stability [4, 5]. Given these principles, imaging algorithms for assessing abdomino-pelvic symptoms, and especially in pregnant patients and young patients, should begin with ultrasound, when appropriate, given that this modality is relatively ubiquitous in terms of access, is less expensive, and generally has adequate sensitivity and specificity for the diagnosis of many common acute abdominal and pelvic conditions [6]. However, in equivocal situations, in patients where ultrasound is not the imaging modality of choice (e.g., ischemic bowel evaluation), or when symptoms are discordant, MRI or CT is important for establishing a clear diagnosis.

Although there are many diagnostic tools and references available for emergency radiologists (these will be covered in subsequent chapters of this book), there are still many research questions waiting to be answered.

1.2 Perceived Barriers to Research in the Emergency Department

Patients present to the emergency department (ED) with a wide range of symptoms, signs, and underlying medical conditions. The level of acuity in this patient population varies: In many patients, urgent or emergent imaging is required, often reducing or eliminating the time needed for obtaining consent. Some patients may not be able to give consent due to reduced level of consciousness. For example, poly-trauma patients may be unconscious or hemodynamically unstable, and therefore unable to provide consent. This critical factor can be a barrier when designing research protocols, particularly for prospective studies.

Emergency departments operate 24 h a day, 365 days a year, and patients with abdominal and pelvic symptoms present at all hours. This can be a challenge to conducting prospective research, as members of the research team, including nurses and specific physicians, who are required to explain the prospective research protocols to potential study candidates, may not be present in the ED at the time consent needs to be obtained to enter a study.

Another potential barrier to research in emergency radiology is that patients who pass through the ED are usually not followed long term in the ED as compared to family practices or with other specialist physicians. The relationship between an emergency physician (EP) and patient is usually not as established as with other physicians. As a result, obtaining adequate follow-up of these patients can be difficult at times. This is particularly relevant for diagnostic accuracy research regarding determination of false-negative interpretations which often require rigorous clinical follow-up [7].

Radiologists working in the ED may either be subspecialized or work part-time in other fields and "pinch hit" in the ED. Those who work part-time in the ED often have other areas of subspecialization to which they may dedicate the majority of their research efforts. Even radiologists who are dedicated in the field of emergency radiology may find it challenging to perform certain types of research due to the nature of shift work associated with emergency radiology, coupled with the pressures of turnaround time for their final reports.

However, as we demonstrate later in this chapter, there are opportunities for research in the field of abdominal and pelvic emergency radiology which can help build upon already existing data in this growing field of imaging and intervention.

1.3 Evidence Currently Available in Emergency Abdominal Radiology

Peer-reviewed articles can be identified on numerous topics through Internet searches including Google Scholar, as well as Pubmed and many others [8, 9]. Previously published research used as supporting evidence in emergency radiology has often dealt with diagnostic accuracy of various imaging modalities to make a particular diagnosis. In some manuscripts the data included non-emergent patients, which can lead to various biases. However, more recently, "emergency-centered" or "emergency-specific" data is being published in various journals, and more recently journals specific to the field of emergency radiology have been established [10]. These publications include various types of research, including systematic reviews and single-center versus multicenter prospective studies, as well as retrospective studies, in addition to some topics which may include review articles and opinion pieces. Becoming familiar with bias in imaging research when critically appraising published articles is important. Many research efforts in emergency radiology are directed at optimizing patient outcomes, creating standardized imaging pathways, improving communication between radiologists and other physicians, as well as increasing efficiency of imaging in this patient population [10, 11].

Several resources are available to assist in assessing the completeness of research reporting and risk of bias; the tool used will depend on the study design. A large portion of imaging research is diagnostic accuracy. For this type of work, STARD 2015 can be used to assess completeness of reporting, while QUADAS-2 can be used to assess risk of bias [2, 12]. This will be described in more detail in the next section of this chapter.

Other forms of information and reference support can be accessed on the Internet. For example, the American College of Radiology (ACR) publishes Appropriateness Criteria related to numerous topics pertinent to the field of radiology which are accessible to everyone free of charge. They have organized, transparent, and reproducible methods to create their final topic development and recommendations [13]. This process utilizes structured iterative meetings of experts in the field who participate in the process of critically appraising available data and synthesizing this to develop guidelines, using the highest quality and up-to-date published data.

Within the ACR appropriateness criteria, not only is the level of supporting evidence described in the body of the text, but also the overall assigned level of appropriateness (from 0 to 9, 9 being the highest) as well as the radiation exposure related to the imaging modality and associated costs are included in tabular form at the top, for a quick overview on each topic. There has been a substantial expansion of the number of topics covered in these criteria in the past decade. They cover acute and chronic conditions, allowing a fairly robust source of support for emergency radiology [14]. For example, this website could be accessed to determine the best imaging for a patient presenting to the ED with abdominal pain and elevated lipase. Often requests for CT may be received from the ED physicians for assessment of a patient presenting with suspected pancreatitis. However, upon review of the ACR Appropriateness Criteria, unless the patient is critically ill, or if a different diagnosis is being entertained (such as ischemic bowel, in addition to pancreatitis), ultrasound is the most appropriate initial examination for imaging the biliary tract to assess for gallstones, cholelithiasis, or choledocholithiasis [15]. This type of evidence-based information helps to guide the most effective imaging for various patient scenarios.

Many other organizations, when creating guidelines or white papers for their various specialties, refer to levels of evidence when making a specific recommendation (e.g., the American Thyroid Association (ATA), the Society of Gynecology of Canada (SOGC)) [16, 17]. Describing specific levels of evidence helps to understand how to weigh different sources of information when making health-care-related decisions. Typically, higher levels of evidence have more rigorous study designs (e.g., systematic reviews rather than case reports), as well as higher quality and reliability of evidence. Creation of guidelines with indications of levels of evidence is an area of potential future work in the field of emergency abdominal and pelvic radiology.

In addition to guidelines and "white papers," various decision-support tools are also being developed through different venues, to help radiologists, clinicians, and surgeons to choose the most appropriate imaging for their patients. Some of these are available online, while others are being integrated into computer physician order-entry programs [18]. Some early publications have shown reduction in overall imaging utilization such as for pulmonary embolism CT, and radiographs of the ankles, when decision-support tools are available for physicians to follow, compared to control groups where these support systems were not available [3]. For example, in the study by Murthy et al., implementation of a clinical decision-support tool led to almost doubling of positive CT scan for assessing suspected pulmonary emboli [19]. The authors found a substantial reduction in the use of CT for this indication when the modified Wells' score was <4. This suggests that development of decision trees and associated support tools has the potential for significant positive impact on patient care. Further study is needed to quantify the direct effects of these tools on patient care, particularly in emergency abdominal and pelvic imaging [19, 20].

1.4 Growth of Evidence-Based Medicine and Tools Available

The number of publications in scientific journals has continued to grow at an increasing pace in the past several decades [21]. However, it has been documented that not all published studies are reproducible or adhere to accepted research standards [22]. There are many factors which have been proposed for this, including ones which pique the public's interest, such as the lack of research ethics approval, conflicts of interest on the part of drug companies, and even fabrication of results. However, a more common aspect of the problem facing legitimate researchers is that for a long time, no specific standards were available [23, 24]. As a result, key information was often poorly reported, thus diminishing potential usefulness of a research project.

As a goal of improving quality of medical publications, the concept of evidence-based medicine was pioneered at McMaster University in Canada and Oxford University in the UK in the mid-1990s and also applied to evidence-based imaging studies [24]. This concept incorporates research evidence, along with clinical expertise as well as patient values. The process of evidence-based medicine (and imaging) is based on five steps:

1. Ask a clinically relevant and answerable question
2. Search relevant medical literature and identify publications relevant to the topic
3. Critically appraise this literature
4. Summarize the evidence
5. Apply this evidence to clinical and imaging practices [25]

However, even with these steps in place, the various methods employed to answer a particular question have often been difficult to confidently determine. Also, the type of information to include in the methods sections and results is not always clear. It is very important that all published research, including research in the realm of emergency radiology, be reported fully, and transparently to allow readers to assess the strengths and weaknesses of the investigation. Given these various barriers that have existed for a long time, efforts have recently been made to address some of the concerns: specifically, various standards have now been developed and enhanced over time. Two such examples, which are particularly pertinent to imaging research, are STARD and PRISMA [26–28].

Many journals with high-impact factors, including Radiology and the Journal of Magnetic Imaging Resonance, now strongly encourage and in some cases even require authors to fill out checklists according to standardized tools, including STARD and PRISMA, before submitting a manuscript for review [26, 29, 30]. Reviewers use these templates to ensure completeness of the reporting such that all important factors that might contribute to bias be evident. It is therefore essential for radiologists to be familiar with these systems.

The STARD (Standards for Reporting of Diagnostic Accuracy) statement was initially developed to improve the quality of reporting diagnostic accuracy results, such as are often being evaluated in radiology publications. This tool consists of a checklist of 30 items, and a flow diagram which authors can use to ensure that all relevant information is present [26]. These items consist of essential elements of diagnostic accuracy research (e.g., index test, in sufficient detail to allow replication; whether reader of the index test was blinded to the reference standard) which allow for assessment of risk of bias and applicability.

PRISMA (Preferred Reporting Items for Systematic Reviews and Meta-Analyses) was developed as a tool for authors who are reporting systematic reviews and meta-analyses [28]. A systematic review attempts to collate all empirical evidence that fits prespecified eligibility criteria to answer a specific research question. This type of work should use explicit and systematic methods with the goal of minimizing bias. A properly conducted systematic review should provide reliable findings from which conclusions can be drawn and decisions made. This type of manuscript is considered high level of evidence as per the Cochrane Library. This is currently considered the preferred way of reporting items for systematic reviews and meta-analyses. Like STARD, PRIMSA also has a specific checklist to follow; this one includes 27 items which help guide creation and reporting of systematic reviews. Since many imaging systematic reviews are related to diagnostic accuracy, and these have particular methodologic challenges, a forthcoming extension of PRISMA for test accuracy systematic reviews (PRISMA-DTA) may be of particular relevance [31–33].

QUADAS-2 (Quality Assessment of Diagnostic Accuracy Studies) is another tool that can be used to assess the quality of and bias in primary diagnostic accuracy studies, if systematic reviews on a topic are not available [2]. This tool comprises four domains including patient selection, choosing the index test, choosing a reference standard, and optimizing flow and timing. Each domain is assessed in terms of risk of bias, and the first three domains are also assessed in terms of concerns regarding applicability. Signalling questions are included to help judge the risk of bias. The main signalling questions include the following:

1. Did the manuscript adhere to predefined objectives and eligibility criteria?
2. Were the eligibility criteria appropriate for the question being evaluated?
3. Were the eligibility criteria clearly described and unambiguous as well as appropriate based on the question being evaluated [34]?

Keeping this in mind, when reviewing and designing a study, these questions should be reflected upon to ensure that the risk of bias in results is minimized.

The QUADAS-2 tool is applied in four phases: summarize the review question, tailor the tool and produce review-specific guidance, construct a flow diagram for the primary study, and judge bias and applicability. The goal of this tool is to increase transparent rating of bias, and thereby allow better quality assessment of applicability of primary diagnostic accuracy studies [2].

For more information on reporting guidelines in general, readers are encouraged to visit the EQUATOR (Enhancing the QUAlity and Transparency Of health Research) group's website [31].

It is important to note the existence of so-called predatory journals. These are publishing business models that exploit researchers by charging publication fees to authors without providing the editorial and publishing services associated with legitimate journals [35]. It can sometimes be challenging to know which journals are in this category, both for those submitting manuscripts for potential publication and for those critically appraising literature found online. Of note, there are various websites available which publish lists of predatory journals, although these are not always kept up to date, and can change over time. One simple method to determine if a publication is from a non-predatory journal is to check if it indexed on Pubmed or Medline. Shamseer et al. published a recent article which identified 13 potential ways differentiating predatory journals from legitimate scientific publications (e.g., spelling mistakes on the website, article submission by e-mail) [36].

1.5 Setting Up a Research Project in Abdominal and Pelvic Emergency Radiology

Given the relative youth of emergency radiology as a specialty, there is a wide range of research projects which can be undertaken. This includes retrospective reviews, quality assurance and quality initiative projects, prospective studies as well as systematic reviews, meta-analyses, and smaller PICO (patient, intervention, comparison, outcome) projects. For radiology, the more pertinent construct, rather than PICO, may be diagnostic accuracy terminology of patients, index test, target condition, reference standard [37]. These various types of studies can be undertaken in a single center, or to increase sample size (and thus precision of estimate) as well as generalizability can involve multiple centers.

With respect to prospective studies, a way to ensure high quality of adherence to research standards, including development of primary and secondary outcomes, is the registration of prospective clinical trials at the outset of the study in the United States [38]. At this time there is a requirement, by law, for only certain types of studies to be registered before they start. Specifically, Section 801 of the United States Food and Drug Administration Amendments Act requires registration submission of summary results of clinical trials with ClinicalTrials.gov for certain clinical trials of drugs (including biological products) and medical devices [38]. Observational studies, such as those often performed in imaging, are not required by USA law to be preregistered, though it is still strongly encouraged. However, the International Committee of Medical Journal Editors (ICMJE) now requires trial registration

Table 1.1 Reasons for registering a research project and resultant beneficiaries

Role and purpose of registering project	Beneficiaries
Ethical obligations to participants and the research community are made public and fulfilled. Allows research boards additional information when making their recommendations about a project	Patients, research community, research ethics boards, the public at large
Provide information to potential participants and referring clinicians, so that a larger patient population can be encouraged to join a study	Patients, clinicians/ researchers
Reduce publication bias	Users of the medical literature
Clarify the context of the study, including results to journal editors prior to assigning formal reviewers	Journal editors, users of the medical literature
Promote efficient allocation of research funds, and reduce accidental repetition of a study already under way	Granting agencies, researchers

as a condition of the publication of research results generated by a clinical trial [38, 39]. ClinicalTrials.gov is a registry where organizations and individuals can provide the World Health Organization (WHO) Trial Registration Data Set required by the ICMJE, though others are also considered acceptable including www.anzctr.org.au, www.ISRCTN.org, www.umin.ac.jp/ctr/index/htm, www.trialregister.nl, and https://eudract.ema.europa.eu [38, 40–43].

There are purported benefits of such a registry, even when not mandatory, as outlined below in Table 1.1.

1.6 Areas of Current and Future Potential Research in Emergency Radiology

In emergency radiology, there are not only established tenets but also developing facets of research, all of which can also be areas of focus for future research endeavors. Many are interconnected and can be associated with various levels of evidence. Several examples, which tie into the subsequent topics covered in this book, include the following:

1. *Research investigating the value of radiology*: These areas of growing research include issues related to increasing throughput (e.g., investigations of CT protocols which do not need enteric contrast), decreasing costs (e.g., risk/benefit ratios of cross-sectional imaging of patients in the emergency department), and imaging algorithms that reduce the need for exploratory surgery or additional future imaging or intervention [44, 45].
2. *Standardization of reports and structured reporting*: This is an area of research growth throughout radiology but of particular interest to emergency radiology. Current investigations are looking to determine if structured reporting leads to faster turnaround time, if reports answer specific questions, and if they can reduce the need for additional, unnecessary follow-up imaging [46]. More research is needed to determine if this is helpful in both acute and follow-up scenarios.

Within this broad topic is the specific issue of communicating the risks of radiation from CT. This poses a particular challenge in the ED. However, the ED is a location of utmost importance to effectively and accurately discuss these risks with patients. Up to one-third of CT scans performed are ordered from the ED. Some data suggest that lifetime malignancy risk from CT may be as high as 1%, while other data are less clear [47]. Communicating the possible risks of radiation from CT to patients is therefore an important topic for emergency radiology. This poses opportunities, challenges, and avenues of work for clinical and research endeavors in emergency radiology.

Some of the barriers to effective communication of radiation risks in the ED include the urgency of cases, lack of a long-term physician–patient relationship, as well as lack of communication between emergency physicians (EPs) and radiologists. Challenges of communicating the potential risks of radiation-induced complications are substantial, both between radiologists and referring EPs, as well as to patients. Robey et al. showed that while 74% of EPs felt that radiation exposure should be discussed with patients, EPs only reported doing so with an average of 24% of patients [47]. Both patients and EPs felt that easier access to information regarding the risks of radiation is required. Data has shown that EPs and patients should discuss radiation more often in the ED. As physician uncertainty and knowledge are often primary barriers, radiologists may help to improve communication regarding radiation by helping to educate EPs [47]. A structured method to communicate these risks may help to ameliorate these barriers and could be a valuable tool.

3. *Sustainability of radiology in the era of competition with other specialties and potential changes arising from artificial intelligence (AI)* [48]*:* This includes topics of providing 24/7 coverage, including effects on patient outcomes, turnaround times, and overall costs to the health-care system, as well as sustainability within a radiology department, particularly when it is a smaller department.
4. *Investigation of new technologies pertinent to emergency radiology:* There are many areas with emerging and exciting new technologies. These include use of dual-energy CT, and MRI in acute abdominal conditions. MRI is being increasingly used in pregnant women for assessment of possible appendicitis, as well as for a growing list of intra-abdominal, gynecologic, and obstetric-related suspected diagnoses, especially if initial ultrasound is nondiagnostic.

Dual-energy CT (DECT): This topic of growing interest includes both prospective and retrospective research in the field of dual-energy CT [49].

Dual-energy CT is an emerging technique with useful applications for pathology in the abdomen and pelvis which may present to the ED. Dual-energy CT acquires images at two different energy levels simultaneously, using attenuation differences at those energy levels to obtain additional information. Some applications include virtual non-enhanced images, artifact suppression, and ability to determine composition of various materials (such as renal calculi). Several applications of DECT in emergency abdominal and pelvic radiology will be described in greater detail in other chapters of this textbook.

With DECT, the low-kilovoltage images increase contrast, resulting in decreased contrast usage and decreased radiation. This can be particularly useful in CT angiography, for the identification of subtle enhancement such as endoleaks. In addition, DECT has the benefit of reducing metallic artifact, which can be useful in imaging of patients with grafts [49, 50].

One of the emerging uses of dual-energy CT includes assessment of acute aortic syndrome. Some protocols acquire non-enhanced series, in order to more easily identify hyperdense intramural hematoma, or intimal calcifications, followed by intravenous, contrast-enhanced images. The non-enhanced images add additional radiation exposure. The virtual non-enhanced images obtained from DECT are diagnostic in approximately 95% of patients [50, 51]. The same dose reduction strategy can be applied to assessment for endoleaks in patients with prior endovascular aortic repair. While the virtual non-enhanced images are noisier, the diagnostic accuracy appears sufficient to have the potential to reduce radiation dose in the ED.

Other uses for this technology include assessment of renal calculi composition and evaluation of cystic versus solid renal masses. For example, this is particularly useful for calculi composed specifically of uric acid, which can be treated with urine alkalinization. These will be described in more detail in subsequent chapters.

5. *Reduced imaging utilization intensity, based on campaigns such as "Imaging Wisely" and "Image Gently"* [4, 5]: As introduced earlier in this chapter, this area of growing research looks at the strength of evidence to determine links between radiation exposure from imaging and future cancer development. For example, how can decision-support tools help physicians when deciding about the need for imaging of patients with acute abdominal and pelvic symptoms?

Optimization of existing technologies to reduce or limit radiation exposure is an area of ongoing research in abdominal and pelvic radiology. This includes only areas of interest in the images as well as the use of lower dose CT protocols. In terms of limiting the area of interrogation, this can be considered in young patients with suspected appendicitis, when initial ultrasound is unable to identify the appendix: although this topic is still controversial in the literature, a CT following a nondiagnostic ultrasound can be optimized to reduce radiation dose in this patient population by excluding the upper aspects of the abdomen which are not of clinical interest based on the presentation symptoms [52].

1.6.1 Lower Radiation Dose CT in Emergency Radiology

Lower dose CT (LDCT) may play an important role in the ED, due to the high volume of CT, and the young age of some of the patient population. One of the greatest barriers to LDCT is the lower signal-to-noise ratio, with resulting decreased confidence of interpreting radiologists. Some areas in which LDCT has shown promise include assessment for acute appendicitis. One study showed high specificity and positive predictive value for acute appendicitis [53]. Lower radiation dose renal colic CT scans are now being used relatively routinely in the ED [54].

Various radiation dose reduction strategies for CT imaging will be further elaborated upon in subsequent chapters of this book.

Summaries of already accrued evidence, including some of the associated strengths and weaknesses of current research evidence, will be covered in subsequent chapters, based on intra-abdominal and pelvic organs of concern. When interpreting currently published research however, it is important to maintain a critical thought process and evaluate the quality of the evidence provided.

Conclusion

The most up-to-date evidence related to imaging of acute abdominal and pelvic conditions in the emergency setting will be explained in subsequent chapters. As outlined in this chapter, there are new and growing areas where research in the ED setting has potential to grow. Although potential barriers to research exist in particular in emergency radiology compared to other subspecialties in imaging, with the use of organized and meticulous methodology to set up a research project, these can be completed successfully in ED radiology.

References

1. Bossuyt PM, Reitsma JB, Bruns DE, Gatsonis CA, Glasziou PP, Irwig L, et al. STARD 2015: an updated list of essential items for reporting diagnostic accuracy studies. Clin Chem. 2015;61(12):1446–52.
2. Whiting PF, Rutjes AW, Westwood ME, Mallett S, Deeks JJ, Reitsma JB, et al. QUADAS-2: a revised tool for the quality assessment of diagnostic accuracy studies. Ann Intern Med. 2011;155(8):529–36.
3. Modica MJ, Kanal KM, Gunn ML. The obese emergency patient: imaging challenges and solutions. Radiographics. 2011;31(3):811–23.
4. www.imagewisely.org. Accessed 1 Jun 2017.
5. www.imagegently.org. Accessed 1 Jun 2017.
6. Patel SJ, Reede DL, Katz DS, Subramaniam R, Amorosa JK. Imaging the pregnant patient for nonobstetric conditions: algorithms and radiation dose considerations. Radiographics. 2007;27(6):1705–22.
7. Deeks JJ, Macaskill P, Irwig L. The performance of tests of publication bias and other sample size effects in systematic reviews of diagnostic test accuracy was assessed. J Clin Epidemiol. 2005;58(9):882–93.
8. https://scholar.google.ca. Accessed 30 May 2017.
9. www.ncbi.nlm.nih.gov/pubmed/. Accessed 3 Jun 2017.
10. link.springer.com/journal/10140. Accessed 3 Jun 2017.
11. Loy CT, Irwig L. Accuracy of diagnostic tests read with and without clinical information: a systematic review. JAMA. 2004;292(13):1602–9.
12. Bossuyt PM, Cohen JF, Gatsonis CA, Korevaar DA, Group S. STARD 2015: updated reporting guidelines for all diagnostic accuracy studies. Ann Transl Med. 2016;4(4):85.
13. www.acr.org/~/media/ACR/Documents/AppCriteria/TopicDevelopmentProcess.pdf?la=en. Accessed 3 Jun 2017.
14. www.acr.org/Quality-Safety/Appropriateness-Criteria. Accessed 30 May 2017.
15. acsearch.acr.org/docs/69468/Narrative/. Accessed 6 Jun 2017.
16. https://sogc.org/wp-content/uploads/2013/01/135E-CPG-October2003.pdf. Accessed 6 Jun 2017.
17. http://online.liebertpub.com/doi/pdf/10.1089/thy.2015.0020. Accessed 6 Jun 2017.

18. http://www.health.gov.on.ca/en/pro/programs/ecfa/quality/standards/hsp_mrict_tool.aspx Accessed 6 Jun 2017.
19. Murthy C, Davis R, Koegelenberg CF, Irusen EM, Pitcher RD. The impact of an electronic clinical decision support for pulmonary embolism imaging on the efficiency of computed tomography pulmonary angiography utilisation in a resource-limited setting. S Afr Med J. 2015;106(1):62–4.
20. Hunt DL, Haynes R, Hanna SE, Smith K. Effects of computer-based clinical decision support systems on physician performance and patient outcomes: a systematic review. JAMA. 1998;280(15):1339–46.
21. Larsen PO, von Ins M. The rate of growth in scientific publication and the decline in coverage provided by Science Citation Index. Scientometrics. 2010;84(3):575–603.
22. Hong JP, Korevaar DA, McGrath TA, Ziai H, Frank R, Alabousi M, et al. Reporting of imaging diagnostic accuracy studies with focus on MRI subgroup: adherence to STARD 2015. J Magn Reson Imaging. 2017;in press.
23. Glasziou P, Altman DG, Bossuyt P, Boutron I, Clarke M, Julious S, et al. Reducing waste from incomplete or unusable reports of biomedical research. Lancet. 2014;383(9913):267–76.
24. Evidence-based health care: a new approach to teaching the practice of health care. Evidence-Based Medicine Working Group 1994 [updated Aug. 1994/08/01:[648–53].
25. Staunton M. Evidence-based radiology: steps 1 and 2--asking answerable questions and searching for evidence. Radiology. 2007;242(1):23–31.
26. Bossuyt PM, Reitsma JB, Bruns DE, Gatsonis CA, Glasziou PP, Irwig L, et al. STARD 2015: an updated list of essential items for reporting diagnostic accuracy studies. Radiology. 2015;277(3):826–32.
27. Cohen JF, Korevaar DA, Altman DG, Bruns DE, Gatsonis CA, Hooft L, et al. STARD 2015 guidelines for reporting diagnostic accuracy studies: explanation and elaboration. BMJ Open. 2016;6(11):e012799.
28. http://www.prisma-statement.org. Accessed 6 Jun 2017.
29. http://onlinelibrary.wiley.com/journal/10.1002/(ISSN)1522-2586/homepage/JMRI_04105_IFFA.pdf. Accessed 8 Jun 2017.
30. http://pubs.rsna.org/page/radiology/pia/checklists. Accessed 2 Jun 2017.
31. https://www.equator-network.org/library/reporting-guidelines-under-development. Accessed 22 May 2017.
32. McGrath TA, McInnes MD, Korevaar DA, Bossuyt PM. Meta-analyses of diagnostic accuracy in imaging journals: analysis of pooling techniques and their effect on summary estimates of diagnostic accuracy. Radiology. 2016;281(1):78–85.
33. Tunis AS, McInnes MD, Hanna R, Esmail K. Association of study quality with completeness of reporting: have completeness of reporting and quality of systematic reviews and meta-analyses in major radiology journals changed since publication of the PRISMA statement? Radiology. 2013;269(2):413–26.
34. http://www.bristol.ac.uk/media-library/sites/social-community-medicine/robis/robisguidancedocument.pdf. Accessed 2 Jun 2017.
35. Johal J, Ward R, Gielecki J, Walocha J, Natsis K, Tubbs RS, et al. Beware of the predatory science journal: a potential threat to the integrity of medical research. Clin Anat. 2017;30(6):767–73.
36. Shamseer L, Moher D, Maduekwe O, Turner L, Barbour V, Burch R, et al. Potential predatory and legitimate biomedical journals: can you tell the difference? A cross-sectional comparison. BMC Med. 2017;15(1):28.
37. McInnes MD, Bossuyt PM. Pitfalls of systematic reviews and meta-analyses in imaging research. Radiology. 2015;277(1):13–21.
38. https://clinicaltrials.gov. Accessed 2 Jun 2017.
39. www.icmje.org/about-icmje/faqs/icmje-recommendations. Accessed 3 Jun 2017.
40. www.anzctr.org.au. Accessed 3 Jun 2017.
41. www.umin.ac.jp/ctr/index/htm. Accessed 3 Jun 2017.
42. www.trialregister.nl. Accessed 3 Jun 2017.
43. https://eudract.ema.europa.eu. Accessed 3 Jun 2017.
44. Kielar AZ, Patlas MN, Katz DS. Oral contrast for CT in patients with acute non-traumatic abdominal and pelvic pain: what should be its current role? Emerg Radiol. 2016;23(5):477–81.
45. Gunderman RB, Boland GW. Value in radiology. Radiology. 2009;253(3):597–9.
46. Flusberg M, Ganeles J, Ekinci T, Goldberg-Stein S, Paroder V, Kobi M, et al. Impact of a structured report template on the quality of CT and MRI reports for hepatocellular carcinoma diagnosis. J Am Coll Radiol. 2017;14(9):1206–11.
47. Robey TE, Edwards K, Murphy MK. Barriers to computed tomography radiation risk communication in the emergency department: a qualitative analysis of patient and physician perspectives. Acad Emerg Med. 2014;21(2):122–9.
48. Blum A, Zins M. Radiology: is its future bright? Diagn Interv Imaging. 2017;98(5):369–71.
49. Aran S, Daftari Besheli L, Karcaaltincaba M, Gupta R, Flores EJ, Abujudeh HH. Applications of dual-energy CT in emergency radiology. Am J Roentgenol. 2014;202(4):W314–24.
50. Vlahos I, Chung R, Nair A, Morgan R. Dual-energy CT: vascular applications. Am J Roentgenol. 2012;199(5_supplement):S87–97.
51. Dick EA, Varma D, Kashef E, Curtis J. Use of advanced imaging techniques during visits to emergency departments--implications, costs, patient benefits/risks. Br J Radiol. 2016;89(1061):20150819.
52. Ahn S. LOCAT (low-dose computed tomography for appendicitis trial) comparing clinical outcomes following low- vs standard-dose computed tomography as the first-line imaging test in adolescents and young adults with suspected acute appendicitis: study protocol for a randomized controlled trial. Trials. 2014;15:28.
53. Joo SM, Lee KH, Kim YH, Kim SY, Kim K, Kim KJ, et al. Detection of the normal appendix with low-dose non-enhanced CT: use of the sliding slab averaging technique. Radiology. 2009;251(3):780–7.
54. Bhatt K, Monga M, Remer EM. Low-dose computed tomography in the evaluation of urolithiasis. J Endourol. 2015;29(5):504–11.

Radiation Dose Reduction Strategies for Acute Abdominal and Pelvic CT

2

Samad Shah, Faisal Khosa, and Savvas Nicolaou

Abstract

Since the inception of CT, its use in the emergency department (ED) has increased rapidly, raising concerns about potential risks of radiation exposure to patients, particularly the pediatric population. Therefore, radiologists should adhere to the ALARA principle, to ensure that imaging examinations are clinically indicated and to keep the radiation dose to a minimum. A substantial radiation dose reduction in abdominal and pelvic CT performed in emergency patients is achievable using the strategies described below while maintaining an acceptable level of diagnostic image quality.

Keywords

CT · Radiation exposure · Strategies · CT parameters · Iterative reconstruction

2.1 Introduction

The introduction of computed tomography (CT) has transformed diagnostic radiology. Since the inception of CT in the 1970s, its use has increased rapidly for all body parts and across all ages. CT use has increased by nearly 600% in the past decade, including its use in the emergency department (ED) setting [1, 2]. It is an increasingly utilized imaging modality for ED patients with abdominal and/or pelvic pain, in an estimated 8% of adult and adolescent ED visits [1, 3]. However, with diagnostic power comes the potential risk associated with ionizing radiation exposure. Although controversial, models implicate CT-related radiation in up to 2% of cancers in the USA, and the estimated lifetime attributable cancer mortality from abdominal CT is 1 in 700 at birth, and 1 in 5000 by age 35 [3]. Therefore, radiologists should adhere to the ALARA ("as low as reasonably achievable") principle, which is particularly important in the pediatric population. The primary components of the ALARA principle in CT are to ensure that the examination is clinically indicated, and to keep the radiation dose as low as possible, without compromising diagnostic quality. Examples of organ doses from various imaging examinations, including CT, are shown in Table 2.1.

In response to concerns about medical radiation, radiologists and manufacturers have implemented many examination protocols, software, and hardware modifications to reduce CT radiation dose [4, 5]. The purpose of this chapter is to describe the techniques used to manage and minimize abdominal and pelvic CT radiation dose in clinical practice.

S. Shah, M.D. • F. Khosa, M.D., F.R.C.P.C
S. Nicolaou, M.D., F.R.C.P.C (✉)
Vancouver General Hospital, University of British Columbia, Vancouver, BC, Canada
e-mail: savvas.nicolaou@vch.ca

M. Patlas et al. (eds.), *MDCT and MR Imaging of Acute Abdomen*,
https://doi.org/10.1007/978-3-319-70778-5_2

Table 2.1 Typical organ radiation doses from various imaging examinations

Study type	Relevant organ	Relevant organ dose (mGy)
PA chest radiograph	Lung	0.01
Screening mammography	Breast	3
Adult abdominal CT	Stomach	10
Neonatal abdominal CT	Stomach	20

2.2 Strategies

2.2.1 Before the Scan

2.2.1.1 Clinical Decision Rules

Acute abdominal/pelvic pain can be due to multiple causes [6], including appendicitis, bowel obstruction and/or ischemia, diverticulitis, cholecystitis, renal colic, pancreatitis, and gynecological disorders. The medical history, physical examination findings, and laboratory tests are the starting point, and are usually enough to diagnose and treat patients with milder signs and symptoms. In the remaining patients, they can give clues as to the nature and location of the causal process; however, they often yield nonspecific differential diagnoses which need to be narrowed or confirmed with imaging [6]. Such tests should ideally provide either substantial positive or negative information for therapeutic decisions. A positive result establishes a diagnosis, and/or its etiology and location, and it allows for staging of its severity. A reliable negative result promotes an early discharge from the ED, avoiding admissions and unnecessary expenses.

Educating referring providers and patients about the appropriate indications for an abdominal/pelvic CT examination is a critical aspect of the ALARA principle. Recent literature calls into question the use of CT in a variety of contexts, including seizures, chronic headaches, and suspected pulmonary embolism without a moderate-to-high pretest probability, and particularly questioning its use as a primary diagnostic tool for the acute abdomen in children [3]. Several educational tools are available on the Internet that can help guide referring clinicians in ordering the most appropriate imaging examinations, particularly the American College of Radiology (ACR) Appropriateness Criteria [7].

Radiologic consultation and decision support tools may help clinicians order CT for a particular clinical indication, or help recommend alternative imaging examinations including ultrasonography (US) or magnetic resonance (MR) imaging, which do not use ionizing radiation. Web-based computerized radiology order entry systems with real-time decision support for referring physicians [8] provide an appropriateness score based on clinical indications when the clinician submits a request for a relatively expensive imaging examination (MRI, CT, and nuclear cardiology). This has been shown to decrease the growth of outpatient CT volume despite an increase in outpatient clinical visits [9].

2.2.1.2 Patient Transfer and Duplicate Studies

Often duplicate imaging examinations are ordered at the time of patient transfer from one hospital to another. At Vancouver General Hospital, where the authors of this chapter work, examinations performed at outside hospitals (OHs) are imported into a patient's medical record, which usually obviates the need to immediately repeat the examination. Software programs, including Newton, LifeImage, and Mass, allow outside CT examinations to be imported into a patient's medical record. Sodickson et al. showed that importing image CDs at the time of transfer to a level I trauma center led to a 29% reduction in repeat CT examinations compared with historical controls [10].

In case of pediatric trauma, CT examinations should not be performed at an OH when a patient is being transferred for treatment, according to the Advanced Trauma Life Support (ATLS) recommendations [11–13]. Many pediatric patients already have had CT examinations performed at OHs before being transferred to a level I pediatric trauma center for specialized care [14, 15]. These examinations are often repeated at level I facilities for reasons including poor image quality, inadequate imaging, inability to upload the images to the computer system, or change in a patient's clinical condition [16]. Liepert and Cochran (2011) found that 61% of transferred trauma patients have CTs performed at both an OH and then at level I facilities. Forty-eight percent of these were of the same body area [16]. Ultimately, repeat imaging is usually associated with delays in patient care, increased cost, and increased exposure to ionizing radiation [13].

2.2.1.3 Use of Other Imaging Modalities Based on Location of Pain

Diagnostic management of acute abdominal and pelvic differs from one country or institution to another, with two major trends: early use of CT or clinical examination, complemented with radiography and/or US, with CT on request [17, 18]. Although the former option seems to improve diagnostic accuracy, prospective studies have not shown any significant differences compared with other measures [18]. Most clinical guidelines indicate that the most appropriate imaging examination depends on the location of the pain, with ultrasound being the primary choice for the right upper quadrant and the pelvis, and CT for the remaining quadrants. Laméris et al. attained maximum sensitivity with minimal radiation dose, beginning with abdominal radiography, followed by US and CT in patients with uncertain diagnoses [17].

The location of pain or tenderness is usually a helpful starting point. The American College of Radiology (ACR) has developed Appropriateness Criteria to aid physicians in ordering the most appropriate imaging examinations for specific clinical conditions.

Right Upper Quadrant

Acute cholecystitis is the primary diagnostic consideration in this patient group. The ACR Appropriateness Criteria recommend US as the initial imaging examination for patients presenting with right upper quadrant pain [19]. Although cholescintigraphy has been shown to have slightly higher sensitivity and specificity for diagnosis, US is preferred as the initial examination due to greater availability, shorter examination time, absence of ionizing radiation, morphologic evaluation, confirmation of the presence or absence of gallstones, evaluation of the bile ducts, and identification or exclusion of alternative diagnoses. CT or MRI may be helpful in equivocal patients, and may be used to identify complications of acute cholecystitis. In pregnant patients, when ultrasound findings are inconclusive, MRI is the preferred next examination [19].

Right Lower Quadrant

Acute appendicitis (AA) is the most common cause of acute right lower quadrant (RLQ) pain requiring surgery [20]. The ACR Appropriateness Criteria recommend CT as the initial imaging examination of choice for nonpregnant adult patients presenting with RLQ pain [20]. However, in children, US is the preferred initial examination. In pregnant women, US is favored initially, with MRI as the next imaging examination when US is inconclusive, which is the vast majority of such patients [20].

Left Upper Quadrant

CT is currently the primary modality used for imaging patients with acute left upper quadrant (LUQ) pain [21]. The subperitoneal compartment and peritoneal spaces of the LUQ are vital anatomic features in understanding the imaging appearance of acute diseases in this region. Disorders of the stomach, spleen, pancreatic body and tail, and colonic splenic flexure are encountered in patients with acute LUQ pain.

Left Lower Quadrant

Acute sigmoid diverticulitis is the most common cause of acute left lower quadrant (LLQ) pain in adults. Diverticulitis is often diagnosed clinically without imaging, but imaging should be considered if the diagnosis is unclear or if complications (e.g., abscess, fistula, obstruction, or perforation) are suspected. The ACR recommends CT as the initial imaging examination for the evaluation of LLQ pain [22].

2.2.1.4 Adult Females

US is the imaging modality of choice for the evaluation of pelvic pain in female patients, especially

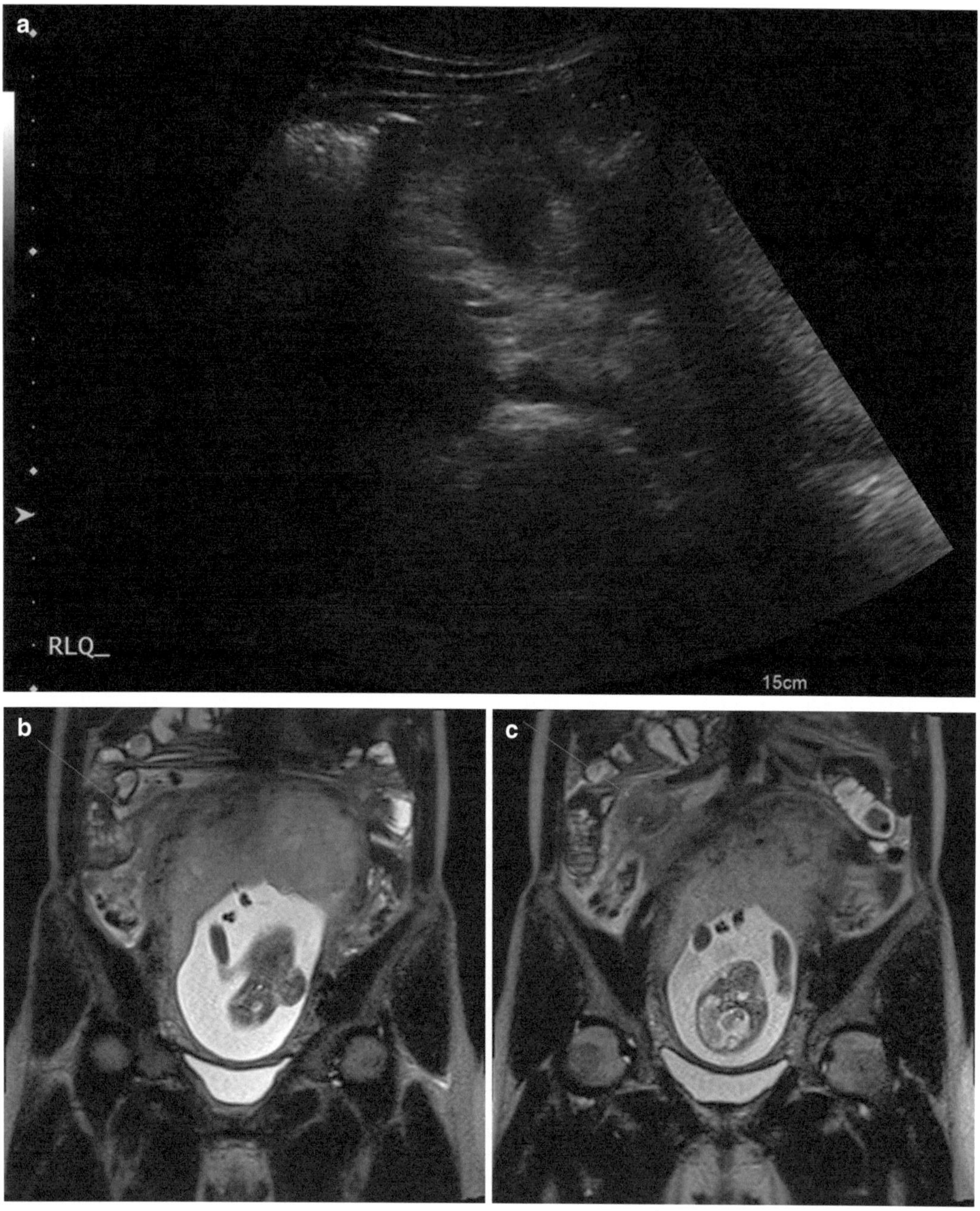

Fig. 2.1 (**a**) US of the RLQ in a 20-week pregnant woman. The appendix was not visualized. Subsequently, MRI of the abdomen was performed. (**b**) Coronal T2 fat-saturation images show a dilated appendix arising from the cecum with adjacent fat stranding (orange arrows), representing acute appendicitis. 20-week intrauterine gestation is also noted

if gynecological pathology is suspected. MRI is being increasingly used as a problem-solving tool in pregnancy (Fig. 2.1), and as a follow-up examination to reduce patient radiation exposure. Occasionally, CT will be performed after equivocal US or after US to further evaluate the findings [23].

2.2.1.5 Pediatric Population

The recent increase in the use of CT in the pediatric population is largely caused by the advent of fast helical and then multi-detector CT [24], which reduces the need for sedation [25]. Pediatric patients represent a relatively small fraction of the overall number of patients undergoing CT examinations. The combination of higher radiation doses to children for a given CT examination, and a much larger lifetime risk per unit dose of radiation, could potentially result in a significantly higher lifetime cancer mortality compared to adults. In the USA, at least 600,000 abdominal/pelvic and head CT examinations per year are performed on children less than 15 years old, and of these individuals approximately 500 may, at least theoretically, eventually die from a cancer attributable to the radiation from the CT [26]. The dose delivered in most pediatric CT examinations could be reduced by decreasing the milliampere-seconds (mAs), either manually or automatically, and by increasing the pitch [26].

2.2.1.6 Role of Conventional Radiography (CR)

CR is widely available and has been the initial imaging examination of choice for the evaluation of patients with abdominal and/or pelvic pain. However, recent studies have shown that it has limited diagnostic value for assessing abdominal/pelvic pain, and that the results infrequently change patient management [27]. Conventional radiography is appropriate for a select group of patients. It has been shown to have good accuracy for the diagnosis of suspected bowel obstruction, perforated viscus, and foreign bodies [28].

2.2.2 During the Scan

Once the decision has been made to perform a CT examination, there are many available strategies to reduce radiation exposure.

2.2.2.1 Eliminate Unnecessary Phases

It is vital to critically examine the significance of each phase in a given CT protocol. For instance, in patients with undifferentiated abdominal pain, many practices have historically performed additional pyelographic phase scans of the kidneys with the rationale that this provides additional free information. This additional acquisition usually adds approximately 30% of the radiation dose from full abdomen/pelvis scan, for very low incremental clinical yield. Similarly, in protocols for suspected mesenteric ischemia, non-contrast phase could also be eliminated, thereby eliminating this additional radiation exposure [4].

2.2.2.2 Patient Size

Small patients absorb fewer of the incident X-rays than larger patients, so to maintain similar image quality lower X-ray tube output is needed in smaller patients. The pediatric radiology community is the forerunner in this concept [29], but the general principle also holds for adult patients, as well as for imaging various body parts, particularly the extremities.

2.2.2.3 External Shielding

If used, radiation shields must be placed after the planning scout views. Otherwise, the placement of shields before the scouts causes the scanner to compensate by increasing X-ray output to penetrate the additional detected attenuation. Proponents point to substantive dose reduction from the use of overlying shields, whereas opponents argue that the shields introduce noise and artifacts [4].

2.2.2.4 CT Parameters

Automatic Tube Current Modulation

Longitudinal (z-axis): Increasing tube current or duration of an examination (mAs) results in a proportional increase in radiation dose to the patient. Tube current modulation allows the tube current to be actively modulated during the scan along the z-axis, to more efficiently apply radiation to the patient instead of using a fixed tube current. The scanner will produce fewer X-ray photons in regions of lower attenuation (caudal chest), and will modulate higher values of tube current in regions of higher attenuation (pelvis). Modulating tube current has been reported to provide up to 40% dose reduction per examination [30]. Additionally, it is used for consistency of image quality.

Axial (x-y-axis): Axial or in-plane modulation adjusts the X-ray tube output as the gantry rotates around the patient, typically increasing mAs for lateral projections, where there is more tissue to penetrate, and decreasing mAs for frontal projections, where there is less tissue to penetrate [30]. Tube output variation can be derived using heuristic estimation methods from a single orthogonal scout view.

Tube Voltage Modification

Unlike tube current, kV has a nonlinear relationship with radiation exposure. For example, a 14% decrease in tube voltage from 140 to 120 kV will decrease radiation dose by up to 30–35% [31]. Reducing tube voltage from 120 to 100 or 80 kV often permits overall reduced exposure technique, and is advised for small- and average-sized patients [31, 32]. However, a single tube voltage level is chosen for each CT examination because current CT technology does not allow real-time modulation during the exam.

Lowering tube voltage can improve image contrast for CT angiograms, as well as other high-contrast structures, including renal and ureteral calculi, since lower voltage examinations depict the presence of iodine with a greater contrast-to-noise ratio [33, 34]. However, lowering tube voltage increases image noise, which degrades image quality. Recently, automated tube voltage-assist technology has been introduced by CT manufacturers. This software aids tube voltage selection based on the patient's attenuation profile from the CT localizer and the user's chosen examination type. Importantly, the reduced tube voltage values were found to provide diagnostically acceptable image quality [35].

Reducing *z*-Axis

When evaluating a specific diagnosis such as acute appendicitis (AA), a focused CT which is limited to the lower abdomen and pelvis rather than a complete abdominal and pelvic CT scan is one way to limit radiation exposure. Several studies in adults suggest that focused CT examinations have similar diagnostic results compared to complete CT examinations while substantially reducing the overall amount of radiation to which the patient is exposed [36]. However, CT targeted to the tender region of the abdomen or pelvis may potentially have an unacceptably high rate of misdiagnosis [37]. Further prospective study is warranted to determine the diagnostic utility of partially visualized pathology, and clinical outcomes.

2.2.2.5 Low-Radiation-Dose CT

It is possible to tolerate increased levels of image noise when assessing intrinsically high-contrast structures, including renal and ureteral calculi as noted, in which reduced mA can be used. Interestingly, studies have also shown suitability of low-dose CT for assessment of low-contrast disorders, including suspected diverticulitis and AA [38–42]. However, CT is often acquired to assess or exclude many other differential diagnoses in clinical practice. In addition, these examinations had severely compromised image quality compared to standard-dose CT and did not evaluate diagnostic performance.

Subsequently, Othman et al. showed acquisition of high-quality CT images at low radiation doses with comparable diagnostic performance to standard-dose CT images using a combination of 100 kVp imaging, intermediate tube current levels, and model-based iterative reconstruction in the general setting of acute abdominal pain, regardless of the suspected clinical diagnosis [43]. However, prospective evaluations are needed utilizing low-dose CT in routine clinical practice.

2.2.3 After the Scan

2.2.3.1 Image Reconstruction Algorithms

Different mathematical algorithms are used to reconstruct images from the raw CT data. Unlike adjusting CT parameters, including kVp and mAs, reconstruction algorithms do not directly affect radiation dose, but rather help reduce noise, which consequently allows implementation of lower dose.

The first commercial CT scanners used filtered back projection (FBP) techniques because of its faster reconstruction and ease of implementation [44]. However, FBP does not permit reduction of radiation dose while trying to improve image resolution. To address some of these concerns, scanner manufacturers have introduced newer image reconstruction algorithms—namely, iterative reconstruction techniques.

Iterative Reconstruction

Iterative reconstruction techniques iterate the image reconstruction several times to better estimate mathematic assumptions, therefore requiring longer computational time and robust computers. The common endpoint of all current iterative reconstruction algorithms is to produce lower image noise and higher resolution by maintaining edges and lower artifacts [44]. This enables use of reduced-dose CT. Studies have shown lower image noise for abdominal CT at radiation doses lower than FBP [45–47]. Singh et al. showed lower image noise and improved diagnostic confidence for abdominal CT at 8 mGy with adaptive statistical iterative reconstruction (ASIR) compared with a standard dose of 17 mGy with FBP [45].

Third-Generation Iterative Reconstruction

The first and second generations of iterative reconstruction algorithms enabled dose reduction by up to 40–60% compared with FBP techniques for some clinical applications [48, 49].

A new third generation of iterative reconstruction algorithm, the model-based iterative reconstruction (MBIR), was recently developed and offers the possibility of a large reduction in image noise while improving spatial resolution (Fig. 2.2). Recent clinical studies showed MBIR to be useful in abdominal and pelvic CT examinations [50, 51]. A prospective study showed that the use of MBIR allowed a substantial reduction in dose for abdominal CT imaging by approximately 84%, compared with a standard-dose ASIR 50%, without a conspicuous deterioration in image quality [51].

2.2.3.2 Reconstruct with Smoother Kernels

Use of smoother kernels reduces image noise versus bone algorithm. The unavoidable compromise is in the loss of fine edge detail. However, this may be a helpful strategy to salvage noisy images, including those obtained in obese patients [52].

2.2.3.3 Reconstruct at Larger Slice Thickness

Image noise is proportional to the square root of the slice thickness. Therefore, decreasing slice thickness produces more noisy images, and causes automated tube modulation to increase mAs. Therefore, one should use caution in acquiring thinner slices, if they are not truly needed for the diagnostic task at hand [4].

2.3 Dual-Energy CT (DECT)

A few studies have investigated the radiation dose delivered by DECT compared to single-energy CT (SECT), with varying results. Wichmann

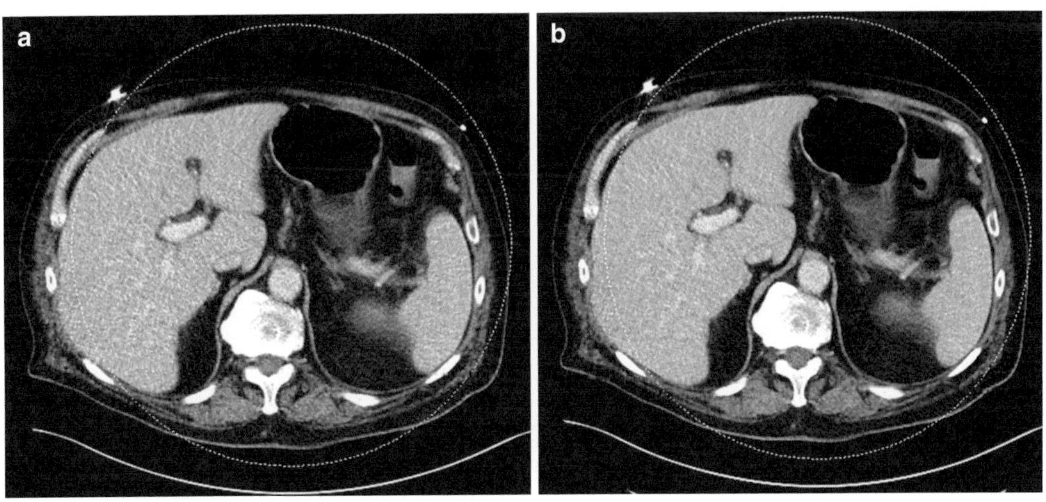

Fig. 2.2 Axial CT images at the level of the right portal vein without (**a**) and with (**b**) advanced modeled iterative reconstruction (ADMIRE). Image **a** is more noisy compared to **b**, subjectively. Both images were acquired using the same CT parameters (mA 149) at 3 mm in soft-tissue kernel

et al. showed that DECT can be performed without radiation dose penalty or impairment of image quality compared to SECT [53]. In contrast, Purysko et al. observed a significant decrease in radiation dose with DECT compared to SECT in patients who underwent abdominal second-generation SECT and DECT for hepatocellular carcinoma screening [54]. Large-scale prospective studies need to be conducted to compare radiation doses between DECT and SECT for various protocols and body parts.

2.4 Monitoring Radiation Doses

It is highly recommended to analyze dose trends with a departmental safety committee composed of radiologists, physicists, and technologists. Many authors now have their CT equipment connected to the ACR dose registry [55]. The ACR issues quarterly reports comparing CT parameters, including CTDIvol and DLP by examination type and scanner for one's institution, and compares a particular practice's averages to US national averages.

Dose tracking software can identify outliers within a department or practice by CT scanner and examination type. By setting alerts if radiation dose thresholds are exceeded, quality metrics can be maintained in a retrospective fashion. If outlier results are identified, then the examination can be reviewed by the site to determine if the protocol was followed and correct technique was used [30]. It is important to create a departmental culture to monitor image quality and examination dose (Fig. 2.3).

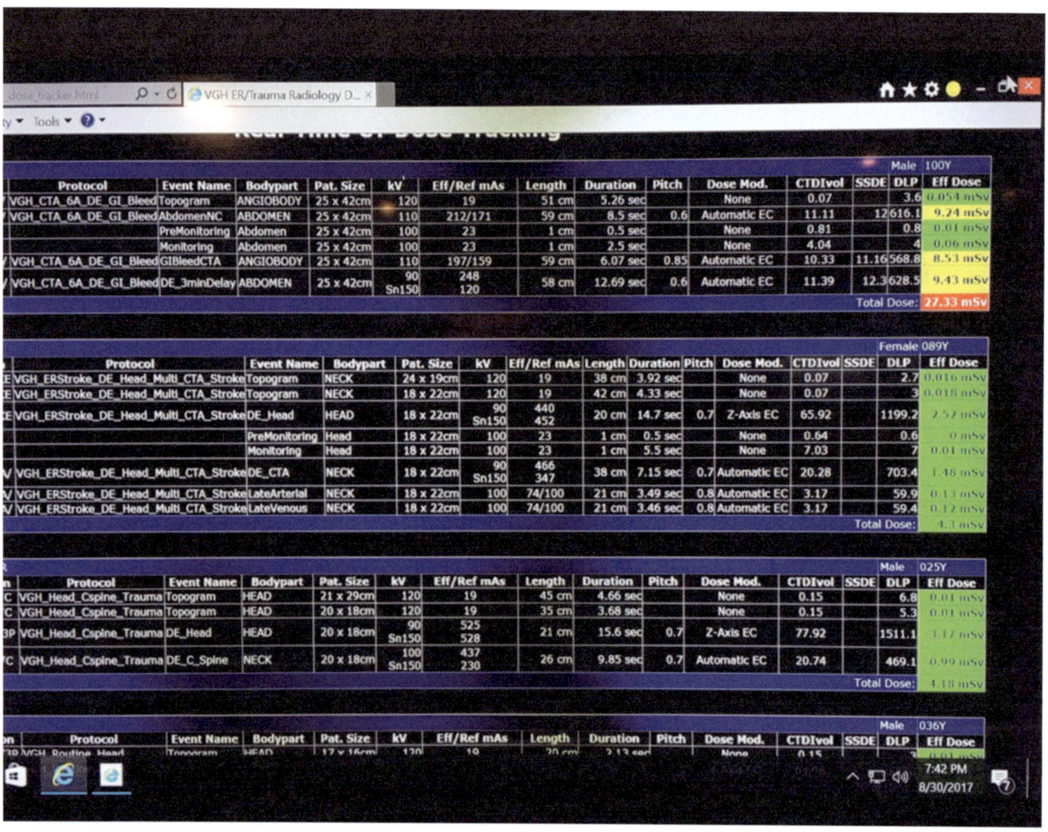

Fig. 2.3 Real-time dose monitor in the emergency radiology consultation room at the authors' institution. For each patient, the number of examinations, patient size, and CT parameters are shown. Left side of the screen containing patient demographics was cropped

Conclusion

A substantial dose reduction of abdominal/pelvic CT performed in emergency patients is achievable using strategies that target simple adjustments (e.g., the number of phases of acquisition), technical optimization (e.g., mAs and kVp reduction), and use of indication-specific protocoling while maintaining an acceptable level of diagnostic image quality. In addition to the above strategies, we must develop and implement training programs for young clinicians, and foster constructive discussion in multidisciplinary sessions, while promoting the role of the radiologist as a consultant.

References

1. Broder J, Warshauer DM. Increasing utilization of computed tomography in the adult emergency department, 2000-2005. Emerg Radiol. 2006;13(1):25–30.
2. Broder J, Fordham LA, Warshauer DM. Increasing utilization of computed tomography in the pediatric emergency department, 2000-2006. Emerg Radiol. 2007;14(4):227–32.
3. Brenner DJ, Hall EJ. Computed tomography—an increasing source of radiation exposure. N Engl J Med. 2007;357(22):2277–84.
4. Sodickson A. Strategies for reducing radiation exposure in multi-detector row CT. Radiol Clin N Am. 2012;50(1):1–14.
5. McCollough CH, Chen GH, Kalender W, Leng S, Samei E, Taguchi K, et al. Achieving routine submillisievert CT scanning: report from the summit on management of radiation dose in CT. Radiology. 2012;264(2):567–80.
6. Gans SL, Stoker J, Boermeester MA. Plain abdominal radiography in acute abdominal pain; past, present, and future. Int J Gen Med. 2012;5:525–33.
7. ACR Appropriateness Criteria®—American College of Radiology. 2017. https://www.acr.org/Quality-Safety/Appropriateness-Criteria.
8. Rosenthal DI, Weilburg JB, Schultz T, Miller JC, Nixon V, Dreyer KJ, et al. Radiology order entry with decision support: initial clinical experience. J Am Coll Radiol. 2006;3(10):799–806.
9. Sistrom CL, Dang PA, Weilburg JB, Dreyer KJ, Rosenthal DI, Thrall JH. Effect of computerized order entry with integrated decision support on the growth of outpatient procedure volumes: seven-year time series analysis. Radiology. 2009;251(1):147–55.
10. Sodickson A, Opraseuth J, Ledbetter S. Outside imaging in emergency department transfer patients: CD import reduces rates of subsequent imaging utilization. Radiology. 2011;260(2):408–13.
11. Chatoorgoon K, Huezo K, Rangel E, François N, Schweer L, Daugherty M, et al. Unnecessary imaging, not hospital distance, or transportation mode impacts delays in the transfer of injured children. Pediatr Emerg Care. 2010;26(7):481–6.
12. Haley T, Ghaemmaghami V, Loftus T, Gerkin RD, Sterrett R, Ferrara JJ. Trauma: the impact of repeat imaging. Am J Surg. 2009;198(6):858–62.
13. Emick DM, Carey TS, Charles AG, Shapiro ML. Repeat imaging in trauma transfers: a retrospective analysis of computed tomography scans repeated upon arrival to a level I trauma center. J Trauma Acute Care Surg. 2012;72(5):1255–62.
14. Newgard CD, McConnell KJ, Hedges JR, Mullins RJ. The benefit of higher level of care transfer of injured patients from nontertiary hospital emergency departments. J Trauma. 2007;63(5):965–71.
15. Gupta R, Greer SE, Martin ED. Inefficiencies in a rural trauma system: the burden of repeat imaging in interfacility transfers. J Trauma. 2010;69(2):253–5.
16. Liepert AE, Cochran A. CT utilization in transferred trauma patients. J Surg Res. 2011;170(2):309–13.
17. Laméris W, van Randen A, van Es HW, van Heesewijk JPM, van Ramshorst B, Bouma WH, et al. Imaging strategies for detection of urgent conditions in patients with acute abdominal pain: diagnostic accuracy study. BMJ. 2009;338:b2431.
18. Sala E, Watson CJE, Beadsmoore C, Groot-Wassink T, Fanshawe TR, Smith JC, et al. A randomized, controlled trial of routine early abdominal computed tomography in patients presenting with non-specific acute abdominal pain. Clin Radiol. 2007; 62(10):961–9.
19. Yarmish GM, Smith MP, Rosen MP, Baker ME, Blake MA, Cash BD, et al. ACR appropriateness criteria right upper quadrant pain. J Am Coll Radiol. 2014;11(3):316–22.
20. Smith MP, Katz DS, Lalani T, Carucci LR, Cash BD, Kim DH, et al. ACR appropriateness criteria® right lower quadrant pain--suspected appendicitis. Ultrasound Q. 2015;31(2):85–91.
21. Ecanow JS, Gore RM. Evaluating patients with left upper quadrant pain. Radiol Clin N Am. 2015;53(6):1131–57.
22. ACR Appropriateness Criteria® left lower quadrant pain—suspected diverticulitis. National guideline clearinghouse. 2017. https://www.guideline.gov/summaries/summary/48282.
23. Vandermeer FQ, Wong-You-Cheong JJ. Imaging of acute pelvic pain. Clin Obstet Gynecol. 2009; 52(1):2–20.
24. Frush DP, Donnelly LF. Helical CT in children: technical considerations and body applications. Radiology. 1998;209(1):37–48.
25. White KS. Invited article: helical/spiral CT scanning: a pediatric radiology perspective. Pediatr Radiol. 1996;26(1):5–14.

26. Brenner D, Elliston C, Hall E, Berdon W. Estimated risks of radiation-induced fatal cancer from pediatric CT. AJR Am J Roentgenol. 2001;176(2):289–96.
27. Kellow ZS, MacInnes M, Kurzencwyg D, Rawal S, Jaffer R, Kovacina B, et al. The role of abdominal radiography in the evaluation of the nontrauma emergency patient. Radiology. 2008;248(3):887–93.
28. Stoker J, van Randen A, Laméris W, Boermeester MA. Imaging patients with acute abdominal pain. Radiology. 2009;253(1):31–46.
29. Pediatric radiology & imaging – Radiation safety – image gently. 2017. http://www.imagegently.org/.
30. Mayo-Smith WW, Hara AK, Mahesh M, Sahani DV, Pavlicek W. How I do it: managing radiation dose in CT. Radiology. 2014;273(3):657–72.
31. Huda W, Mettler FA. Volume CT dose index and dose-length product displayed during CT: what good are they? Radiology. 2011;258(1):236–42.
32. Yu L, Li H, Fletcher JG, McCollough CH. Automatic selection of tube potential for radiation dose reduction in CT: a general strategy. Med Phys. 2010;37(1):234–43.
33. Hough DM, Fletcher JG, Grant KL, Fidler JL, Yu L, Geske JR, et al. Lowering kilovoltage to reduce radiation dose in contrast-enhanced abdominal CT: initial assessment of a prototype automated kilovoltage selection tool. AJR Am J Roentgenol. 2012;199(5):1070–7.
34. Winklehner A, Goetti R, Baumueller S, Karlo C, Schmidt B, Raupach R, et al. Automated attenuation-based tube potential selection for thoracoabdominal computed tomography angiography: improved dose effectiveness. Investig Radiol. 2011;46(12):767–73.
35. Goetti R, Winklehner A, Gordic S, Baumueller S, Karlo CA, Frauenfelder T, et al. Automated attenuation-based kilovoltage selection: preliminary observations in patients after endovascular aneurysm repair of the abdominal aorta. AJR Am J Roentgenol. 2012;199(3):W380–5.
36. Corwin MT, Chang M, Fananapazir G, Seibert A, Lamba R. Accuracy and radiation dose reduction of a limited abdominopelvic CT in the diagnosis of acute appendicitis. Abdom Imaging. 2015;40(5):1177–82.
37. Broder JS, Hollingsworth CL, Miller CM, Meyer JL, Paulson EK. Prospective double-blinded study of abdominal-pelvic computed tomography guided by the region of tenderness: estimation of detection of acute pathology and radiation exposure reduction. Ann Emerg Med. 2010;56(2):126–34.
38. Kim SH, Yoon J-H, Lee JH, Lim Y-J, Kim OH, Ryu JH, et al. Low-dose CT for patients with clinically suspected acute appendicitis: optimal strength of sinogram affirmed iterative reconstruction for image quality and diagnostic performance. Acta Radiol. 2015;56(8):899–907.
39. Karabulut N, Kiroglu Y, Herek D, Kocak TB, Erdur B. Feasibility of low-dose unenhanced multidetector CT in patients with suspected acute appendicitis: comparison with sonography. Clin Imaging. 2014;38(3):296–301.
40. Remer EM, Herts BR, Primak A, Obuchowski NA, Greiwe A, Roesel DM, et al. Detection of urolithiasis: comparison of 100% tube exposure images reconstructed with filtered back projection and 50% tube exposure images reconstructed with sinogram-affirmed iterative reconstruction. Radiology. 2014;272(3):749–56.
41. Poletti P-A, Platon A, Rutschmann OT, Schmidlin FR, Iselin CE, Becker CD. Low-dose versus standard-dose CT protocol in patients with clinically suspected renal colic. AJR Am J Roentgenol. 2007;188(4):927–33.
42. Laqmani A, Veldhoen S, Dulz S, Derlin T, Behzadi C, Schmidt-Holtz J, et al. Reduced-dose abdominopelvic CT using hybrid iterative reconstruction in suspected left-sided colonic diverticulitis. Eur Radiol. 2016;26(1):216–24.
43. Othman AE, Bongers MN, Zinsser D, Schabel C, Wichmann JL, Arshid R, et al. Evaluation of reduced-dose CT for acute non-traumatic abdominal pain: evaluation of diagnostic accuracy in comparison to standard-dose CT. Acta Radiol. 2017;13:028418511770315.
44. Padole A, Ali Khawaja RD, Kalra MK, Singh S. CT radiation dose and iterative reconstruction techniques. Am J Roentgenol. 2015;204(4):W384–92.
45. Singh S, Kalra MK, Hsieh J, Licato PE, Do S, Pien HH, et al. Abdominal CT: comparison of adaptive statistical iterative and filtered back projection reconstruction techniques. Radiology. 2010;257(2):373–83.
46. Singh S, Kalra MK, Do S, Thibault JB, Pien H, O'Connor OJ, et al. Comparison of hybrid and pure iterative reconstruction techniques with conventional filtered back projection: dose reduction potential in the abdomen. J Comput Assist Tomogr. 2012;36(3):347–53.
47. Gervaise A, Naulet P, Beuret F, Henry C, Pernin M, Portron Y, et al. Low-dose CT with automatic tube current modulation, adaptive statistical iterative reconstruction, and low tube voltage for the diagnosis of renal colic: impact of body mass index. AJR Am J Roentgenol. 2014;202(3):553–60.
48. Gervaise A, Osemont B, Louis M, Lecocq S, Teixeira P, Blum A. Standard dose versus low-dose abdominal and pelvic CT: comparison between filtered back projection versus adaptive iterative dose reduction 3D. Diagn Interv Imaging. 2014;95(1):47–53.
49. McLaughlin PD, Murphy KP, Hayes SA, Carey K, Sammon J, Crush L, et al. Non-contrast CT at comparable dose to an abdominal radiograph in patients with acute renal colic; impact of iterative reconstruction on image quality and diagnostic performance. Insights Imaging. 2014;5(2):217–30.
50. Pickhardt PJ, Lubner MG, Kim DH, Tang J, Ruma JA, del Rio AM, et al. Abdominal CT with model-based iterative reconstruction (MBIR): initial results of a prospective trial comparing ultralow-dose with

standard-dose imaging. AJR Am J Roentgenol. 2012;199(6):1266–74.

51. Yasaka K, Katsura M, Akahane M, Sato J, Matsuda I, Ohtomo K. Model-based iterative reconstruction for reduction of radiation dose in abdominopelvic CT: comparison to adaptive statistical iterative reconstruction. Springerplus. 2013;2(1):209.
52. Modica MJ, Kanal KM, Gunn ML. The obese emergency patient: imaging challenges and solutions. Radiographics. 2011;31(3):811–23.
53. Wichmann JL, Hardie AD, Schoepf UJ, Felmly LM, Perry JD, Varga-Szemes A, et al. Single- and dual-energy CT of the abdomen: comparison of radiation dose and image quality of 2nd and 3rd generation dual-source CT. Eur Radiol. 2017;27(2):642–50.
54. Purysko AS, Primak AN, Baker ME, Obuchowski NA, Remer EM, John B, et al. Comparison of radiation dose and image quality from single-energy and dual-energy CT examinations in the same patients screened for hepatocellular carcinoma. Clin Radiol. 2014;69(12):e538–44.
55. Dose index registry - American College of Radiology. 2017. https://www.acr.org/Quality-Safety/National-Radiology-Data-Registry/Dose-Index Registry.

3 Dual-Energy CT in Patients with an Acute Abdomen

HeiShun Yu, David D. B. Bates, and Dushyant V. Sahani

Abstract

Over the past two decades, multidetector computed tomography (CT) has become a powerful diagnostic tool in emergency medicine relied upon for a variety of conditions. More recently, the development of dual-energy CT technology has enhanced the ability of radiologists to diagnose and distinguish between a variety of conditions, improving accuracy and patient care. The ability to separate material density pairs allows for highly specific observations, and helps to avoid diagnostic pitfalls. Dual-energy CT has benefits in diagnosing conditions of the liver, gallbladder, kidneys, adrenals, pancreas, large and small bowel, as well as vascular structures. It also has benefits in diagnostic evaluation of patients in the setting of trauma. When its benefits are harnessed, dual-energy CT has the potential to significantly improve patient care in the emergency department.

H. Yu, M.D.
Brigham and Women's Hospital, Boston, MA, USA

D. D. B. Bates, M.D.
Memorial Sloan Kettering Cancer Center, New York, NY, USA

D. V. Sahani (✉)
Massachusetts General Hospital, Boston, MA, USA
e-mail: DSAHANI@mgh.harvard.edu

3.1 Introduction

Use of computed tomography in the evaluation of patients in the emergency department (ED) has grown markedly in recent years [1]. The percentage of patients being seen in the ED who undergo CT as part of their ED visit increased from 2.8% in 1995 to 13.9% by 2007 [2]. The increase in imaging volume has been possible because of several technological advances, namely the widespread use of multi-detector CT (MDCT) scanners, and computer hardware and software which enables rapid multi-planar reformatting. The rapid acquisition and processing have led to the use of CT as a primary modality for the evaluation of a number of acute conditions, both traumatic and nontraumatic. In body imaging, CT is used extensively to evaluate a wide variety of conditions affecting the vasculature, genitourinary, biliary, digestive, and musculoskeletal systems.

Dual-energy CT (DECT) has emerged as a very useful tool in emergency radiology, and has many potential applications in body imaging. Conventional single-energy CT creates images based on the X-ray attenuation properties of anatomic structures from a single energy source. DECT is able to provide the same information as single-energy CT, but has the added benefit of being able to separate materials based on their material density, as different materials demonstrate different attenuation properties when there is a change in the kilovoltage peak (kVp).

M. Patlas et al. (eds.), *MDCT and MR Imaging of Acute Abdomen*,
https://doi.org/10.1007/978-3-319-70778-5_3

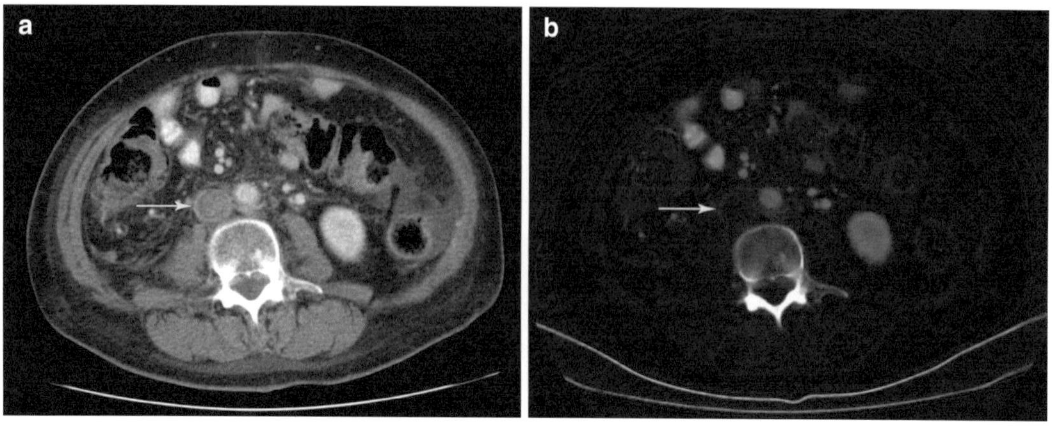

Fig. 3.1 64-year-old woman with a history of cholangiocarcinoma with liver metastases presents with progressive abdominal pain. (**a**) Axial IV contrast-enhanced CT image performed with dual-energy technique demonstrates heterogeneous hypoattenuation in the inferior vena cava (arrow), which may be interpreted as contrast mixing, bland thrombus, or tumor thrombus. (**b**) On the corresponding axial iodine image, the finding is more apparent. The iodine image offers additional information as the absence of iodine within the thrombus (arrow) is more consistent with bland thrombus, rather than tumor thrombus

In this chapter, the technical aspects of DECT are discussed, along with a variety of conditions for which DECT may be useful to the emergency radiologist. The potential benefits of DECT in the ED are very substantial, both for assisting in the diagnosis of acute conditions, and for problem solving when encountering incidental findings which require characterization (Fig. 3.1).

3.2 Technique

Conventional single-energy computed tomography utilizes a single polychromatic X-ray beam, with peak energy levels ranging from 80 to 140 kVp, emitted from a single X-ray tube to a single detector. In contrast, dual-energy CT (DECT) acquires images utilizing two energy spectra. Typically, low-energy images are acquired using 80 kVp, while high-energy images acquired using 140 kVp [3–6]. Some scanners (e.g., Somatom Force, Siemens Healthcare) allow variations (e.g., low energy 100 kVp, and high energy 150 kVp).

There are three DECT platforms which are currently commercially available: dual-source DECT, single-source (rapid kV switching) DECT, and detector-based spectral CT. Dual-source DECT (Siemens Healthcare) utilizes two perpendicular X-ray tubes and two corresponding sets of detectors for image acquisition. Rapid kV switching DECT, available from several CT vendors, utilizes a single X-ray tube which rapidly alternates (0.5 msc) between low and high energies, along with a single detector. The third mechanism (referred to as "spectral" CT; Philips Healthcare) involves utilization of a single X-ray tube, with a detector with a top layer which absorbs low energy, and a deep layer which absorbs high-energy X-rays [4, 7].

Image contrast is dependent on attenuation of X-ray photons by varying materials, which is in turn influenced by the photon energy level in relation to the k-edge of the material. The k-edge refers to the K-shell electron-binding energy. As photon energy level approaches the k-edge of a given material, there is a sharp increase in the attenuation coefficient [8, 9]. By obtaining information of a tissue at two different energies, dual-energy CT technology can generate image datasets with attenuation information at several virtual monochromatic (VMC) X-ray energy levels, ranging from 40 to 140 kiloelectron volts (keV). Selection of VMC energy level can be used to optimize image contrast. For example, 40–70 keV VMC images can be reconstructed for the purpose of accentuating iodine enhancement [7, 10]. Significant gain in iodine attenuation on 40–60 keV images has been used to reduce iodine dose on DECT exams. Previous investigations have reported 50–70% reduction in iodine doses for CT angiography by using 40–50 kev VMC images from DECT [10–13]. Despite a current controversy over post-contrast acute kidney injury (AKI), there is still concern about its existence. Therefore, using minimal iodine dose is desirable, especially in the emergency setting, particularly when a patient's renal function may be unknown. This is particularly relevant in the setting of vascular injury, where a subsequent angiogram may be necessary. Contrast-media dose reduction must be accompanied with adjustments in injection rate in order to yield homogeneous vascular enhancement. Total iodine dose reduction can be achieved with both high- and low-concentration contrast media (CM). Low-concentration CM enable higher volumes on low-contrast computed tomography angiography (CTA) examinations. However, high-concentration CM needs to be mixed with saline to preserve volume [11].

On the other end of the spectrum, 80–140 keV images can also be generated to help reduce beam hardening and photon starvation artifacts related to metallic prostheses or foreign bodies [14, 15]. These artifacts are typically seen on conventional CT as a result of attenuation of low-energy photons in a polychromatic X-ray. Similarly, these images can be used to decrease the pseudo-enhancement which is relatively commonly seen in smaller cysts and soft-tissue nodules [4, 16].

Besides virtual monochromatic images, knowledge of the attenuation characteristics of a tissue at different X-ray energies also allows the creation of material-specific images. Given that different materials have different absorb X-ray photons in a unique way, several material density (MD) images can be created to analyze the composition of various tissues. Currently, the most commonly used MD images are MD-I images (iodine maps) and water-density (virtual non-enhanced) images. MD-I images exclusively show iodine contribution within the image, and do not take into account the inherent attenuation of the tissue. Therefore, iodine maps are helpful for detection of iodine content or enhancement within a nodule or mass [4, 5]. In the emergency setting, this is useful for the appropriate "triaging" of incidental nodules or masses. This will be discussed in further detail.

Virtual non-enhanced (VNE) images can be helpful for detecting the presence of calcium in a nodule or mass. A common misconception is that DECT imparts higher radiation doses than conventional CT. While this may have been true early in the development of DECT, this is not the case with current DECT technology [12]. On the contrary, current DECT technology may allow for radiation dose savings as VNE images can be constructed, which may in turn forgo the need for a conventional non-enhanced acquisition [16] (Table 3.1).

Table 3.1 Summary of emergency applications of dual-energy computed tomography in abdominal imaging

Gallbladder	
Gallstone disease	Lower energy scans may reveal cholesterol stones, which may be inapparent on conventional CT images
Acute cholecystitis	Increased sensitivity for detection of gangrenous cholecystitis; improved characterization of gallbladder wall enhancement and intraluminal membranes
Pancreas	
Acute pancreatitis	Increased sensitivity to diagnose gallstone pancreatitis
	Detection of necrotizing or hemorrhagic pancreatitis
	Potential reduced radiation exposure
Kidney	
Nephrolithiasis	Increased detection of renal calculi on IV contrast-enhanced CT, when contrast may opacify collecting system/ureters
	Characterize calculus composition
Incidental focal renal mass	Distinguished incidental enhancing renal masses from hyperdense cysts and pseudo-enhancement
Obstructing urothelial mass	Increased conspicuity of enhancing urothelial mass causing obstruction

(continued)

Table 3.1 (continued)

Adrenal	
Incidental adrenal nodule	Characterize incidental adrenal nodule/mass using VNE images
Bowel	
Acute gastrointestinal hemorrhage	Increased sensitivity to detect and localized acute GI bleeding
Bowel ischemia	Lower kVp increases conspicuity of early bowel ischemia
Aorta	
Traumatic aortic injury	Detection of intramural aortic hematoma using VNC images
	Increased detection of leaks from repaired aortic aneurysms
Traumatic solid visceral injury	Increased conspicuity of solid visceral lacerations
	Improved visualization of contrast extravasation
Traumatic musculoskeletal injury	Increased detection of subtle non-displaced fractures
	Characterize spinal compression fractures as acute or chronic based on the presence of bone marrow edema and/or hemorrhage

VNE virtual non-enhanced

3.3 Gallbladder

3.3.1 Gallstone Disease

Gallstone disease is a common cause for right upper quadrant pain leading to an emergency department visit. Of patients that have gallstone disease, 10–15% will pass calculi into the central bile ducts leading to biliary obstruction, and frequently to subsequent acute cholecystitis or cholangitis [17, 18].

While CT is helpful for detection of hyperattenuating and hypoattenuating calculi, many calculi are essentially isoattenuating to bile within the gallbladder, and are therefore difficult to identify on conventional CT. This can be particularly true when calculi isoattenuating to bile are lodged in the common duct. Dual-energy CT can be helpful in these patients, for calculus detection and characterization (Fig. 3.2). With regard to detection, studies have shown that acquiring imaging with a lower energy (i.e., 40 keV) increases sensitivity for detection of gallstones [18, 19] (Fig. 3.2).

In addition to detection of cholelithiasis, a possible application of DECT is to determine the gallstone composition, as calculi of higher cholesterol content have been shown to have relatively lower attenuation [20, 21]. Given that these calculi may be treated conservatively, prospective characterization may lead clinicians to a more conservative approach [18].

3.3.2 Acute Cholecystitis

Acute cholecystitis is readily diagnosed using conventional CT, with reported sensitivity and specificity greater than 90% [22]. Gangrenous cholecystitis, however, presents a diagnostic challenge. The sensitivity for diagnosing gangrenous cholecystitis on CT is significantly lower at 29% [22]. The implications for missing this diagnosis are potentially serious, as it carries a higher morbidity and mortality. On conventional CT, the main findings suggestive of gangrenous cholecystitis include gas in the wall, intraluminal membranes, and discontinuous or irregular wall and mural striation [22]. While intramural gas in the gallbladder wall is easily detected on conventional CT, the other findings are often more difficult to detect [22]. Dual-energy CT can be helpful in these patients, particularly with iodine maps as areas of enhancement and relative hypoenhancement are easily detected. This may help accentuate areas of wall discontinuity. Intraluminal membranes may also be accentuated by evaluating intraluminal contents with low-keV images, which increases the contrast between the sloughed membranes and the surrounding infected biliary fluid. It may also be easier to see intramural hematoma in the gallbladder wall using VNE images with DECT.

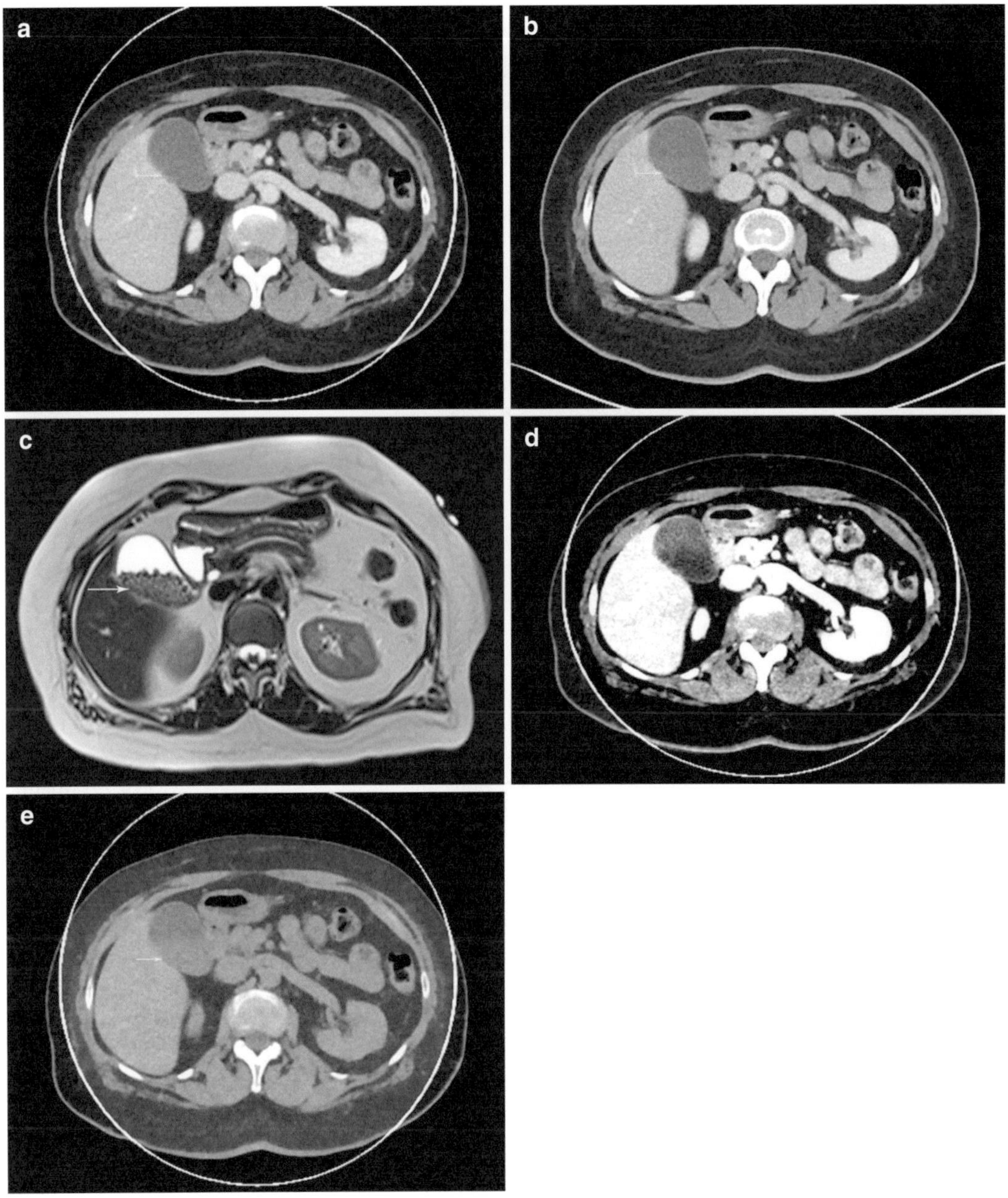

Fig. 3.2 68-year-old man with noncalcified gallstones which are isodense to bile on axial 70 keV (**a**) and mixed images (**b**) on dual-energy CT. The presence of calculi is confirmed on an axial T2-weighted single-shot fast spin-echo MR image (**c**). The calculi decrease in attenuation using virtual monochromatic images at 40 keV (**d**), and increase in attenuation at 190 keV (**e**), with corresponding increase in conspicuity relative to surrounding bile. The dependent gallstones have the lowest HU values at 40 keV (**d**), are isoattenuating at 70 keV (**a**), and are hyperattenuating at 190 keV (**e**)

3.4 Pancreas

3.4.1 Acute Pancreatitis

Acute pancreatitis is one of the most commonly encountered conditions in the emergency setting. Most commonly, the etiology is alcohol induced or gallstone related. In the latter scenario, DECT may be helpful in identifying choledocholithiasis. Because low-keV images can be used to increase conspicuity of certain types of calculi (i.e., cholesterol stones), DECT may increase sensitivity for gallstone detection [23], enabling a faster diagnosis of gallstone pancreatitis without having to then perform MR cholangiopancreatography.

Dual-energy CT may also be helpful in the setting of acute pancreatitis, because it can be used to identify complications, including pancreatic necrosis and hemorrhage. Pancreatic necrosis can be difficult to detect on conventional CT, as areas of hypoenhancement may be subtle. When identified, it is often unclear whether these areas represent areas of necrosis or ischemia. Using DECT, iodine maps can be constructed to help detect areas of subtle enhancement, which suggest ischemia rather than necrosis [4, 14]. Necrotic regions appear as areas without any iodine uptake (Fig. 3.3). Patients with necrotizing pancreatitis are generally managed more aggressively, so the distinction is pertinent [4].

Hemorrhagic pancreatitis can also be accurately diagnosed with the aid of DECT. On conventional contrast-enhanced CT, hyperattenuating regions may represent hemorrhage or enhancing pancreatic parenchyma. In such patients, review of non-enhanced images would be required to distinguish the two. However, this would require an additional acquisition, which is not routinely performed and would increase radiation dose. Review of VNE images on DECT scans can help to characterize these regions, as hyperattenuating foci on these images would stand out relative to non-enhancing parenchyma, which is consistent with hemorrhage rather than enhancement [4].

An additional benefit of DECT is the reduced radiation dose associated with the examination. Younger patients with acute pancreatitis and its complications often require repeated follow-up imaging examinations [7]. As previously suggested, these patients may undergo DECT, which would obviate the need for a non-contrast scan, as VNE images can be constructed.

3.5 Renal

3.5.1 Nephrolithiasis

Nephrolithiasis is a common condition in the United States, affecting approximately 1 out of 11 adults [1]. There is a slightly higher risk in men than in women, and it is known that dietary factors play a role, namely dehydration and dietary salt intake [24]. When renal calculi become obstructive in the renal pelvis, ureter, or ureterovesical junction, the experience is notoriously painful, and often brings patients to the ED. Additionally, approximately half of patients presenting with symptoms related to kidney calculi will have another episode in the next decade [24].

Over two decades, CT has been recognized as the modality of choice when evaluating patients with clinically suspected nephrolithiasis, or obstructing calculi in the urinary tract [25]. In direct comparison, CT has been shown to be more effective at revealing urolithiasis than ultrasound [26, 27]. Although non-enhanced CT is highly effective in the diagnosis of acute conditions related to urinary tract calculi, there are two areas in which DECT may have additional benefits.

First, many CT examinations of the abdomen and pelvis are acquired with intravenous contrast in the ED. Depending on the protocol for a given scan, and whether or not the patient recently received intravenous contrast for another examination, material density separation may be used to isolate radiodense urinary calculi from iodinated contrast in the collecting system or ureters. A high degree of accuracy is achieved by using material density separation to create VNE images to detect renal or ureteral calculi [28]. Thus, even in patients whose symptoms may not be typical for obstructing calculi and therefore undergo an IV contrast-enhanced examination, the correct diagnosis can still be made using DECT.

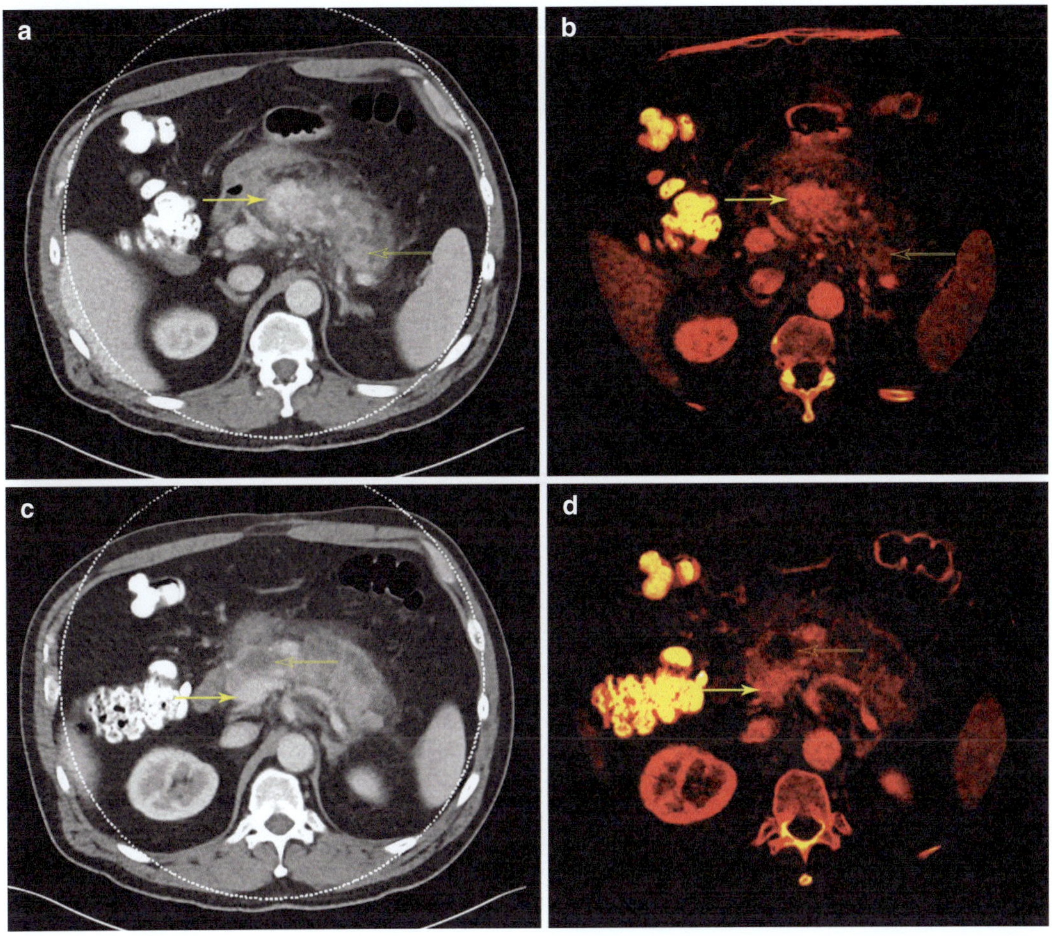

Fig. 3.3 54-year-old man with acute epigastric pain. (**a**) Axial IV contrast-enhanced CT image through the pancreas demonstrating acute pancreatitis with patchy areas of normal enhancement (solid arrow) and hypoenhancing parenchyma (open arrow). On these images, it is unclear whether the hypoenhancement represents ischemia or necrosis. (**b**) On the corresponding iodine image, there is an area of normal iodine uptake (solid arrow). The hypoenhancing area on CT (open arrow) does demonstrate iodine uptake, suggesting ischemia rather than necrosis. (**c**) In the same patient, the IV contrast-enhanced image demonstrates a separate area of normal enhancement (solid arrow) and hypoenhancement (open arrow). (**d**) On the corresponding iodine image, there is an area of normal iodine uptake (solid arrow). The hypoenhancing area on CT (open arrow) demonstrates no iodine uptake, suggesting necrosis rather than ischemia

Second, dual-energy CT has reliably shown the ability to characterize urinary calculus composition in multiple publications [29–35]. Specifically, DECT enables the radiologist to determine whether calculi are predominantly made of calcium oxalate, uric acid, or cysteine (Fig. 3.4). The implications for patient therapy are substantial.

Per the 2014 guidelines from the American Urologic Association, hydration is essential regardless of the type of urinary calculus [24]. For calcium oxalate calculi, recommendations on the dietary intake of sodium, calcium, oxalate, fruits/vegetables, and protein depend on urinary levels of calcium, oxalate, and citrate. Additional pharmacologic therapies may be indicated, such as thiazide diuretics for patients with calcium oxalate calculi or thiol drugs which bind cysteine when dietary modifications fail, or if there is a substantial stone burden. Lastly, differentiating uric acid (UA) calculi from non-uric acid

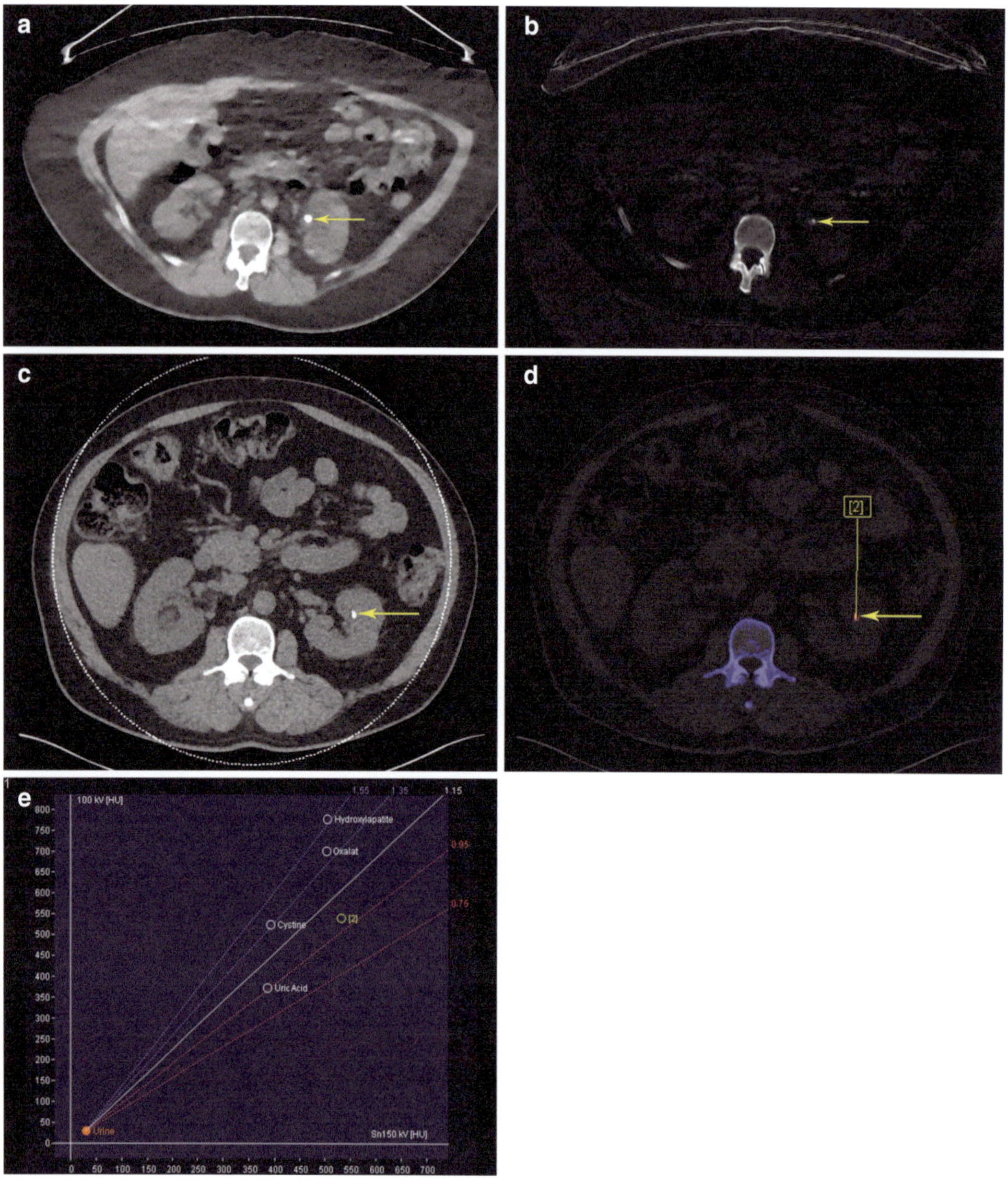

Fig. 3.4 Two different patients with renal calculi. (**a**) Axial VNE CT image through the level of the kidneys demonstrating a left renal calculus (solid arrow). (**b**) The corresponding iodine image again demonstrates the left renal calculus (solid arrow). Given the persistent finding on both images, these findings represent a calcified calculus. In contrast, a uric acid calculus will be present on the VNE image but not on the iodine image. (**c**) In a separate patient, axial non-contrast image through the kidneys demonstrating a left renal calculus (solid arrow). (**d**) Corresponding color overlay DECT image again demonstrating a left renal calculus (solid arrow). (**e**) Graph demonstrating dual-energy indexes for different calculus composition. Renal calculus composition can be determined by comparing the ratio of attenuation on low- versus high-kVp images

calculi is useful, as uric acid stones may be treated with alkalization of urine [36]. Because UA calculi have increased attenuation at higher peak kVp compared to non-UA calculi which have higher attenuation at lower peak kVp, this distinction is possible with DECT [36].

3.5.2 Focal Renal Mass

Focal renal masses are a commonly encountered entity in abdominal imaging. It is estimated that over half of the adults over 50 years old will be shown to have at least one renal mass on cross-sectional imaging [37]. Fortunately, the vast majority of incidentally encountered renal masses are simple cysts, and can be characterize as such by the absence of enhancement on IV contrast-enhanced examinations. However, a clinical dilemma arises when a focal renal mass is encountered which is not clearly a simple cyst, namely masses with attenuation greater than 20 HU. In this scenario, the most common explanations for a hyperattenuating focal renal mass include a hemorrhagic or proteinaceous cyst, so-called pseudo-enhancement of a renal cyst under 2 cm in diameter, or a solid renal mass. Because the management for these diagnoses is considerably different, it is important to correctly characterize these incidentally encountered renal masses.

Although the majority of abdominopelvic CT scans in the ED are acquired with intravenous contrast in a single phase (portal venous), separation of material density pairs with post-processing enables characterization of incidentally encountered renal masses with VNE [38]. Furthermore, after many investigators have struggled to eliminate pseudo-enhancement of small renal masses [37], DECT has been shown to reliably overcome pseudo-enhancement on virtual monochromatic images [37]. By making the distinction between solid enhancing renal masses and other differential diagnoses, unnecessary follow-up examinations may be avoided, reducing cost, radiation exposure, and patient anxiety.

3.5.3 Detection of Urothelial Masses

Detection of urothelial masses can be difficult, particularly when they grow in a plaque-like manner along the course of the urinary tract. In patients presenting with new hydronephrosis without an obstructing renal calculus, radiologists in the ED may be charged with locating a urothelial mass. DECT urography has been described, and shows promise as a way to evaluate patients with hematuria while possibly reducing radiation exposure [39, 40]. With dual-energy CT, it is possible to use separation of material density pairs to better appreciate the enhancement of urothelial masses which may have caused signs and/or symptoms which have brought the patient to the ED. Although the enhancing masses will commonly be primary transitional cell carcinoma, metastases from other malignancies, including prostate, pancreas, and breast, are also possible.

3.6 Adrenal

3.6.1 Incidental Adrenal Nodules

As the use of cross-sectional imaging has increased markedly over the past 20 years, radiologists working in the emergency department often encounter incidental nodules and masses which are of indeterminate significance. The frequency of incidentally discovered adrenal nodules larger than 1 cm in size, in particular, is estimated to be between 3 and 7% in adults [41]. Adrenal nodules discovered incidentally therefore present one of the common challenges facing radiologists in this setting. In those adult patients without a history of malignancy, the vast majority of adrenal nodules will ultimately prove benign. In one study of 973 patients, with a total of 1049 adrenal nodules, none proved malignant [42]. While the clinical context is important in ascertaining whether further workup is required, such as a history of malignancy or comparison with a prior imaging examination, a certain number of patients will remain indeterminate on the initial evaluation. In this group there is a role for new technology, which can help triage patients with incidental adrenal nodules, possibly avoiding unnecessary further workup.

Because of the inherent ability of dual-energy CT to separate different material densities, VNE images can be created by separating iodine and water components from IV contrast-enhanced images. In recent years, a number of studies have attempted to characterize indeterminate renal mass using DECT [43–47].

Slebocki et al. assessed a group of 63 patients undergoing CT angiography after endovascular repair of an abdominal aortic aneurysm who were evaluated with both pre-contrast CT and single-phase CTA. Of those patients, six had adrenal abnormalities detected, and an excellent correlation was found between the true non-contrast (TNC) and VNE mean attenuation values (12.8 vs. 12.4 HU) [46]. Glazer et al. also found that VNE images can help triage adrenal nodules, and reported excellent interobserver agreement (*kappa* = 0.92) among multiple radiologists [43]. Gnannt et al. showed that there was no difference in the mean attenuation of adrenal nodules between VNE and TNC images acquired in the portal venous phase of IV contrast-enhanced CT [44]. Botsikas et al. reported a slightly higher mean HU for VNE images made from portal venous-phase images (4.02 HU higher for VNE), but no significant difference from VNE made from 15-min images [45]. Mileto et al. showed that VNE images may be better than TNC images for characterizing lipid-poor adrenal adenomas [47].

In summary, by using material density pairs, a radiologist in the ED can reliably characterize many incidental adrenal nodules on IV contrast-enhanced CT scans. This is true at a variety of kVp settings, and works in both the portal venous and arterial phases of acquisition (Fig. 3.5).

3.7 Bowel

3.7.1 Acute Gastrointestinal Hemorrhage

Detection and localization of acute gastrointestinal hemorrhage present a diagnostic challenge for the practicing radiologist. The presence of high-density material within the bowel lumen (i.e., positive oral contrast or other ingested material) may confound CT findings which indicate the presence of acute blood products. Upper endoscopy and optical colonoscopy are essential diagnostic tools in the setting of acute gastrointestinal hemorrhage, and have the additional benefit of providing an opportunity for therapeutic intervention, either through clipping of a bleeding vessel or injection of a sclerosing agent. However, a number of factors, including the presence of a large amount of blood within the bowel lumen, may limit the ability of the gastroenterologist to detect and localize the source of acute bleeding.

As the technology of multi-detector computed tomography (MDCT) has advanced over the past two decades, MDCT has emerged as a valid diagnostic tool in the evaluation of patients with acute gastrointestinal hemorrhage [48–53]. Some challenges are inherent to the interpretation of MDCT examinations for the assessment of known or suspected acute gastrointestinal hemorrhage, namely the presence of intrinsically high-density material within the bowel lumen, which may confound the interpretation of a scan. Because of the ability of dual-energy computed tomography (DECT) to separate elements of different attenuation, and therefore to determine the iodine contribution to an image, there is an emerging role for the use of DECT in the evaluation of acute gastrointestinal hemorrhage in the ED setting [48–53].

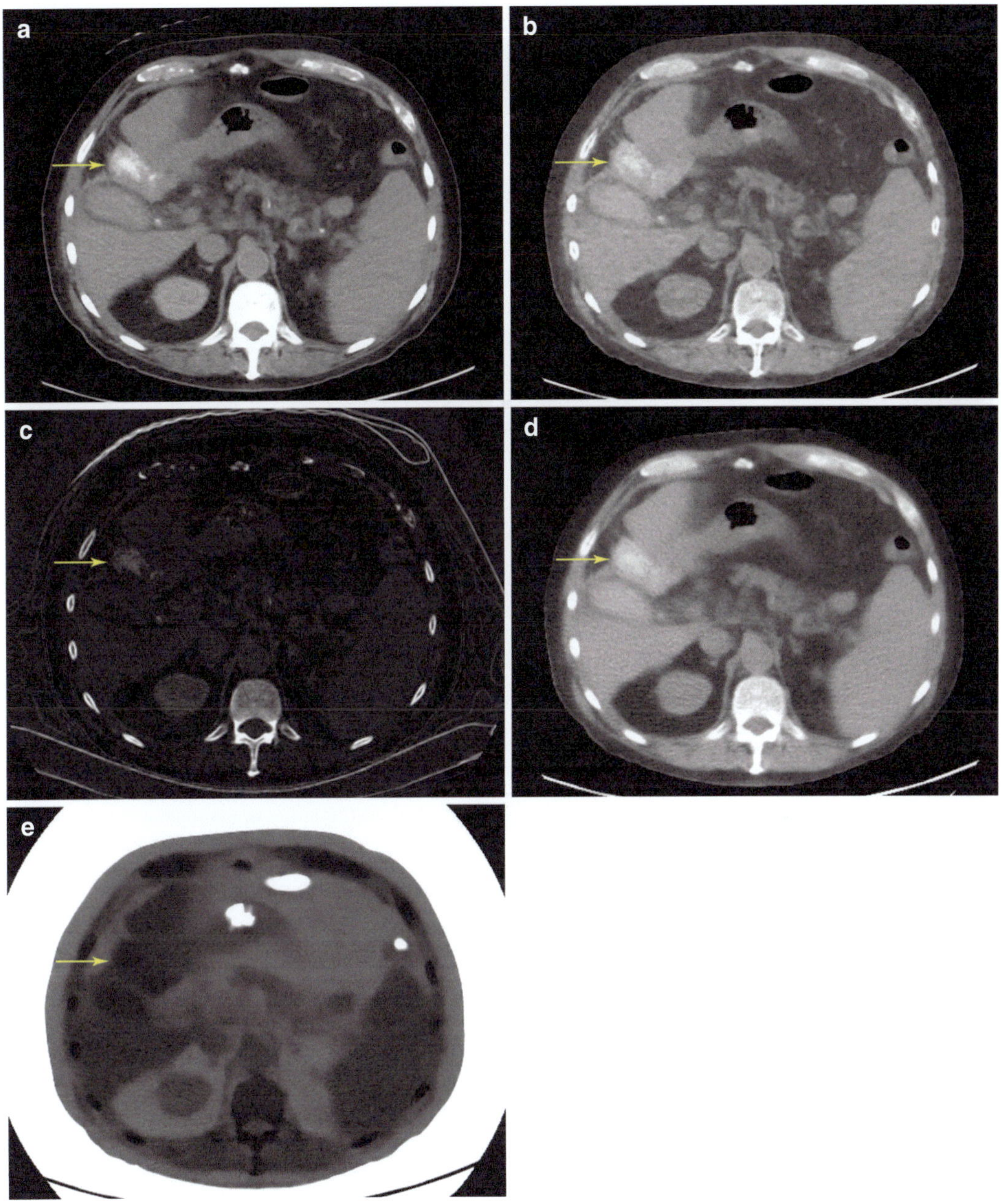

Fig. 3.5 79-year-old man with abdominal pain. (**a**) Axial non-contrast CT image demonstrating a hyperattenuating subhepatic collection (solid arrow). Given that enteric contrast was previously administered, it was unclear whether this collection represented leakage of contrast. (**b**) Corresponding axial VNE image shows the same subhepatic collection (solid arrow). (**c**) Corresponding axial iodine image also demonstrates the same subhepatic collection (solid arrow). (**d**) Axial calcium image also demonstrates the hyperattenuating subhepatic collection (solid arrow). (**e**) On the corresponding non-calcium image, the same collection is hypoattenuating (solid arrow). The interpreting radiologist was unable to elicit a history to explain the findings, but the calcification within the collection indicates that it is chronic

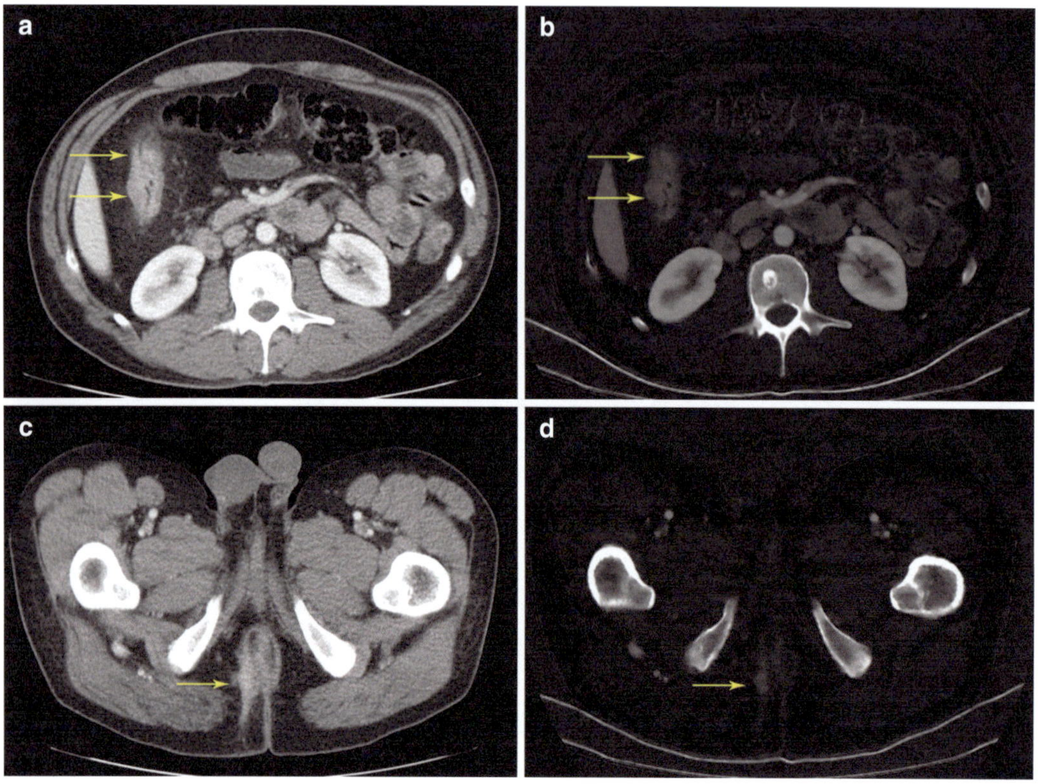

Fig. 3.6 37-year-old man with a history of Crohn disease presents with abdominal and rectal pain. (**a**) Axial IV contrast-enhanced CT image demonstrating wall thickening and enhancement involving the hepatic flexure of the colon (*arrows*). (**b**) Iodine image at a similar level demonstrating increased conspicuity of the finding (*arrows*). (**c**) IV contrast-enhanced CT image demonstrating a right perianal fistula extending towards the right gluteal cleft (*arrow*). (**d**) As before, an iodine image at a similar level also shows increased conspicuity of the same finding (*arrow*)

3.7.2 Bowel Inflammation

Patients with inflammatory bowel disease (IBD) may present to the ED with acute or worsening abdominal pain. Some of the CT findings associated with bowel inflammation include hyperenhancement, bowel dilation, and bowel wall thickening, as well as secondary signs of mesenteric fat stranding. By separating material density pairs to create iodine maps, areas of bowel wall hyperenhancement may become more conspicuous and thus may be more readily detected (Fig. 3.6). Iodine maps may be beneficial in common conditions of bowel inflammation including inflammatory bowel disease, acute appendicitis, and diverticulitis [54]. There is ample opportunity for further research in this area.

3.7.3 Bowel Ischemia

Acute bowel ischemia often presents a diagnostic challenge in the ED. Patients presenting with bowel ischemia usually have abdominal pain, signs of a systemic illness such as tachycardia, and/or hematochezia. These symptoms may appropriately prompt an IV contrast-enhanced CT of the abdomen and pelvis. However, "conventional" MDCT may lend to missing as many as 34% of acute mesenteric ischemia [55]. DECT may be useful in acute mesenteric ischemia. In animal models, it has been shown that DECT using a low kVp increases attenuation differences between normally perfused bowel and early ischemic bowel. The authors found this difference to be statistically significant for a lower kVp (51 keV) when compared to conventional 120 kVp images, but also saw improved

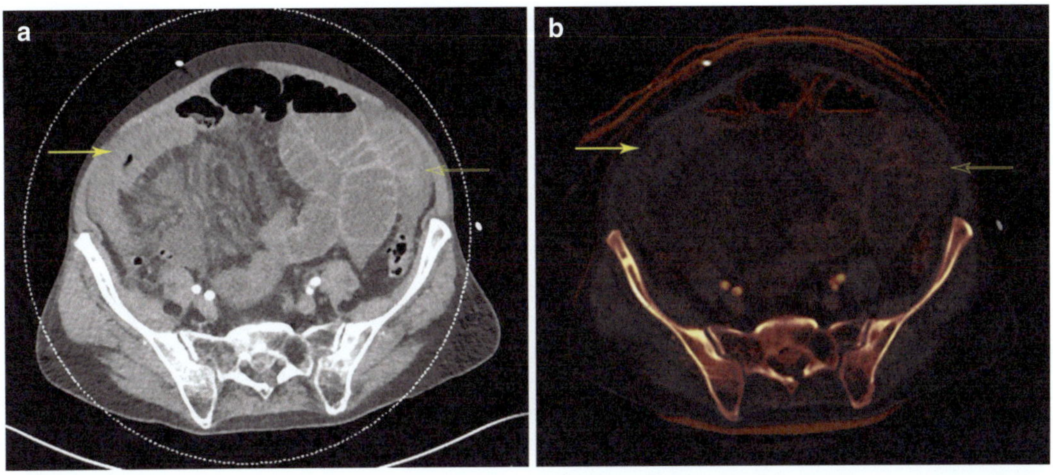

Fig. 3.7 68-year-old man with cirrhosis, with increasing abdominal pain. (**a**) Axial IV contrast-enhanced CT image through the abdomen demonstrates right lower quadrant small bowel loops with wall thickening (solid arrow) and dilated small bowel loops in the left lower quadrant (open arrow). (**b**) Corresponding axial iodine image demonstrates absence of iodine uptake in the right lower quadrant small bowel loops (solid arrow), strongly suggesting ischemic bowel. In contrast, the left lower quadrant small bowel loops have normal iodine uptake (open arrow)

conspicuity of early bowel ischemia when the kVp was 65 and 70 keV [56] (Fig. 3.7).

3.8 Trauma

Abdominopelvic trauma is common, and is a leading cause of morbidity and mortality among younger patients in the emergency setting. CT plays a crucial role in the workup of all hemodynamically stable trauma patients [57]. Portal venous-phase imaging is standard on abdominopelvic CT imaging. However, depending on the severity and mechanism of trauma, protocols can be tailored to the clinical history to include additional phases, i.e., arterial phase or delayed images [57]. In all patients with trauma, it is important to emphasize the need to be highly accurate while minimizing radiation dose to the patient. In this regard, DECT is an ideal technology that can be used to accomplish both of these goals without compromises.

3.8.1 Aortic Injury and Endoleak

In the setting of trauma, the aorta is best evaluated with multiphase imaging, typically including arterial and delayed phases. Non-enhanced images are not routinely acquired at most institutions, but can be helpful for the identification of intramural hematoma. Dual-energy CT can be helpful in these patients as VNE images can be created instead of the conventional non-enhanced acquisition, thus reducing radiation dose. While these images are noisier than the conventional non-enhanced images, they are of diagnostic quality in 95% of patients [6]. Additionally, with further development of DECT technology, image quality has been significantly improved such that the images currently closely resemble acquired non-enhanced images.

Another scenario where DECT has been shown to be helpful is for detection of endoleaks. Endovascular aneurysm repair is a commonly performed procedure for abdominal aortic aneurysms. A common complication of the procedure is subacute to chronic endoleak, which allows for filling of the aneurysm sac, and which is associated with an increased risk of rupture [58]. As previously suggested, CT with arterial and delayed phases is highly sensitive and specific for detection of endoleaks. Unlike in acute aortic injury, non-enhanced images are usually routinely acquired, particularly on the initial post-procedure CT scans. However, sensitivity, specificity, and accuracy may be further increased by using dual-energy technique. This is possible by using lower kVp images, which increases the attenuation of intravenously

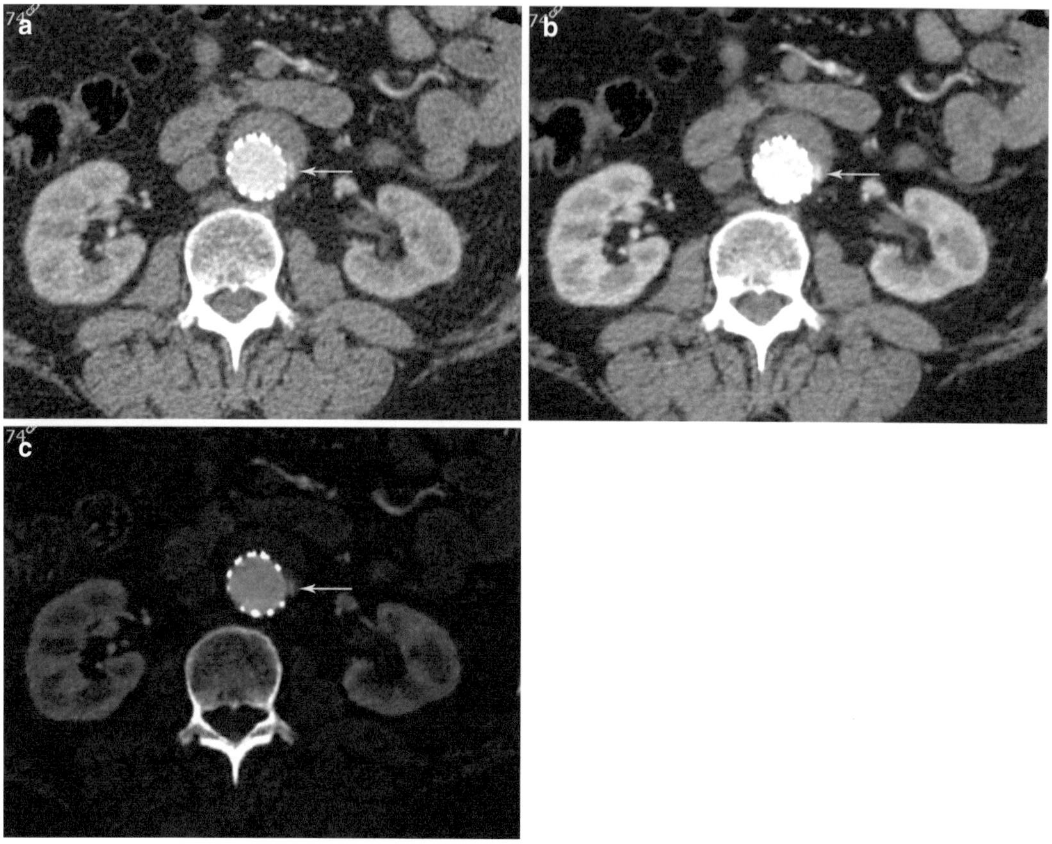

Fig. 3.8 70-year-old man following remote endovascular abdominal aortic aneurysm repair, with clinical concern for a graft endoleak. (**a**) CT angiogram axial image demonstrating endoleak along the left lateral aspect of the stent graft (arrow). (**b**) Low-keV image demonstrates increased conspicuity of the same finding despite the same window and level values (arrow). Also note the differences in attenuation on the low-keV images, best seen in the aorta. Intravenous contrast appears brighter on low-keV images. (**c**) The same finding on the iodine image is much more apparent (arrow)

administered contrast (Fig. 3.8). In one study of 22 patients, endoleaks were shown to be more conspicuous on 80 kVp images when compared to images using 120 kVp [59].

3.8.2 Solid Organ Injury

Solid organ injury is very common in the setting of trauma. In order of frequency, the most commonly injured organs are spleen, liver, and kidney, with bowel and bladder less commonly injured [57]. The American Association for the Surgery of Trauma (AAST) has developed grading scales for injuries of the solid organs, taking into account size of hematomas and depth of lacerations. CT is an invaluable tool for early detection of these injuries. Typical CT trauma protocols include portal-venous-phase images through the abdomen and pelvis, with or without delayed images [57].

On CT images, lacerations appear as linear areas of hypoattenuation. While these findings may be detected on conventional CT, DECT is useful as it can accentuate the findings (Fig. 3.9). Iodine images can also be constructed to highlight areas of perfusion and areas of hypoenhancement [16, 60]. Other important findings on CT include subcapsular hematoma/hemoperitoneum, active extravasation of contrast, and pseudoaneurysm formation. All of these findings can be made more conspicuous on DECT images.

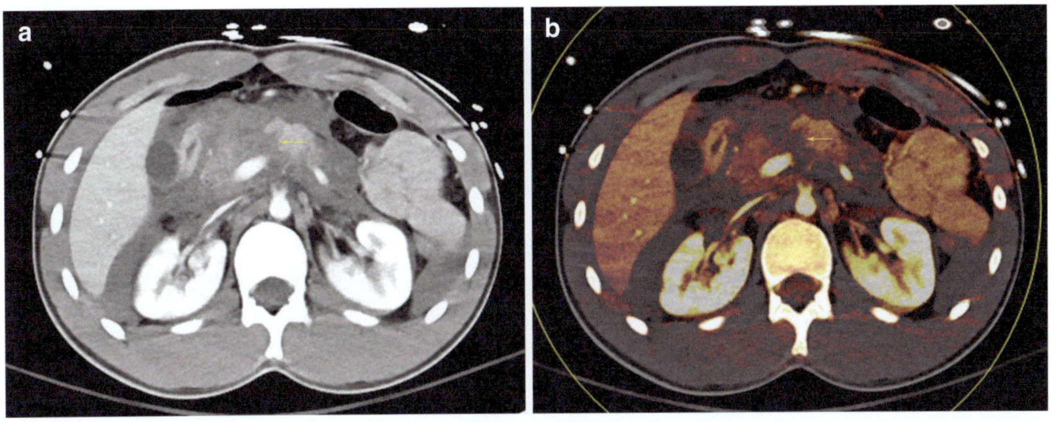

Fig. 3.9 40-year-old man brought to the emergency department after a motor vehicle collision. (**a**) Axial IV contrast-enhanced CT image through the abdomen at the level of the pancreas demonstrates heterogeneous enhancement in the pancreatic head and neck (solid arrow), as well as hemoperitoneum and flattening of the inferior vena cava. (**b**) The iodine image confirms the presence of a laceration through the pancreatic neck (solid arrow)

As previously suggested, trauma CT protocols typically do not include non-enhanced images. While this is sufficient in most patients, there are situations where non-enhanced images can provide valuable information. In the setting of trauma, non-enhanced images may demonstrate subcapsular hematomas of the spleen or liver as a layer of hyperattenuating material overlying and conforming to the contour of the injured organ [60]. Similarly, hemoperitoneum can be subtle, particularly when there are only small amounts adjacent to enhancing bowel loops or other hyperattenuating structures. On post-contrast images, the blood products may be isoattenuating relative to the adjacent organ. Given that non-contrast images are not routinely acquired, these findings can potentially be missed on "routine" IV contrast-enhanced images. However, review of VNE images on DECT will demonstrate increased contrast differentiation between hematoma and adjacent injured organ [60] (Fig. 3.10).

IV contrast extravasation is a critical finding to identify on CT, as it strongly suggests the need for more invasive management, i.e., angiographic intervention or surgical management. Active arterial (and occasionally venous) contrast extravasation appears as blush of contrast within or adjacent to solid organs or bowel, which should change its morphology and density on delayed images [57]. As these findings can be subtle, DECT can be used to increase conspicuity [60]. Subtle hyperattenuating foci can be more easily detected on iodine images or low-keV images.

A diagnostic dilemma occurs on a single-phase CT examination. In this setting, a single image demonstrating a hyperdense focus may represent contrast extravasation, vascular or gastrointestinal, or other intrinsically hyperdense material. This is further complicated if the finding is seen in the vicinity of a comminuted fracture with osseous fragments or calcified atherosclerotic plaque potentially mimicking contrast extravasation. Dual-energy CT can be very helpful in this scenario, as review of VNE in conjunction with iodine images can help to differentiate between the two. Calcium will be present on both VNE and iodine images. However, extravasated contrast will only be seen on iodine images, and not on VNE images [60] (Fig. 3.11).

3.8.3 Musculoskeletal Injury

Fractures are commonly seen in the emergency setting. This is true even in the absence of trauma, given that elderly patients can present with insufficiency fractures. While displaced fractures are easily detected on conventional CT images, non-displaced and minimally dis-

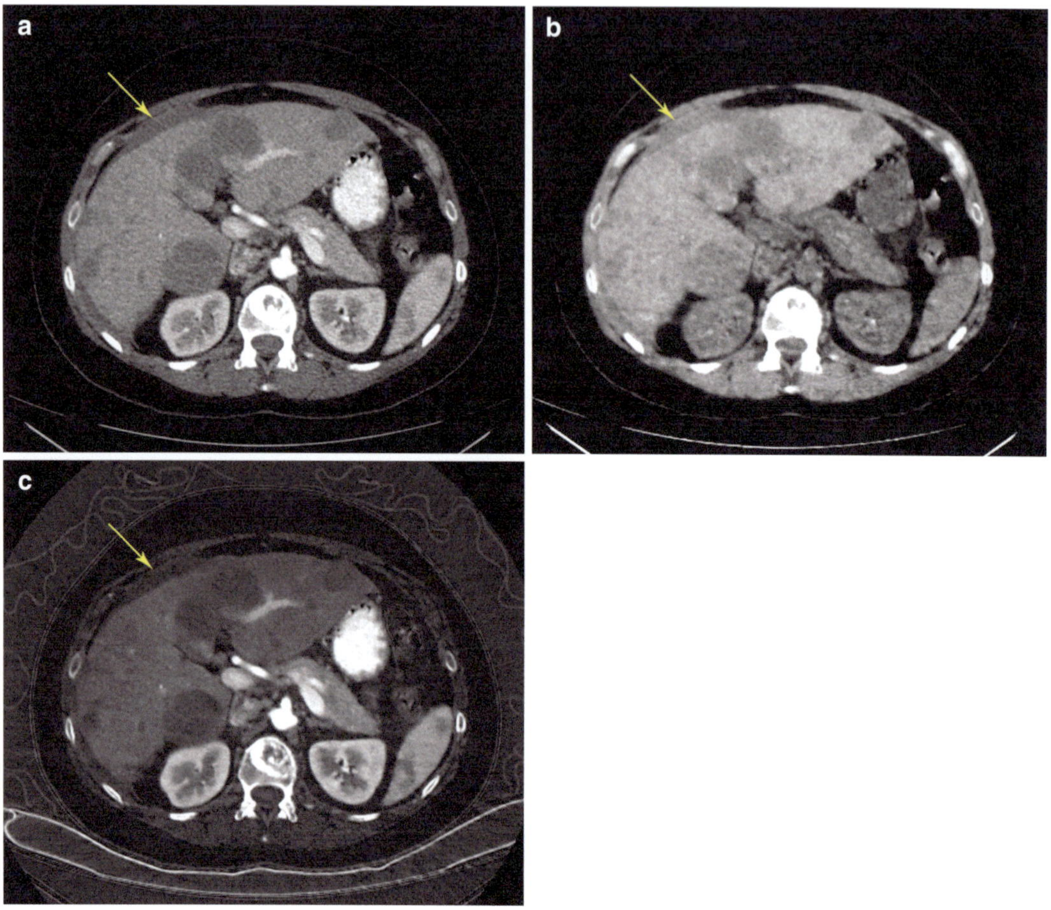

Fig. 3.10 46-year-old woman with known metastatic melanoma presents to the emergency department with abdominal pain. (**a**) Axial IV contrast-enhanced CT image demonstrating hypoattenuating material layering anterior to the liver (solid arrow). (**b**) On the corresponding VNE image, the collection appears hyperattenuating (solid arrow), using the fluid seen in the stomach as an internal reference. (**c**) On the corresponding iodine image, there is no iodine uptake in the collection (solid arrow). This collection represents hemoperitoneum from hepatic melanoma metastases

placed fractures can often be difficult to detect. In these patients, clinicians typically order MRI for detection of bone marrow edema [61]. While MRI is an excellent tool, it is relatively expensive, time consuming, and sometimes technically difficult to perform in the inpatient setting. An alternative approach is to use DECT, which can be used to subtract calcium from the image. This process removes trabecular bone from the image, allowing bone marrow to be visualized. On the resulting virtual non-calcium images, hyperattenuation in the marrow represents marrow edema and/or hemorrhage [7, 10, 14]. Aside from detection, this technique can also be helpful for characterization of fractures. As previously suggested, elderly patients are often incidentally noted to have spinal compression fractures on CT examinations. In the absence of prior imaging examinations for comparison, these fractures are often interpreted as age indeterminate, leading clinicians to then order MRI or nuclear bone scan for further characterization. As with fracture detection, DECT can be used in these patients to characterize the fractures. In these patients, the presence of marrow edema or hemorrhage is consistent with acute

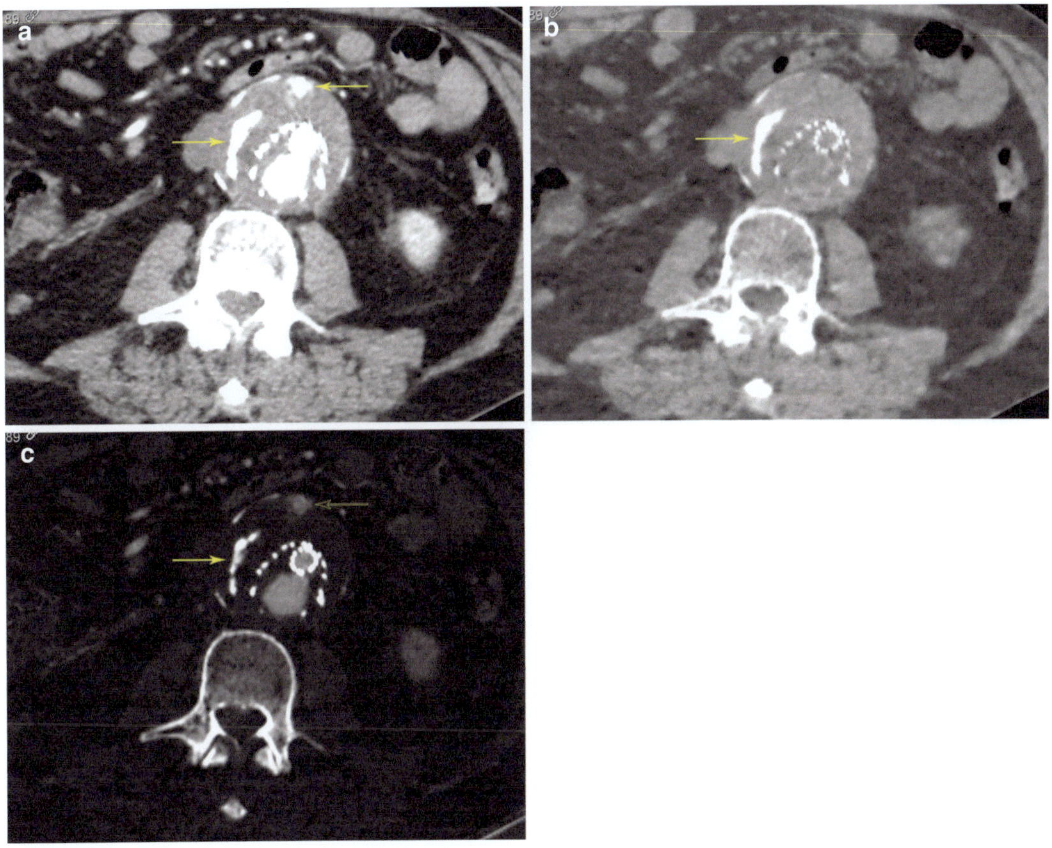

Fig. 3.11 69-year-old man after endovascular abdominal aortic aneurysm repair with concern for endoleak. (**a**) Axial CT angiogram image clearly depicts two areas of hyperattenuation (arrows) within the aneurysm sac—a curvilinear structure on the right and an amorphous structure anteriorly. It is unclear whether these findings represent an endoleak or atherosclerotic calcification. (**b**) VNE image demonstrating the curvilinear structure in the right side of the aneurysm sac (arrow), but not the hyperattenuating material anteriorly. (**c**) Iodine images demonstrate both areas of hyperattenuation. There is curvilinear calcification along the right side of the aneurysm sac (arrow), and an endoleak anteriorly (open arrow)

to subacute fracture, while their absence suggests chronicity.

Conclusion

Dual-energy CT has a wide range of applications in diagnostic imaging in the emergency department. Familiarity with the role of DECT in the evaluation of the gallbladder, pancreas, kidneys, bowel, vasculature, and musculoskeletal system can enable timely and accurate diagnoses while frequently eliminating the need for further diagnostic imaging workup.

References

1. Scales CD Jr, Smith AC, Hanley JM, Saigal CS, Urologic Diseases in America. Prevalence of kidney stones in the United States. Eur Urol. 2012;62(1):160–5.
2. Larson DB, Johnson LW, Schnell BM, Salisbury SR, Forman HP. National trends in CT use in the emergency department: 1995-2007. Radiology. 2011;258(1):164–73.
3. Uyeda JW, Sahani DV. Dual-energy CT in the acute abdomen. Curr Radiol Rep. 2015;3:20.
4. Silva AC, Morse BG, Hara AK, Paden RG, Hongo N, Pavlicek W. Dual-energy (spectral) CT: applications in abdominal imaging. Radiographics. 2011;31(4):1031–46. discussion 1047-1050

5. Karcaaltincaba M, Aktas A. Dual-energy CT revisited with multidetector CT: review of principles and clinical applications. Diagn Interv Radiol. 2011;17(3):181–94.
6. Vlahos I, Chung R, Nair A, Morgan R. Dual-energy CT: vascular applications. AJR Am J Roentgenol. 2012;199(5 Suppl):S87–97.
7. Patino M, Prochowski A, Agrawal MD, Simeone FJ, Gupta R, Hahn PF, et al. Material separation using dual-energy CT: current and emerging applications. Radiographics. 2016;36(4):1087–105.
8. Heye T, Nelson RC, Ho LM, Marin D, Boll DT. Dual-energy CT applications in the abdomen. AJR Am J Roentgenol. 2012;199(5 Suppl):S64–70.
9. Marin D, Boll DT, Mileto A, Nelson RC. State of the art: dual-energy CT of the abdomen. Radiology. 2014;271(2):327–42.
10. Grajo JRPM, Prochowski A, Sahani DV. Dual energy CT in practice: basic principles and applications. Appl Radiol. 2016;45(7):6–12.
11. Agrawal MD, Oliveira GR, Kalva SP, Pinho DF, Arellano RS, Sahani DV. Prospective comparison of reduced-iodine-dose virtual monochromatic imaging dataset from dual-energy CT angiography with standard-iodine-dose single-energy ct angiography for abdominal aortic aneurysm. AJR Am J Roentgenol. 2016;207(6):W125–32.
12. Foley WD, Shuman WP, Siegel MJ, Sahani DV, Boll DT, Bolus DN, et al. White paper of the society of computed body tomography and magnetic resonance on dual-energy CT, Part 2: radiation dose and iodine sensitivity. J Comput Assist Tomogr. 2016;40(6):846–50.
13. Shuman WP, Chan KT, Busey JM, Mitsumori LM, Koprowicz KM. Dual-energy CT aortography with 50% reduced iodine dose versus single-energy CT aortography with standard iodine dose. Acad Radiol. 2016;23(5):611–8.
14. Aran S, Daftari Besheli L, Karcaaltincaba M, Gupta R, Flores EJ, Abujudeh HH. Applications of dual-energy CT in emergency radiology. AJR Am J Roentgenol. 2014;202(4):W314–24.
15. Lewis M, Reid K, Toms AP. Reducing the effects of metal artefact using high keV monoenergetic reconstruction of dual energy CT (DECT) in hip replacements. Skelet Radiol. 2013;42(2):275–82.
16. Yeh BM, Shepherd JA, Wang ZJ, Teh HS, Hartman RP, Prevrhal S. Dual-energy and low-kVp CT in the abdomen. AJR Am J Roentgenol. 2009;193(1):47–54.
17. Kim JE, Lee JM, Baek JH, Han JK, Choi BI. Initial assessment of dual-energy CT in patients with gallstones or bile duct stones: can virtual nonenhanced images replace true nonenhanced images? AJR Am J Roentgenol. 2012;198(4):817–24.
18. Shoheiber O, Biskupiak JE, Nash DB. Estimation of the cost savings resulting from the use of ursodiol for the prevention of gallstones in obese patients undergoing rapid weight reduction. Int J Obes Relat Metab Disord. 1997;21(11):1038–45.
19. Uyeda JW, Richardson IJ, Sodickson AD. Making the invisible visible: improving conspicuity of noncalcified gallstones using dual energy CT. Abdom Radiol. 2017;42(12):2933–9.
20. Barakos JA, Ralls PW, Lapin SA, Johnson MB, Radin DR, Colletti PM, et al. Cholelithiasis: evaluation with CT. Radiology. 1987;162(2):415–8.
21. Hickman MS, Schwesinger WH, Bova JD, Kurtin WE. Computed tomographic analysis of gallstones. An in vitro study. Arch Surg. 1986;121(3):289–91.
22. Bennett GL, Rusinek H, Lisi V, Israel GM, Krinsky GA, Slywotzky CM, et al. CT findings in acute gangrenous cholecystitis. AJR Am J Roentgenol. 2002;178(2):275–81.
23. Chen AL, Liu AL, Wang S, Liu JH, Ju Y, Sun MY, et al. Detection of gallbladder stones by dual-energy spectral computed tomography imaging. World J Gastroenterol. 2015;21(34):9993–8.
24. Pearle MS, Goldfarb DS, Assimos DG, Curhan G, Denu-Ciocca CJ, Matlaga BR, et al. Medical management of kidney stones: AUA guideline. J Urol. 2014;192(2):316–24.
25. Boridy IC, Nikolaidis P, Kawashima A, Sandler CM, Goldman SM. Noncontrast helical CT for ureteral stones. World J Urol. 1998;16(1):18–21.
26. Ather MH, Jafri AH, Sulaiman MN. Diagnostic accuracy of ultrasonography compared to unenhanced CT for stone and obstruction in patients with renal failure. BMC Med Imaging. 2004;4(1):2.
27. Ulusan S, Koc Z, Tokmak N. Accuracy of sonography for detecting renal stone: comparison with CT. J Clin Ultrasound. 2007;35(5):256–61.
28. Scheffel H, Stolzmann P, Frauenfelder T, Schertler T, Desbiolles L, Leschka S, et al. Dual-energy contrast-enhanced computed tomography for the detection of urinary stone disease. Investig Radiol. 2007;42(12):823–9.
29. Duan X, Li Z, Yu L, Leng S, Halaweish AF, Fletcher JG, et al. Characterization of urinary stone composition by use of third-generation dual-source dual-energy CT with increased spectral separation. AJR Am J Roentgenol. 2015;205(6):1203–7.
30. Kulkarni NM, Eisner BH, Pinho DF, Joshi MC, Kambadakone AR, Sahani DV. Determination of renal stone composition in phantom and patients using single-source dual-energy computed tomography. J Comput Assist Tomogr. 2013;37(1):37–45.
31. Leng S, Huang A, Cardona JM, Duan X, Williams JC, McCollough CH. Dual-energy CT for quantification of urinary stone composition in mixed stones: a phantom study. AJR Am J Roentgenol. 2016;207(2):321–9.
32. Matlaga BR, Kawamoto S, Fishman E. Dual source computed tomography: a novel technique to determine stone composition. Urology. 2008;72(5):1164–8.
33. Ogawa N, Sato S, Ida K, Kato K, Ariyoshi Y, Wada K, et al. Evaluation of urinary stone composition and differentiation between urinary stones and phleboliths using single-source dual-energy computed tomography. Acta Med Okayama. 2017;71(2):91–6.
34. Zhang GM, Sun H, Xue HD, Xiao H, Zhang XB, Jin ZY. Prospective prediction of the major component

of urinary stone composition with dual-source dual-energy CT in vivo. Clin Radiol. 2016;71(11):1178–83.
35. Zilberman DE, Ferrandino MN, Preminger GM, Paulson EK, Lipkin ME, Boll DT. In vivo determination of urinary stone composition using dual energy computerized tomography with advanced post-acquisition processing. J Urol. 2010;184(6):2354–9.
36. Aran S, Shaqdan KW, Abujudeh HH. Dual-energy computed tomography (DECT) in emergency radiology: basic principles, techniques, and limitations. Emerg Radiol. 2014;21(4):391–405.
37. Silverman SG, Israel GM, Herts BR, Richie JP. Management of the incidental renal mass. Radiology. 2008;249(1):16–31.
38. Neville AM, Gupta RT, Miller CM, Merkle EM, Paulson EK, Boll DT. Detection of renal lesion enhancement with dual-energy multidetector CT. Radiology. 2011;259(1):173–83.
39. Ascenti G, Mileto A, Gaeta M, Blandino A, Mazziotti S, Scribano E. Single-phase dual-energy CT urography in the evaluation of haematuria. Clin Radiol. 2013;68(2):e87–94.
40. Chen CY, Hsu JS, Jaw TS, Shih MC, Lee LJ, Tsai TH, et al. Split-bolus portal venous phase dual-energy CT urography: protocol design, image quality, and dose reduction. AJR Am J Roentgenol. 2015;205(5):W492–501.
41. Berland LL, Silverman SG, Gore RM, Mayo-Smith WW, Megibow AJ, Yee J, et al. Managing incidental findings on abdominal CT: white paper of the ACR incidental findings committee. J Am Coll Radiol. 2010;7(10):754–73.
42. Song JH, Chaudhry FS, Mayo-Smith WW. The incidental adrenal mass on CT: prevalence of adrenal disease in 1,049 consecutive adrenal masses in patients with no known malignancy. AJR Am J Roentgenol. 2008;190(5):1163–8.
43. Glazer DI, Maturen KE, Kaza RK, Francis IR, Keshavarzi NR, Parker RA, et al. Adrenal Incidentaloma triage with single-source (fast-kilovoltage switch) dual-energy CT. AJR Am J Roentgenol. 2014;203(2):329–35.
44. Gnannt R, Fischer M, Goetti R, Karlo C, Leschka S, Alkadhi H. Dual-energy CT for characterization of the incidental adrenal mass: preliminary observations. AJR Am J Roentgenol. 2012;198(1):138–44.
45. Botsikas D, Triponez F, Boudabbous S, Hansen C, Becker CD, Montet X. Incidental adrenal lesions detected on enhanced abdominal dual-energy CT: can the diagnostic workup be shortened by the implementation of virtual unenhanced images? Eur J Radiol. 2014;83(10):1746–51.
46. Slebocki K, Kraus B, Chang DH, Hellmich M, Maintz D, Bangard C. Incidental findings in abdominal dual-energy computed tomography: correlation between true noncontrast and virtual noncontrast images considering renal and liver cysts and adrenal masses. J Comput Assist Tomogr. 2017;41(2):294–7.
47. Mileto A, Nelson RC, Marin D, Roy Choudhury K, Ho LM. Dual-energy multidetector CT for the characterization of incidental adrenal nodules: diagnostic performance of contrast-enhanced material density analysis. Radiology. 2015;274(2):445–54.
48. Ernst O, Bulois P, Saint-Drenant S, Leroy C, Paris JC, Sergent G. Helical CT in acute lower gastrointestinal bleeding. Eur Radiol. 2003;13(1):114–7. https://doi.org/10.1007/s00330-002-1442-y.
49. Yamaguchi T, Yoshikawa K. Enhanced CT for initial localization of active lower gastrointestinal bleeding. Abdom Imaging. 2003;28(5):634–6.
50. Rajan R, Dhar P, Praseedom RK, Sudhindran S, Moorthy S. Role of contrast CT in acute lower gastrointestinal bleeding. Dig Surg. 2004;21(4):293–6.
51. Yoon W, Jeong YY, Shin SS, Lim HS, Song SG, Jang NG, et al. Acute massive gastrointestinal bleeding: detection and localization with arterial phase multi-detector row helical CT. Radiology. 2006;239(1):160–7.
52. Jaeckle T, Stuber G, Hoffmann MH, Jeltsch M, Schmitz BL, Aschoff AJ. Detection and localization of acute upper and lower gastrointestinal (GI) bleeding with arterial phase multi-detector row helical CT. Eur Radiol. 2008;18(7):1406–13.
53. Sodhi JS, Zargar SA, Rashid W, Shaheen F, Singh M, Javid G, et al. 64-section multiphase CT enterography as a diagnostic tool in the evaluation of obscure gastrointestinal bleeding. Indian J Gastroenterol. 2012;31(2):61–8.
54. Fulwadhva UP, Wortman JR, Sodickson AD. Use of dual-energy CT and iodine maps in evaluation of bowel disease. Radiographics. 2016;36(2):393–406.
55. Firetto MC, Lemos AA, Marini A, Avesani EC, Biondetti PR. Acute bowel ischemia: analysis of diagnostic error by overlooked findings at MDCT angiography. Emerg Radiol. 2013;20(2):139–47.
56. Potretzke TA, Brace CL, Lubner MG, Sampson LA, Willey BJ, Lee FT Jr. Early small-bowel ischemia: dual-energy CT improves conspicuity compared with conventional CT in a swine model. Radiology. 2015;275(1):119–26.
57. Soto JA, Anderson SW. Multidetector CT of blunt abdominal trauma. Radiology. 2012;265(3):678–93.
58. Hong C, Heiken JP, Sicard GA, Pilgram TK, Bae KT. Clinical significance of endoleak detected on follow-up CT after endovascular repair of abdominal aortic aneurysm. AJR Am J Roentgenol. 2008;191(3):808–13.
59. Chandarana H, Godoy MC, Vlahos I, Graser A, Babb J, Leidecker C, et al. Abdominal aorta: evaluation with dual-source dual-energy multidetector CT after endovascular repair of aneurysms--initial observations. Radiology. 2008;249(2):692–700. https://doi.org/10.1148/radiol.2492080359.
60. Nicolaou S, Eftekhari A, Sedlic T, Hou DJ, Mudri MJ, Aldrich J, et al. The utilization of dual source CT in imaging of polytrauma. Eur J Radiol. 2008;68(3):398–408.
61. Feldman F, Staron R, Zwass A, Rubin S, Haramati N. MR imaging: its role in detecting occult fractures. Skelet Radiol. 1994;23(6):439–44.

Acute Hepatobiliary Imaging

4

Marina C. Bernal Fernandez, Jorge A. Soto, and Christina A. LeBedis

Abstract

Abdominal pain is a common chief complaint in the emergency department, and computed tomography (CT) and ultrasound are useful first-line imaging modalities in the appropriate clinical setting. Both are rapid, low cost, and easily accessible. Magnetic resonance (MR) imaging is increasingly used in equivocal situations, especially for imaging the biliary system and pancreas, in the setting of pregnancy, and in young or relatively young patients with chronic diseases which will require multiple imaging examinations, with the associated exposure of ionizing radiation if repetitive CT is performed. MR has proved particularly useful in the setting of Crohn disease, complications of pancreatitis, suspected appendicitis in pregnant patients, complications from pancreatic injury, choledocholithiasis, and biliary obstruction of indeterminate etiology. Acute abdominal pain related to liver, gallbladder, and biliary etiologies may present as acute infections with hepatitis or cholecystitis, acute obstruction with choledocholithiasis or malignancy, hemoperitoneum from a ruptured liver mass, or trauma/iatrogenic injury.

M. C. Bernal Fernandez, M.D. • J. A. Soto, M.D. (✉)
C. A. LeBedis, M.D.
Department of Radiology, Boston University Medical Center, Boston, MA, USA
e-mail: Jorge.Soto@bmc.org

4.1 Acute Nontraumatic

Abdominal pain is a common chief complaint in the emergency department, and computed tomography (CT) and ultrasound are useful first-line imaging modalities in the appropriate clinical setting. Both are rapid, low cost, and easily accessible. Magnetic resonance (MR) imaging is increasingly used in equivocal situations, especially for imaging the biliary system and pancreas, in the setting of pregnancy, and in young or relatively young patients with chronic diseases which will require multiple imaging examinations, with the associated exposure of ionizing radiation if repetitive CT is performed. MR has proved particularly useful in the setting of Crohn disease, complications of pancreatitis, suspected appendicitis in pregnant patients, complications from pancreatic injury, choledocholithiasis, and biliary obstruction of indeterminate etiology. Acute abdominal pain related to liver, gallbladder, and biliary etiologies may present as acute infections with hepatitis or cholecystitis, acute obstruction with choledocholithiasis or malignancy, hemoperitoneum from a ruptured liver mass, or trauma/iatrogenic injury.

4.2 Liver

4.2.1 Acute Hepatitis

Acute hepatitis of any origin causes edema of the hepatocytes leading to injury. It can manifest as

M. Patlas et al. (eds.), *MDCT and MR Imaging of Acute Abdomen*,
https://doi.org/10.1007/978-3-319-70778-5_4

enlarged liver with no focal signs of disease on imaging. When present, symptoms may include fatigue, weakness, abdominal pain, hepatomegaly, and splenomegaly. Acute hepatitis remains a clinical diagnosis, with generally limited need for imaging evaluation. Etiologies include viral hepatitis—hepatitis A (fecal-oral transmission), hepatitis B and C (IV drug use, sex or blood transfusion transmission), and hepatitis D and E—and drug-induced hepatitis with alcohol or acetaminophen, as well as autoimmune, steatohepatitis, among others.

In acute hepatitis, ultrasound (US) may show either a normal liver or a decreased echogenicity of the parenchyma, and prominence of the portal venous system, which is commonly known as a "starry sky" appearance. In chronic hepatitis, the liver is echogenic. However, this is not specific for hepatitis, and may be seen with any chronic liver disease. Additional nonspecific ultrasound findings seen in hepatitis include gallbladder wall thickening, contraction, and periportal lymphadenopathy. Hepatitis B and C increase the risk of cirrhosis, portal hypertension, and hepatocellular carcinoma. Coarse echotexture and surface nodularity are more specific signs of cirrhosis on US. CT and MR play a limited role in evaluating acute hepatitis, but may show nonspecific findings including hepatomegaly and periportal edema or enhancement [1]. MR may show heterogeneous liver intensity on T2-weighted images, and immediately after intravenous contrast administration. In the setting of equivocal liver enzyme elevation with nonspecific symptoms in a patient suspected of having steatohepatitis, MR

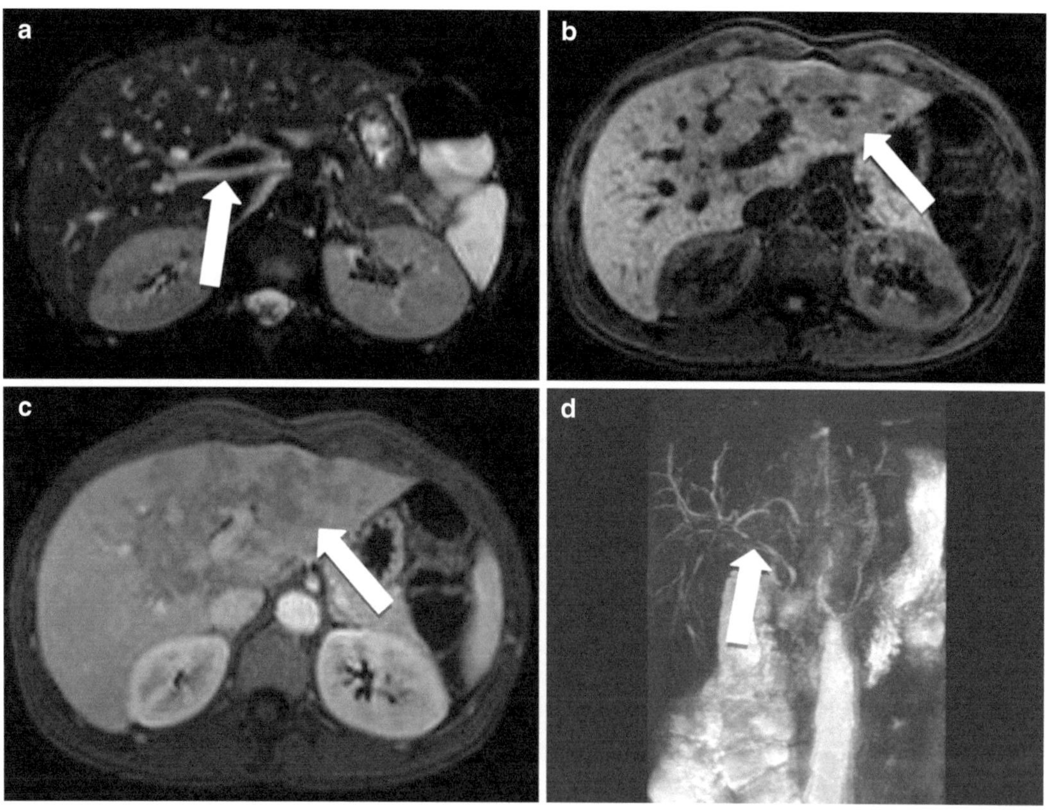

Fig. 4.1 AIDS cholangiohepatitis. 26-year-old man with AIDS and acute transaminitis of unknown etiology. Axial T2-weighted fat-saturated MR image (**a**) shows periportal edema (arrow). Axial T1-weighted fat-saturated pre-contrast (**b**) and post-contrast MR images in the portal venous phase (**c**) demonstrate heterogeneous hepatic parenchymal enhancement (arrow), a nonspecific finding which can be seen in the setting of hepatitis. 3D MRCP image (**d**) reveals multifocal segmental strictures of the intra- and extrahepatic biliary tract (arrow), which given the clinical information is highly consistent with AIDS cholangiopathy

is the examination with the most sensitivity and specificity. MR hepatic perfusion abnormalities may be seen in active liver disease, or in extrinsic inflammatory processes which have blood drainage to the liver, including pancreatitis and bowel inflammatory diseases (Figs. 4.1 and 4.2) [2].

4.2.2 Perihepatitis/Fitz-Hugh-Curtis Syndrome

Fitz-Hugh-Curtis syndrome is characterized by right-sided abdominal pain and perihepatitis due to pelvic inflammatory disease from a variety of organisms, particularly chlamydia and gonorrhea. Infection ascends from the vagina or cervix to the endometrium, fallopian tubes, and contiguous structures, resulting in endometritis, salpingitis, and tubo-ovarian abscess, which, if left untreated, may spread along the right paracolic gutter, resulting in perihepatitis. Typical findings include stringlike adhesions between the anterior surface of the liver and the parietal peritoneum, which are seen on US, CT, or MR as thickening and abnormal enhancement of the anterior liver capsule with peritoneal septations and loculated perihepatic ascites (Fig. 4.3) [3]. Nonspecific findings also include inflammation in the hepatorenal fossa, and gallbladder wall thickening. Clinical history and clinical examination pointing to pelvic inflammatory disease are essential to consider the diagnosis.

4.2.3 Hepatic Abscess

An abscess is a localized collection of necrotic inflammatory tissue caused by bacteria, fungal species, or parasites. Pyogenic liver abscesses usually develop secondary to an intestinal source of bacteria, as with appendicitis or diverticulitis, from recent surgery, or from complications of blunt or penetrating trauma. Clinical presentation is usually insidious, with several days to weeks of low-grade fever and right upper quadrant pain. Complications of liver abscess which may present with acute pain and/or sepsis include subphrenic abscess, peritoneal rupture, and Budd-Chiari syndrome from compression of the inferior vena cava or hepatic veins. Laboratory analysis shows leukocytosis, anemia, and elevated ESR.

US shows complex fluid collections of mixed echogenicity, thick-walled cysts, or cysts with fluid-fluid levels. An abscess may also appear as a solid liver mass, at which time through transmission aids in identifying them as nonsolid [4]. CT or MR may be needed for further characterization. CT demonstrates a peripherally enhancing, centrally hypoattenuating well-defined mass. A "double-target sign" may be seen with a hypodense fluid center, a hyperdense inner ring representing an abscess membrane which persists on delayed imaging, and a hypodense outer ring representing liver edema which only enhances on delayed images. MR classically shows a mass which is hypointense on T1-weighted images, hyperintense on T2-weighted images with thick walls, and internal septations which enhance on early arterial-phase imaging, and demonstrates persistent enhancement on late-phase imaging. An abscess will also show diffusion restriction (Figs. 4.4 and 4.5). MR is useful when a mass is not definitively characterized using CT, as MR gadolinium chelates have a higher sensitivity than CT does using iodinated contrast [5]. Differentiating an abscess from a metastasis with a large necrotic component may be difficult. In the setting of a metastasis, MR may show more progressive, centripetal stromal enhancement, and may have a more nodular, irregular, and thicker rim with a necrotic metastasis than with an abscess.

Fungal abscess may occur in immunocompromised patients, and most commonly caused by *Candida albicans* which concomitantly infects the spleen. Nodules are usually numerous, subcapsular, and small, measuring less than 1 cm. CT may show the classic target nodule in smaller form and peripheral distribution, but often does not show these characteristics convincingly enough to establish definitive diagnosis due to their small size and peripheral distribution. MR sequences with dynamic gadolinium-enhanced gradient-echo and T2-weighted fat-suppressed sequences are more sensitive for the identification of hepatosplenic candidiasis [6, 7]. Chronic

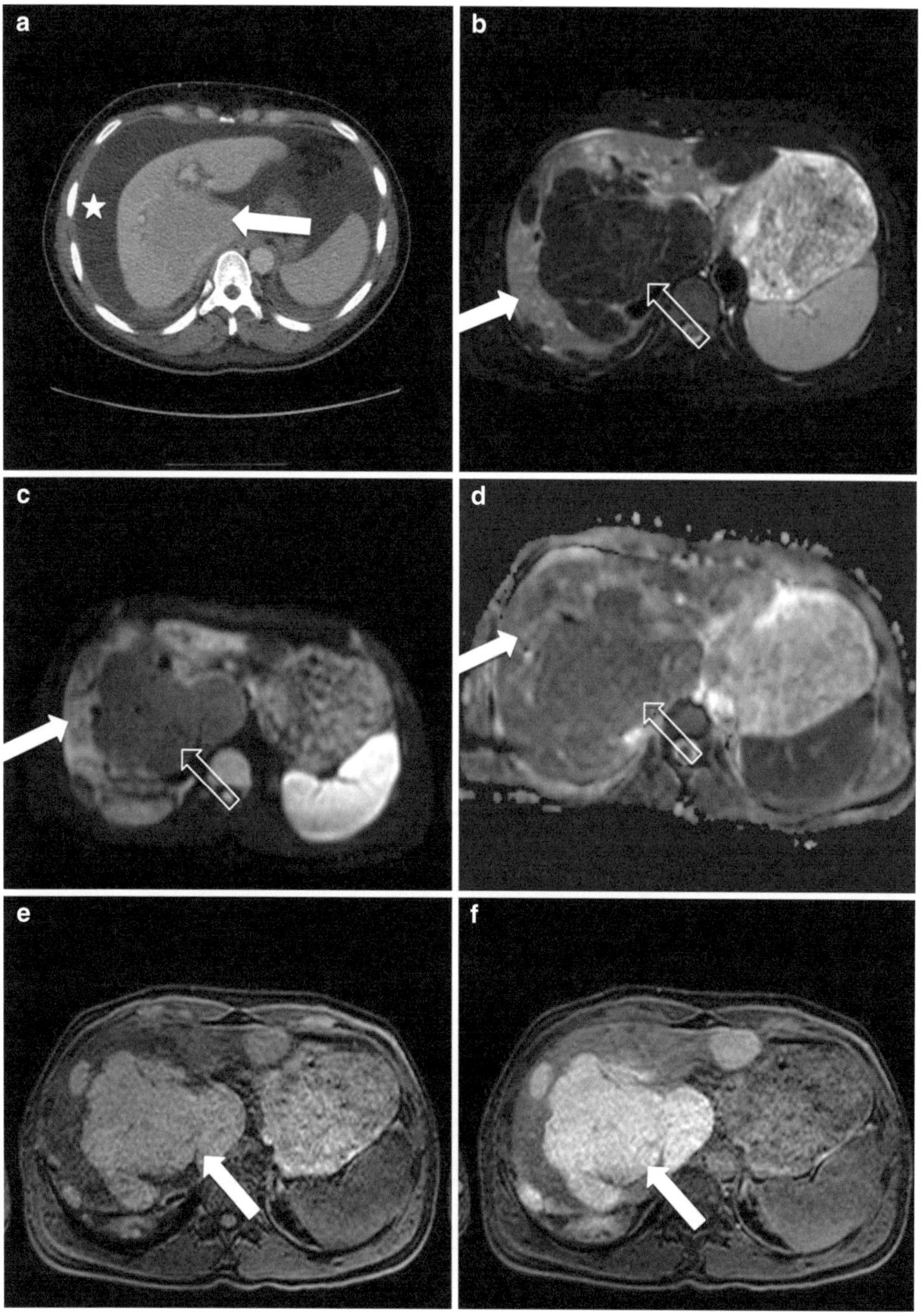

Fig. 4.2 Acute hepatic insult with subsequent nodular regenerative hyperplasia. 38-year-old man with elevated bilirubin, elevated INR, new ascites, and weight loss. Axial IV contrast-enhanced CT image (**a**) demonstrates extensive ascites (star) and a markedly abnormal liver with central hypoenhancement (arrow) and peripheral enhancement which was concerning for a mass. A follow-up MRI was obtained 6 weeks later. Axial T2-weighted fat-saturated MR image (**b**) and B600 diffusion-weighted MR image (**c**) reveal that the periphery of the liver has hyperintense signal (arrows) which does not restrict on the ADC map (arrow, **d**) while the central liver and scattered round foci at the periphery are normal (open arrow on the dominant nodule). T1-weighted fat-saturated pre-contrast (**e**) and 10-min-delay post-contrast (**f**) MR images reveal multiple regenerative nodules, particularly in the central liver (arrow on the dominant nodule), with large regions of hypoenhancement at the periphery of the liver. These findings were sequelae of the acute hepatic insult of unknown etiology that the patient sustained at the time of presentation, and not a tumor

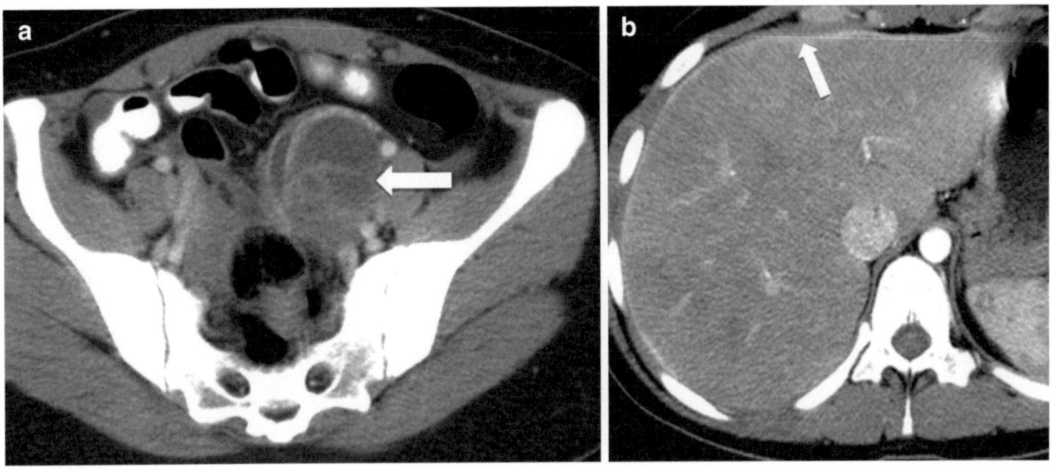

Fig. 4.3 Fitz-Hugh-Curtis syndrome. 25-year-old woman with cervical motion tenderness and right upper quadrant pain. (**a**) Contrast-enhanced axial CT image of the pelvis demonstrates a multi-loculated cyst in the left ovary, consistent with a tubo-ovarian abscess (arrow). (**b**) IV contrast-enhanced axial CT image of the upper abdomen demonstrates capsular enhancement of the liver (arrow), representing perihepatitis. Together, these findings represent Fitz-Hugh-Curtis syndrome

nodules may be seen as irregular shaped foci which are hypointense on T1-weighted images and isointense on T2-weighted images, with negligible enhancement, as they represent scar tissue.

Amebic abscesses result from primary colonic involvement with *Entamoeba histolytica* with seeding through the portal venous drainage, and hence affecting the right hepatic lobe, more commonly. It is thought that abscesses may result from trophosite obstruction in small venules, causing ischemic necrosis and infection [8]. These are indistinguishable from pyogenic abscess, but are more often seen as single masses and in a subdiaphragmatic location, with a thick 5–10 mm capsule which enhances (Fig. 4.6). Complications include intraperitoneal rupture with subsequent peritonitis, and diaphragmatic invasion with pulmonary consolidation and empyema. Conservative medical treatment is effective in most cases, with percutaneous drainage reserved for larger abscesses and abscesses close to the heart.

Other parasitic infections of the liver include echinococcal disease, which presents as a multicystic liver abscess with multiple daughter cysts, and schistosomiasis with ova infecting the portal triads, and causing fibrosis seen as thickened echogenic triads.

4.2.4 Portal Vein Thrombosis/Occlusion

Portal vein thrombosis or occlusion results from either slow flow as in portal hypertension or post-surgery, hypercoagulable states, or intestinal infection/inflammation including appendicitis or pancreatitis, as well as from external compression from tumors or lymphadenopathy. Thrombosis may be well tolerated with no acute symptoms, or may present as acute abdominal pain or variceal bleeding.

US shows an intraluminal filling defect which varies in echogenicity. On color Doppler, flow void or complete lack of intraluminal flow is seen. Sensitivity and specificity are close to 90% [9]. False positive causes include slow portal vein flow. False negative causes include a large periportal collateral which can be confused with a patent portal vein. In the setting of chronic portal vein thrombosis, cavernous transformation is seen as multiple collateral vessels surrounding a thrombosed portal vein (Fig. 4.7).

MR is useful in distinguishing tumor thrombus from bland thrombus and in patients with equivocal US findings. Diagnosis is best achieved by combining black-blood techniques (spin-echo techniques with superior and inferior saturation pulses) or bright-blood technique

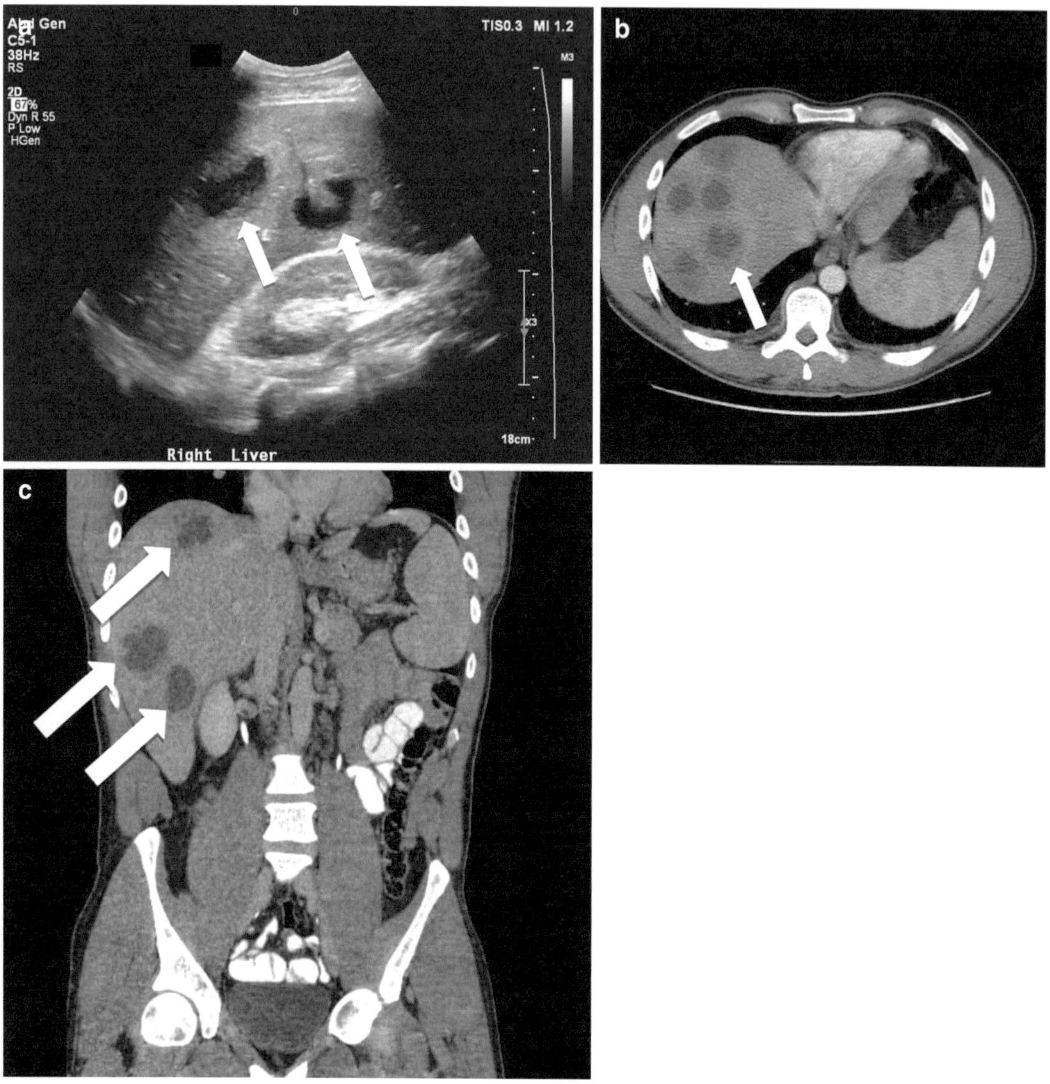

Fig. 4.4 Liver abscesses. 43-year-old man with acute right upper quadrant pain and elevated GGT. Representative longitudinal image from an ultrasound through the liver (**a**) demonstrates multiple hypoechoic hepatic masses with peripheral echogenic rims (arrows). Axial (**b**) and coronal (**c**) IV contrast-enhanced CT images reveal multiple peripherally enhancing, centrally hypoattenuating masses in the liver (arrows), consistent with hepatic abscesses, which were of mixed flora at pathologic analysis via image-guided drainage

(time-of-flight (TOF) gradient echo (GRE) or gadolinium-enhanced gradient echo) [10]. Tumor thrombus is most commonly seen with hepatocellular carcinoma, and shows high signal on T2-weighted images and soft-tissue signal intensity on TOF GRE images, and enhances with intravenous gadolinium. Bland thrombus is seen in cirrhosis, infection, or inflammation, and is low in signal on T2-weighted images and TOF, and does not enhance with gadolinium. If bland thrombus is infected, one may see enhancement of the portal vein wall.

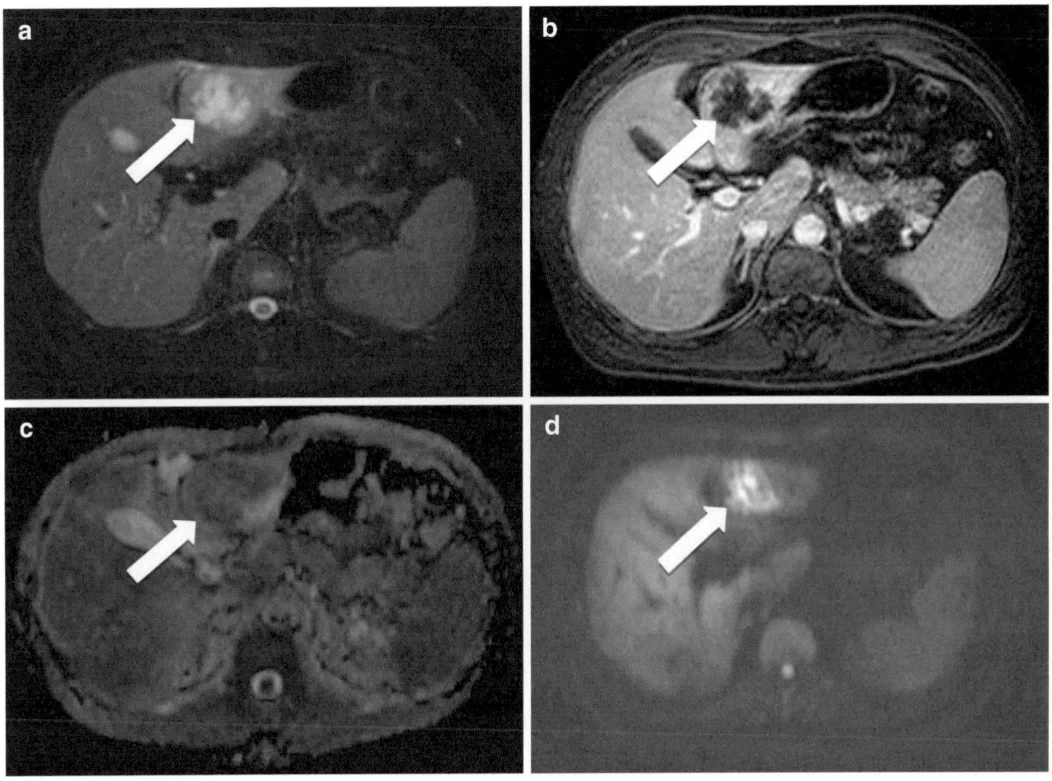

Fig. 4.5 Liver abscess. 45-year-old man with elevated bilirubin, fever, and leukocytosis. Axial T2 fat-saturated image through the liver (**a**) demonstrates an irregular hyperintense mass in segment three (arrow). Axial T1-weighted post-contrast MR image (**b**) in the equilibrium phase shows peripheral enhancement and central hypointensity of this mass, while ADC map (**c**) and B600 (**d**) MR images reveal restricted diffusion in this mass (arrows). Percutaneous sampling proved this to be a *Klebsiella pneumoniae* liver abscess

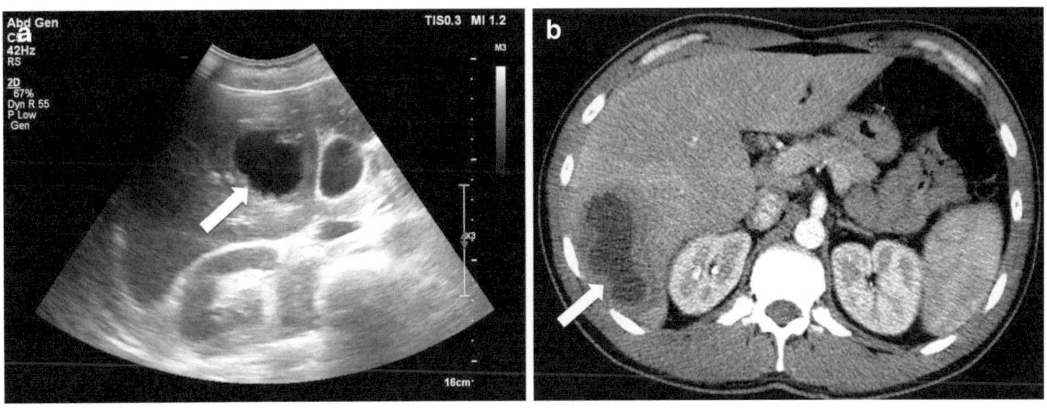

Fig. 4.6 Amebic abscess. 35-year-old woman with abdominal pain, fevers, and chills. Grayscale axial ultrasound image (**a**) demonstrates a large irregular thick-walled cyst in the right hepatic lobe (arrow). Axial IV contrast-enhanced CT image (**b**) reveals a rim-enhancing low-attenuation mass with peripheral edema (arrow) in segment six and associated hyperemia, which proved to be an amebic abscess

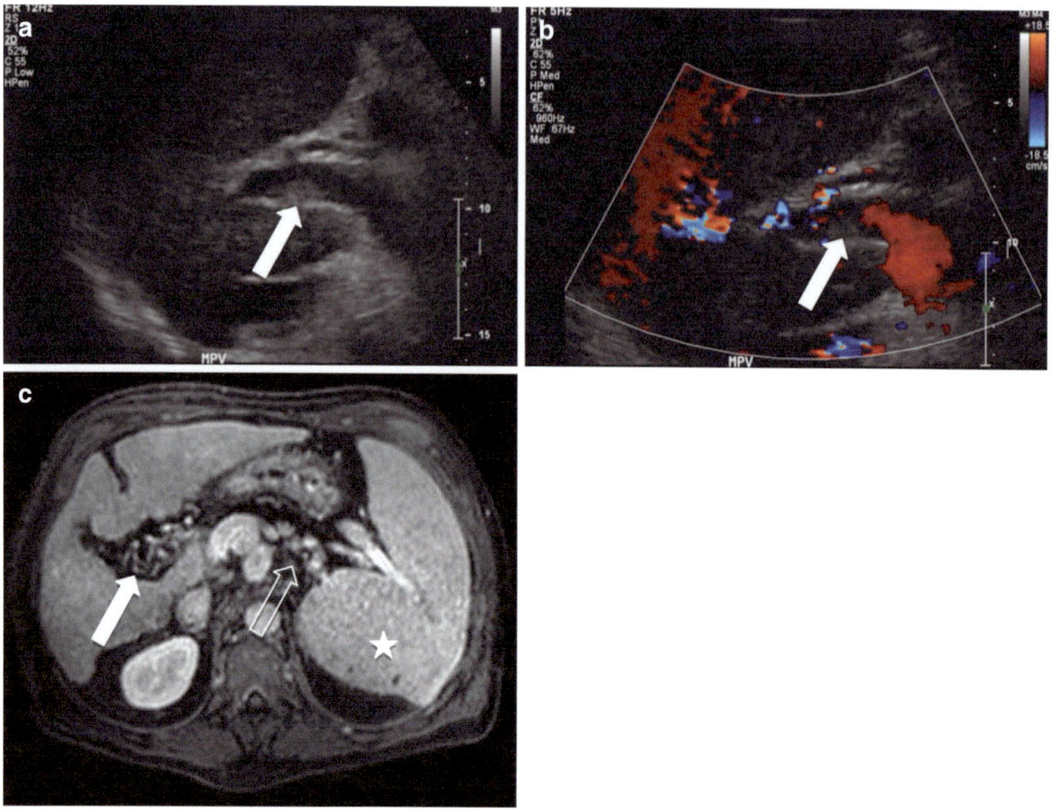

Fig. 4.7 Portal vein thrombosis. 53-year-old man with a history of hepatitis C-related cirrhosis. 2D (**a**) and color Doppler (**b**) longitudinal ultrasound images acquired 8 years prior demonstrate a nonocclusive thrombus (arrows) in the main portal vein. Recent T1-weighted post-contrast axial MR image (**c**) demonstrates cavernous transformation in the porta hepatis (solid arrow) due to interval complete portal vein occlusion since the prior ultrasound. Note is also made of mild splenomegaly (star) and splenorenal shunts (open arrow)

4.2.5 Budd-Chiari Syndrome

Budd-Chiari syndrome is characterized by centrilobular congestion, hepatocellular necrosis, and atrophy from hepatic venous outflow obstruction due to IVC or hepatic vein thrombosis. Common causes of thrombosis include pregnancy, oral contraceptive use, polycythemia vera, chronic fibrosis, webs obstructing the veins, and tumors including HCC, renal cell carcinoma, and adrenal cortical carcinoma. Patients may present clinically with abdominal pain, signs of portal hypertension, and ascites. CT and MR findings in acute Budd-Chiari syndrome include narrowing or non-visualization of the hepatic veins and/or IVC, caudate lobe enlargement, decreased peripheral parenchymal enhancement, and intrahepatic collateral vessels which may be seen as comma-shaped enhancing vessels (Fig. 4.8) [11].

4.2.6 Hepatic Infarction

Because of the dual arterial and portal blood supply to the liver, hepatic infarcts are very uncommon. Hepatic infarction is a grave complication most often seen after liver transplantation, often necessitating repeat transplantation. Acute hepatic infarction appears hypoechoic on US and hypoattenuating on CT. A key imaging feature of hepatic infarction is the preservation of portal tracts, because it differentiates it from other etiologies, including abscess, biloma, and post-biopsy hematoma. A potential pitfall is focal

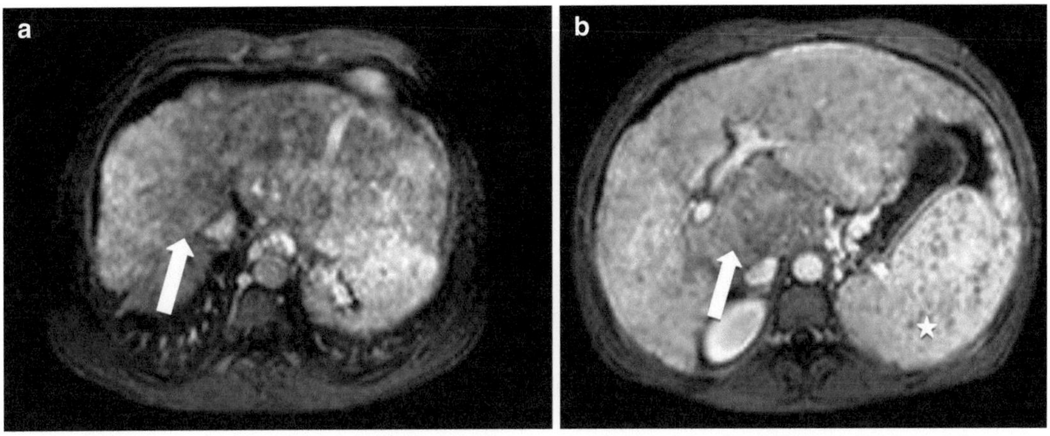

Fig. 4.8 Budd-Chiari syndrome. 26-year-old man from Sudan with a history of giardiasis and amebic infections. T1-weighted post-contrast axial MR image in the portal venous phase (**a**) shows occlusion of the hepatic veins (arrow) in the enlarged and nodular liver. Delayed enhancement of the peripheral liver with central low density and hypertrophy of the caudate lobe (arrow, **b**) is noted on an axial T1-weighted MR image, which is highly consistent with Budd-Chiari syndrome. Note is also made that the spleen is borderline enlarged (star, **b**)

hepatic steatosis. However, this tends to occur in characteristic locations, and normally enhancing vessels course through it [12].

4.2.7 Hepatocellular Carcinoma

Patients with hepatitis or any type of chronic liver disease are at increased risk of hepatocellular carcinoma (HCC). Prevalence is highest in Asia and Africa due to higher rates of viral hepatitis. Nonetheless, incidence has been steadily increasing in the United States. Any liver mass in a patient with chronic liver disease should be further evaluated with dedicated liver imaging, with either a multiphase contrast-enhanced CT liver mass protocol or a dynamic contrast-enhanced MR liver mass protocol. There is consensus that MR is superior to CT for the identification of HCC [13]. US has a sensitivity of 60% and a specificity of 85–90% for the diagnosis of HCC, and is easily accessible and uses no ionizing radiation, hence its use as the primary screening modality. Recent literature has shown the potential usefulness of MR as a screening modality for patients with chronic liver disease at risk of HCC, due to its higher sensitivity and specificity [14].

HCC is the fifth most common malignancy in the world, and accounts for one million deaths annually, with a 5-year survival rate of <5% for untreated, symptomatic HCC [15]. For tumors >2 cm, MR most frequently shows hyperintensity on T2-weighted images and hypointensity on T1-weighted images, with enhancement on arterial phase images, washout on portal venous and delayed images, and late pseudocapsular enhancement (Fig. 4.9). Although usually asymptomatic, HCC may present in the emergency setting as hemoperitoneum from a ruptured mass. Different mechanisms have been described, including tumor expansion leading to subcapsular hemorrhage, and rupture of the liver capsule with associated intraperitoneal hemorrhage. This may present clinically as sudden onset of epigastric or right hypochondrial pain due to Glisson's capsule distention, peritonitis, hypotension, and shock from bleeding. A clinical history of cirrhosis or HCC is essential, or high suspicion in a patient from an endemic area with acute abdominal pain.

CT findings include high-attenuation peritoneal fluid around the liver and spleen in the setting of acute bleeding from a ruptured mass, with change in composition and, hence, density of the hematoma, depending on the age of the blood products, clotting, and layering hematocrit effect [16]. Small volumes of blood may layer in Morrison's pouch or in the pelvis. A classic CT finding, the "sentinel clot"

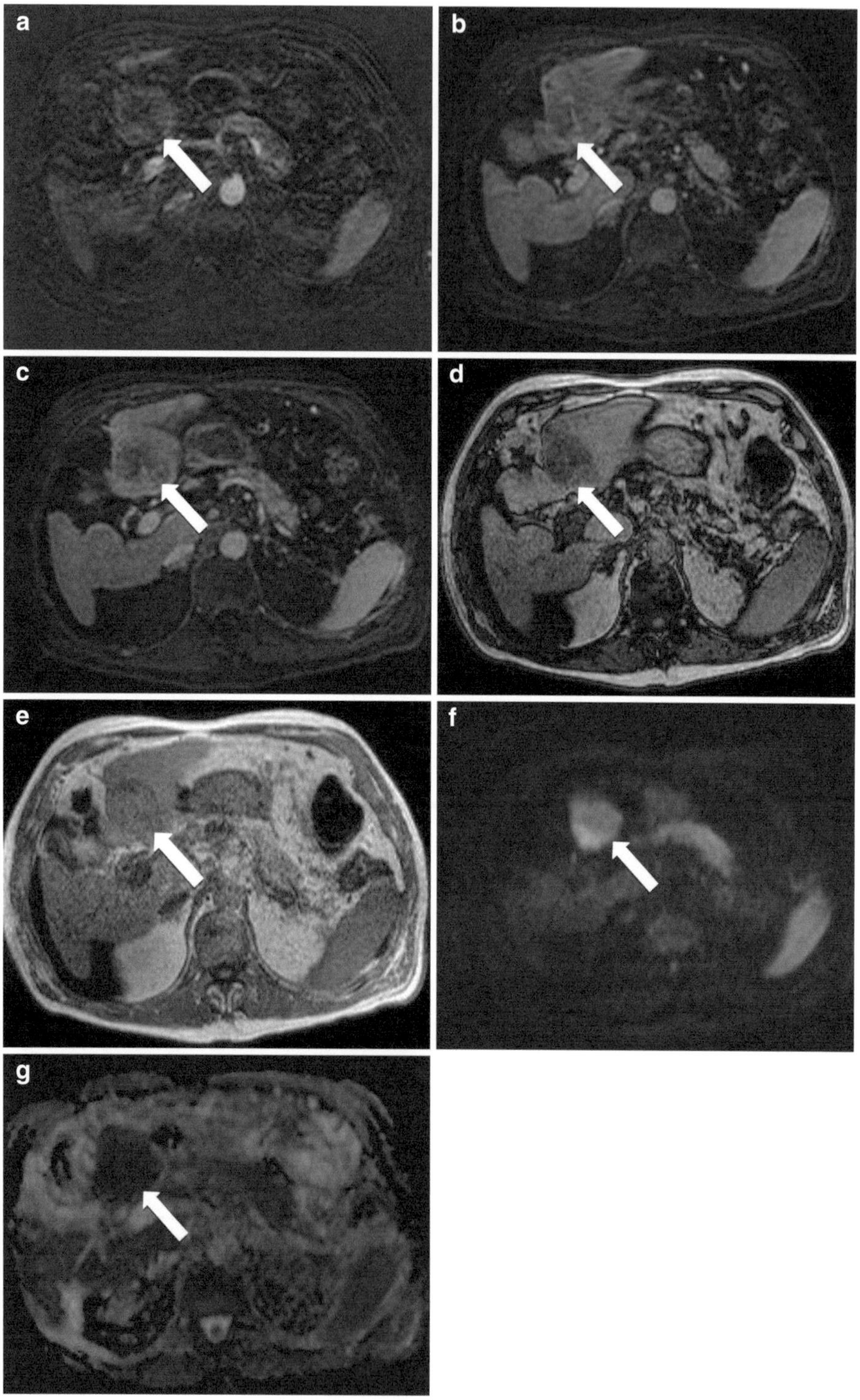

Fig. 4.9 Hepatocellular carcinoma. 79-year-old man with cirrhosis and liver masses detected incidentally on a chest CT done for rectal cancer staging. Axial MR images demonstrate cirrhosis, perihepatic ascites, and a 5.5 cm mass in segment three with arterial enhancement (arrow, **a**), and washout on venous and equilibrium phase T1-weighted fat-saturated images (arrows, **b** and **c**, respectively), signal loss on T1-weighted out-of-phase (arrow, **d**) when compared to T1-weighted in-phase imaging (arrow, **e**), and restricted diffusion on B600 (arrow, **f**) when compared to the ADC map (arrow, **g**), which is highly consistent with a well-differentiated hepatocellular carcinoma

sign, which refers to clotted blood at the site of tissue rupture, which usually has Hounsfield units of 45–60 (Figs. 4.10 and 4.11). Blood spilling into the peritoneal cavity will show Hounsfield units (HU) of acute blood at approximately 45 HU. Mortality is high, and urgent treatment is needed with transcatheter arterial embolization. MR findings are similar to those seen on CT, with signal characteristics of blood varying based on the age of the blood products. By the time most patients get imaged, the majority of the blood products will be high signal on T1-weighted imaging, and mixed or intermediate signal on T2-weighted images [15].

4.2.8 Hepatic Adenoma

Hepatocellular adenoma is a mass composed of normal hepatocytes which produce bile but do not have bile ductules, and are partially or completely enclosed by a pseudocapsule from compressed hepatic parenchyma. It used to be a rare tumor until the introduction of oral contraceptives [17]. Other causes include diabetes, glycogen storage disease, iron overload, and anabolic steroids. Although usually asymptomatic and diagnosed incidentally, patients may present with acute abdominal pain related to intratumoral hemorrhage or, rarely, peritoneal

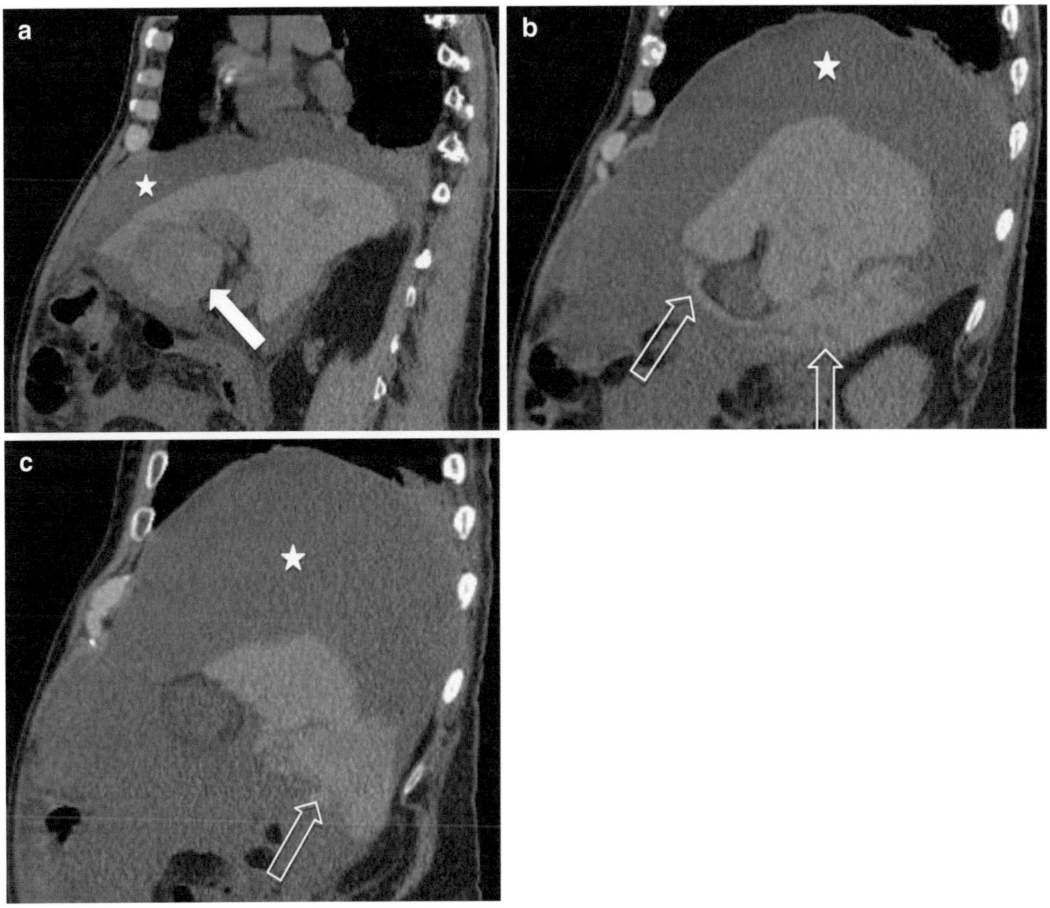

Fig. 4.10 Same patient as in Fig. 4.9. Ruptured hepatocellular carcinoma. 79-year-old man with known hepatocellular carcinoma diagnosed 3 months ago presents with an acute hematocrit drop and grossly bloody ascites on paracentesis after a fall 1 day prior. Sagittal non-contrast CT images demonstrate the known segment three hepatocellular carcinoma (arrow, **a**) and adjacent sentinel clot (open arrows, **b** and **c**) tracking into the right paracolic gutter. Extensive hemoperitoneum is noted (star)

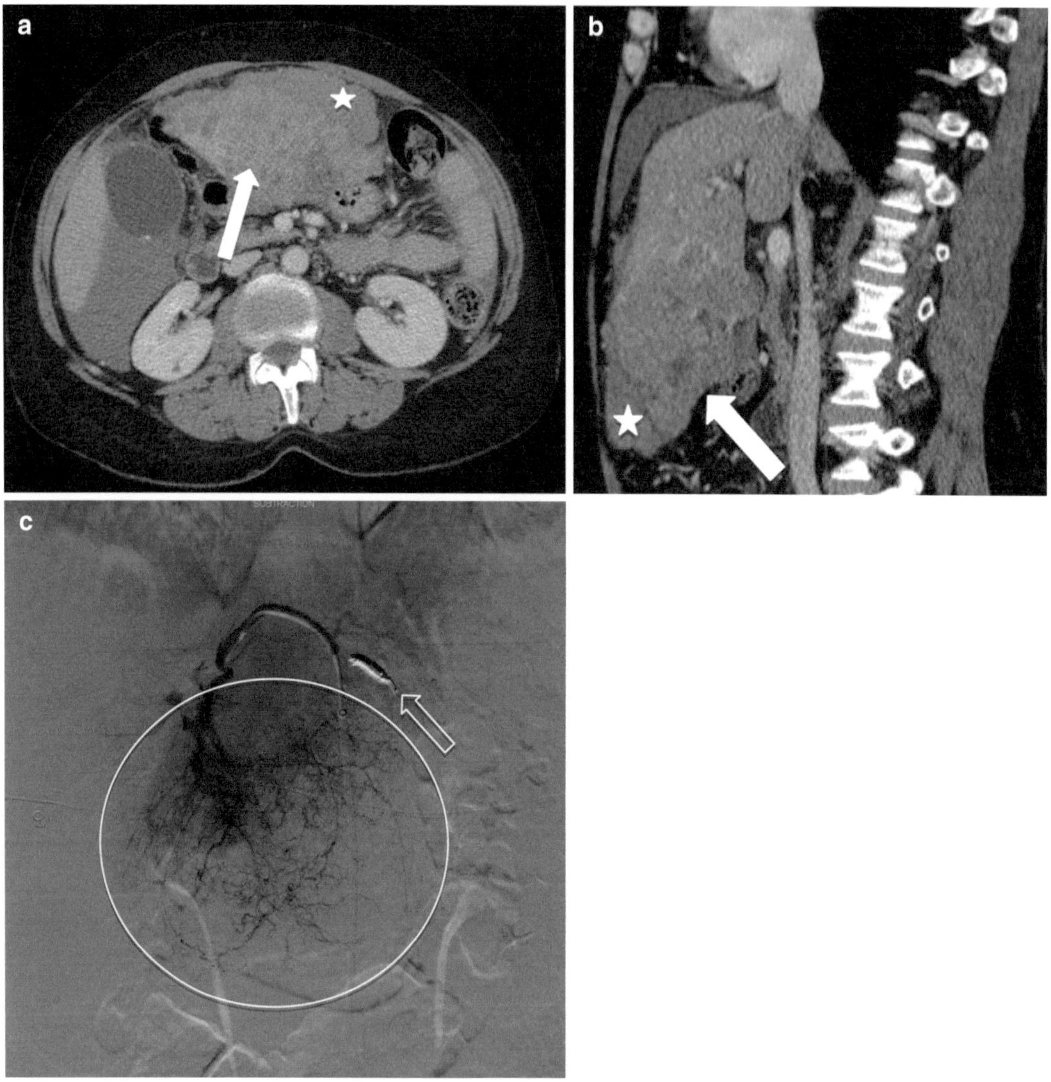

Fig. 4.11 Ruptured hepatocellular carcinoma with subsequent embolization. 54-year-old man with chronic hepatitis C, cirrhosis, and ascites presented with tachycardia and abdominal pain. Axial (**a**) and sagittal (**b**) IV contrast-enhanced CT images show a large heterogeneous mass (arrows) in the left lobe of a cirrhotic liver, with adjacent active hemorrhage (star), representing a ruptured hepatocellular carcinoma. Simple perihepatic ascites is also visualized. Digital subtraction angiographic image (**c**) reveals a large hypervascular tumor arising from the left lobe of the liver (circle). This mass derived its blood supply from a replaced left hepatic artery arising from the left gastric artery. To avoid nontarget embolization of the lesser curvature of the stomach, a large branch of the left gastric artery was embolized using two metallic coils (open arrow). Subsequent bland embolization of the hepatocellular carcinoma was performed

hemorrhage requiring emergent intervention. Malignant transformation is rare.

Because US findings are nonspecific, showing a single mass of variable echogenicity, additional imaging is usually needed for diagnosis. On non-v CT, adenomas are usually isodense to liver, or hypodense if they contain fat (Fig. 4.12). If there is hemorrhage, non-contrast CT shows areas of high attenuation, or heterogeneity if there is old hemorrhage. Intratumoral hemorrhage is seen in 25–40% of adenomas (Fig. 4.13) [18]. If intravenous contrast is given, early homogeneous enhancement

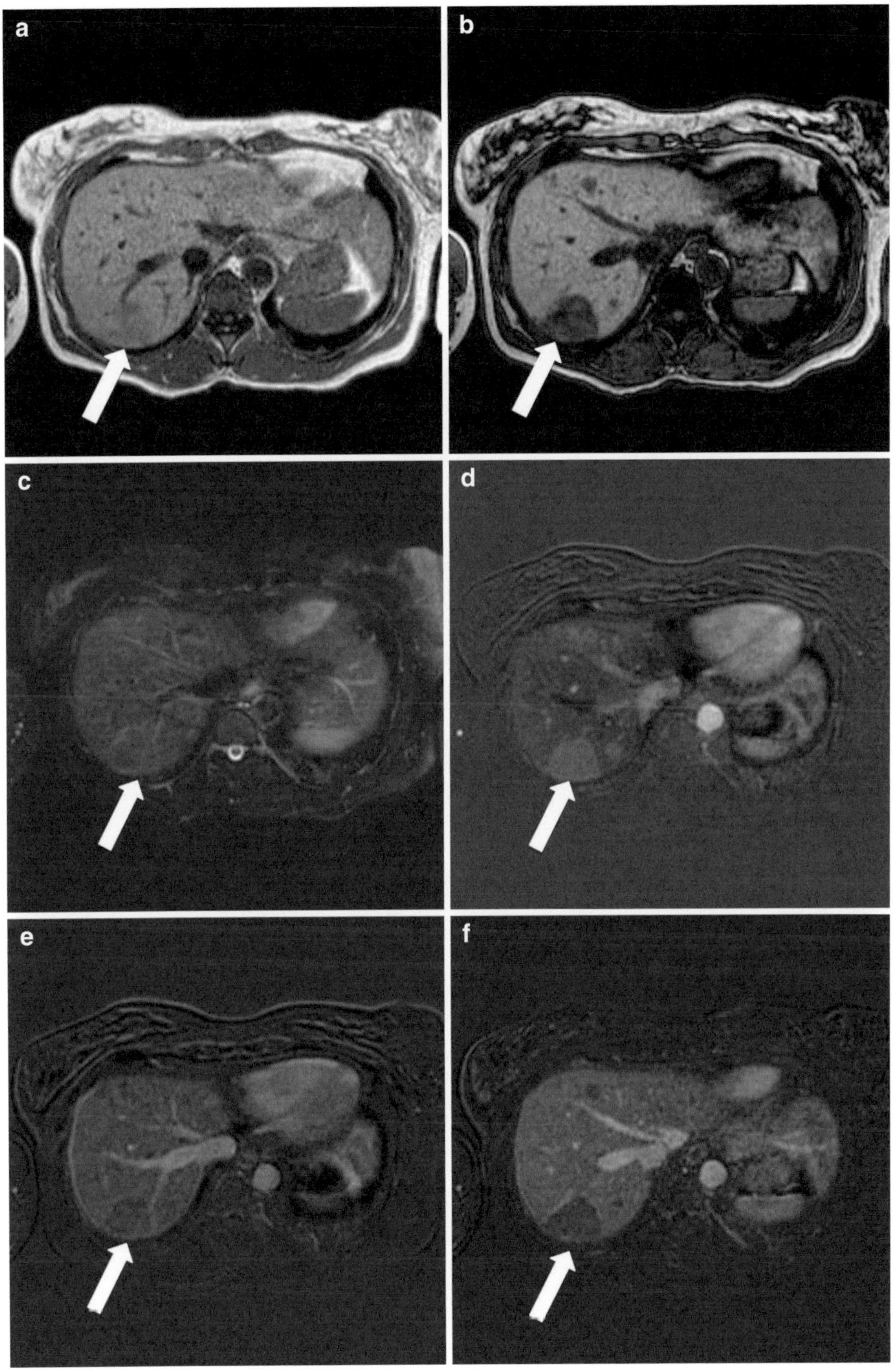

Fig. 4.12 Hepatic adenoma. 51-year-old woman with biopsy-proven hepatic adenomatosis. These masses were incidentally detected on a CT scan of her thorax when she was 36 years old. The largest of the patient's known hepatic adenomas is shown in segment seven on MR imaging. In-phase (**a**) and opposed-phase (**b**) T1-weighted MR images reveal signal loss on the opposed-phase image, consistent with intratumoral fat. This mass is only faintly T2 hyperintense on this T2-weighted fat-saturated image (**c**). Dynamic post-contrast subtraction images reveal arterial enhancement (**d**) followed by rapid washout on the venous phase (**e**), and pseudocapsular enhancement on the equilibrium phase (**f**), classic imaging features for a hepatic adenoma in a non-cirrhotic patient

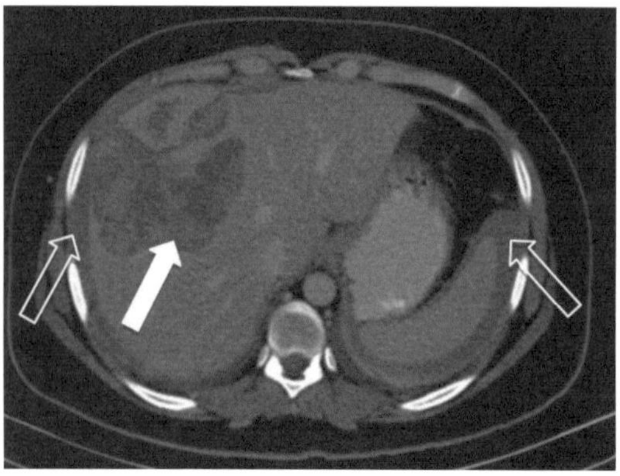

Fig. 4.13 Ruptured hepatic adenoma. 28-year-old woman with a known hepatic adenoma who presents with new-onset acute abdominal pain. Axial IV contrast-enhanced CT image reveals hyperattenuation within the known hepatic adenoma, representing acute hemorrhage (closed arrow). Associated hemoperitoneum is visualized (open arrow)

and isodensity with liver parenchyma in portal venous and delayed phases are seen. Non-bleeding masses are usually managed conservatively if they measure less than 5 cm [19].

MR shows a homogeneous mass with mild hyperintensity on T2-weighted images and hypo- or isointensity on T1-weighted images. Post-contrast images show a transient homogeneous blush which uniformly fades to isointensity with normal liver parenchyma by 1 min [20]. More heterogeneous signal may be seen on T1- and T2-weighted images depending on the amounts of fat, hemorrhage, and necrosis. When the mass shows an intense marble pattern of arterial enhancement, it may be difficult to distinguish it from HCC, but the presence of washout and a capsule in HCC should help make the distinction.

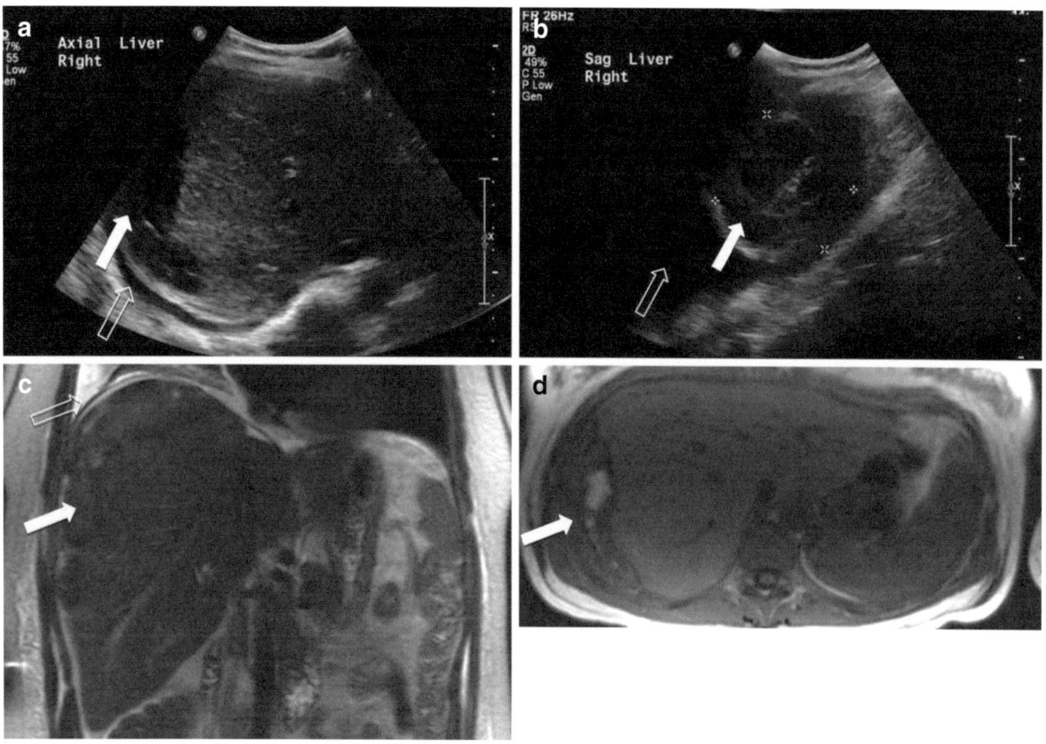

Fig. 4.14 HELLP syndrome. 36-year-old pregnant woman with elevated liver function tests and right upper quadrant pain. Axial (**a**) and longitudinal (**b**) grayscale ultrasound images of the liver demonstrate a heterogeneous perihepatic fluid collection (solid arrows) as well as a right pleural effusion (open arrows). Coronal T2-weighted (**c**) and axial T1-weighted (**d**) images confirm the presence of perihepatic hematoma (solid arrows) in this patient with HELLP syndrome. The right pleural effusion is also seen in C (open arrow) (images courtesy of Dr. Vincent Mellnick)

4.2.9 HELLP Syndrome

HELLP syndrome is an uncommon but serious obstetrical condition characterized by hemolysis (H), elevated liver enzymes (EL), and low platelet count (LP), and occurs in 0.2–0.6% of all pregnancies, and in 10–20% of women with severe preeclampsia [21, 22]. Maternal clinical symptoms are nonspecific and, unfortunately, can masquerade as a variety of other conditions. The pathophysiology of HELLP has not been clearly elucidated to our knowledge; however, altered placental function resulting in ischemia-producing oxidative stress is one proposed etiology [23]. Imaging features of HELLP include perihepatic free fluid, hepatic steatosis, liver enlargement, and a periportal halo which may precede more severe conditions including hepatic hematoma and hepatic rupture with hemoperitoneum (Fig. 4.14), leading to high morbidity and mortality [24].

4.3 Gallbladder

4.3.1 Acute Calculous Cholecystitis

The most common cause of acute cholecystitis is impacted calculi in the cystic duct or common bile duct (95%) [25]. Calculi obstruct bile drainage into the common bile duct, leading to gallbladder overdistention, increased intraluminal pressure, inflammation, and eventually wall ischemia and bacterial superinfection with necrosis, if not treated promptly. Clinical presentation includes a history of colicky pain after a meal of high-fat content, with acute onset of constant, right upper quadrant pain lasting >6 h, with or without fever, chills, and laboratory markers of acute inflammation including leukocytosis. US is the first-line modality for diagnosis, showing cholelithiasis, diffuse wall thickening with pericholecystic fluid and/or hyperemia, gallbladder distention greater than 10 × 4 cm, and a positive sonographic Murphy sign [26].

When initial findings are indeterminate and clinical examination is not definitive for acute cholecystitis, hepatobiliary scintigraphy, CT, or MRI may be used for definitive diagnosis prior to surgery. MR is particularly useful for identifying a different cause for the patient's symptoms, and for identifying a cause for biliary obstruction when calculi are not seen. CT is 85% sensitive for gallstones, less than US, but may show additional findings of stranding of the pericholecystic fat, abnormalities in the gallbladder fossa, and complications including gas in the gallbladder wall as is seen in emphysematous cholecystitis [27]. Additionally, if narrow CT windows are used and/or newer techniques such as dual energy, the yield of CT increases to higher than the aforementioned 85% [28].

A more comprehensive evaluation of cholecystitis, its root cause, and possible complications is achieved with MR. The high sensitivity of T1-weighted fat-saturated contrast-enhanced images makes MR an excellent tool for the diagnosis of cholecystitis, with sensitivity greater than that of ultrasound [29]. Findings are similar to those seen on CT, with mucosal enhancement on early phases, and progressive gallbladder wall enhancement and transient enhancement of surrounding liver parenchyma. On T2-weighted imaging, calculi can be excluded or identified, and pericholecystic fluid and abscesses are revealed if present. MR in conjunction with MRCP increases sensitivity for the diagnosis of exclusion of coexisting choledocholithiasis, can reveal a mass or another cause of obstruction including as stricture, and outlines possible complications, including empyema, perforation, and gangrene, which are not as readily seen on US, CT, or hepatobiliary scintigraphy (Fig. 4.15).

4.3.2 Acute Acalculous Cholecystitis

Acalculous cholecystitis accounts for approximately 5–10% of patients with acute cholecystitis, and has a higher mortality rate than calculous cholecystitis (approaching 50%), and a higher rate of complications including gangrene, emphysema, and perforation [26]. One must consider acute acalculous cholecystitis in patients with prolonged hospitalization, patients with comorbidities includ-

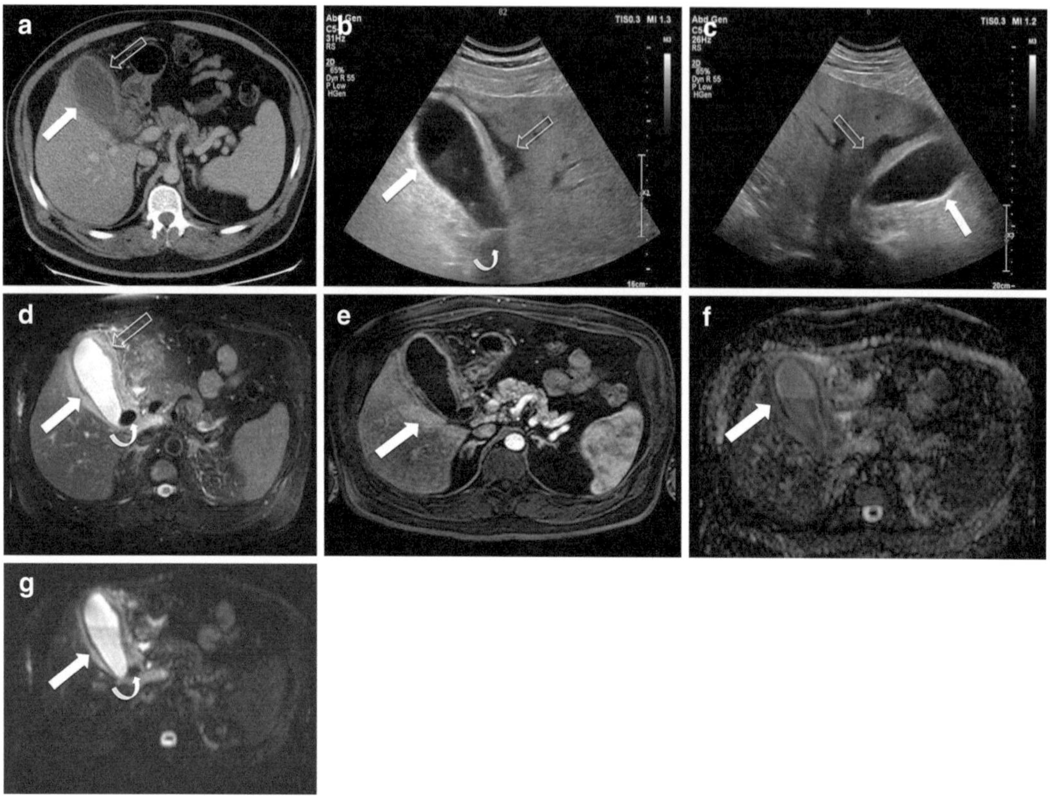

Fig. 4.15 Acute calculous cholecystitis. 53-year-old man with fever and leukocytosis. In the emergency department, an IV contrast-enhanced CT was acquired due to the absence of localizing symptoms. An axial CT image (**a**) demonstrates a distended gallbladder with wall thickening (arrow) and pericholecystic fluid and inflammation (open arrow), which is highly consistent with acute cholecystitis. Subsequent axial (**b**) and longitudinal (**c**) ultrasound images confirmed these findings (solid arrows and open arrows) and also identified a shadowing gallstone (curved arrow). An IV contrast-enhanced MRCP was performed to assess for possible choledocholithiasis and associated findings prior to cholecystectomy. T2-weighted fat-saturated axial image (**d**) again shows gallbladder distention, wall thickening (arrow), calculus (curved arrow), and pericholecystic fluid (open arrow). T1-weighted IV contrast-enhanced arterial phase MR image (**e**) demonstrates gallbladder fossa hyperemia (arrow). ADC (**f**) and B600 (**g**) axial MR images illustrate restricted diffusion of the gallbladder wall edema (arrows) and the calculus (curved arrow)

ing diabetes and sepsis, and patients undergoing mechanical ventilation or parenteral nutrition. Inflammation is not due to cystic duct obstruction, but rather wall ischemia from decreased gallbladder contraction and overdistention, or by direct bacterial infection. Clinical examination is similar to that of acute calculous cholecystitis, but is often masked by other comorbidities.

US, CT, and MR findings of acalculous cholecystitis include a distended gallbladder with wall thickening, intraluminal sludge with no calculi, pericholecystic fluid, and hyperemia of the gallbladder fossa on the arterial phase at CT or MR (Fig. 4.16). These findings are nonspecific, and may be seen with hypoalbuminemia, hepatitis, cirrhosis, and heart failure, making diagnosis difficult. Hepatobiliary scintigraphy may help to confirm the diagnosis by showing non-filling of the gallbladder, but may not reveal the cause for non-filling. MR with MRCP can be used to exclude choledocholithiasis, with a reported negative predictive value of 93% for a normal MRCP, and a probability of 89% of having no CBD calculus demonstrated as well as no readmission due to calculus disease within 6 months following MRCP [30]. MR/MRCP may reduce the amount of unnecessary ERCP procedures and associated complications.

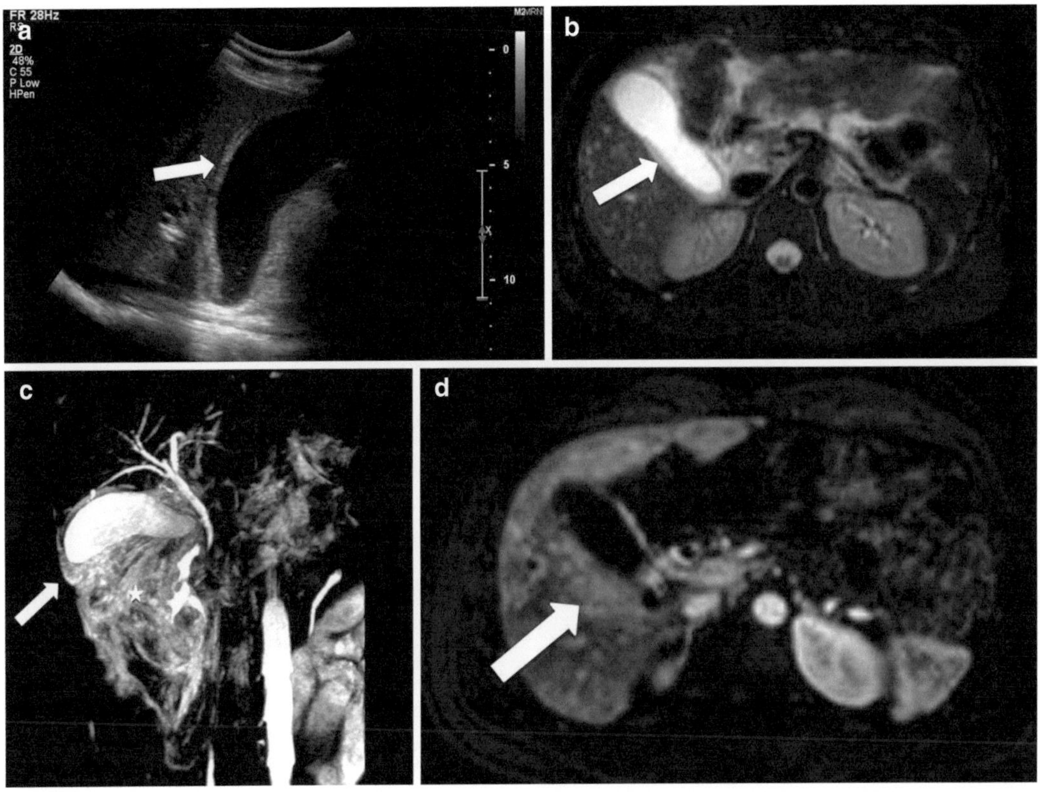

Fig. 4.16 Acute acalculous cholecystitis. 37-year-old man with right upper quadrant pain. Longitudinal ultrasound image (**a**) demonstrates distention and wall thickening of the gallbladder with associated pericholecystic fluid (arrow). No calculi are present. MR/MRCP was subsequently performed to assess for possible choledocholithiasis. Axial T2-weighted fat-saturated MR and 3D MRCP images (**b**, **c**) mirror the ultrasound, with gallbladder distention and wall thickening (arrows) with associated pericholecystic fluid (star on 3D MRCP image). Again, no calculi were seen. T1-weighted axial fat-saturated IV contrast-enhanced arterial phase MR image (**d**) shows hyperemia of the gallbladder fossa (arrow)

4.3.3 Complicated Acute Cholecystitis

Untreated acute cholecystitis may result in perforation, abscess formation, fistula, peritonitis, and gangrenous or emphysematous cholecystitis.

In gangrenous cholecystitis, there is necrosis of the gallbladder wall, which is a surgical emergency. US findings most specific for acute gangrenous cholecystitis include a striated, multilayered appearance of the gallbladder wall, and an irregular gallbladder wall with decreased or absent flow on Doppler [31]. CT and MR show intraluminal membranes, an indistinct wall with non-enhancement of the foci of gangrene, intraluminal blood contents, and pericholecystic abscess (Fig. 4.17) [32].

Emphysematous cholecystitis results from small-vessel ischemia resulting in gallbladder wall inflammation and necrosis with superinfection with gas-forming organisms. This entity is usually seen in diabetic or elderly patients, and carries a high mortality. Gallbladder wall gas is a specific sign readily seen on US and CT (Fig. 4.18). MR may become useful if the diagnosis is unclear, as it can show characteristic signal voids in the gallbladder wall or susceptibility artifact on GRE images. Although the cross-sectional imaging features of gangrenous and emphysematous cholecystitis overlap, the end result is still ischemia and necrosis, with an urgent need for appropriate management.

Additional complications from acute cholecystitis are perforation and/or hemorrhage of

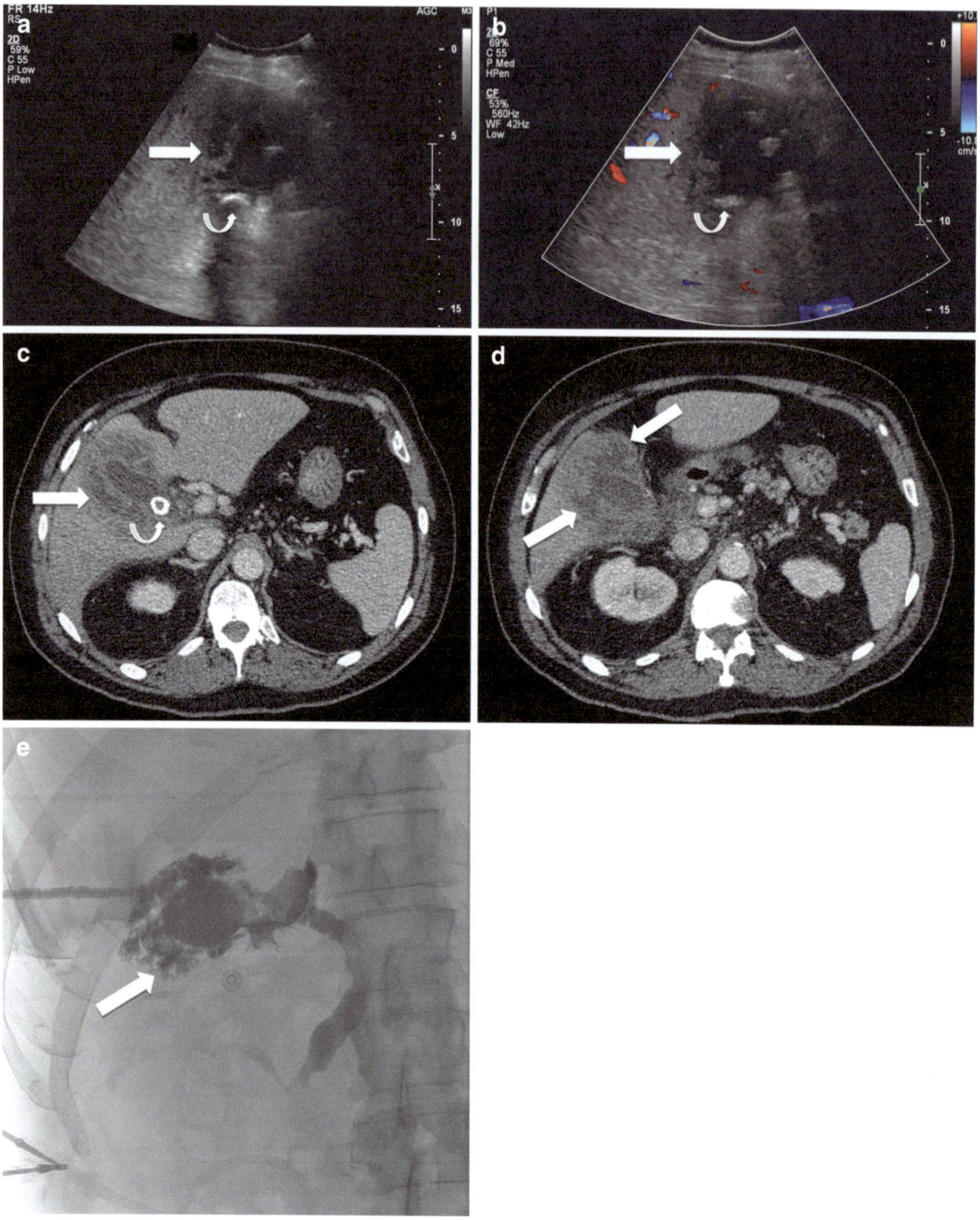

Fig. 4.17 Gangrenous cholecystitis. 70-year-old man with new liver function test elevation and fever. Grayscale (**a**) and color Doppler axial ultrasound images (**b**) reveal a markedly abnormal gallbladder which contains a calculus (curved arrows), and which has an irregular, thickened wall with associated pericholecystic fluid collections (arrows). Axial IV contrast-enhanced CT images (**c**, **d**) show similar findings; however, the discontinuity of the gallbladder wall is more conspicuous (arrows in **d**). A percutaneous cholecystostomy tube was placed, and at a later date a fluoroscopy tube check was performed (**e**), which demonstrates a patent cystic duct and a markedly abnormal gallbladder with a discontinuous wall and opacification of multiple pericholecystic fluid collections (arrow)

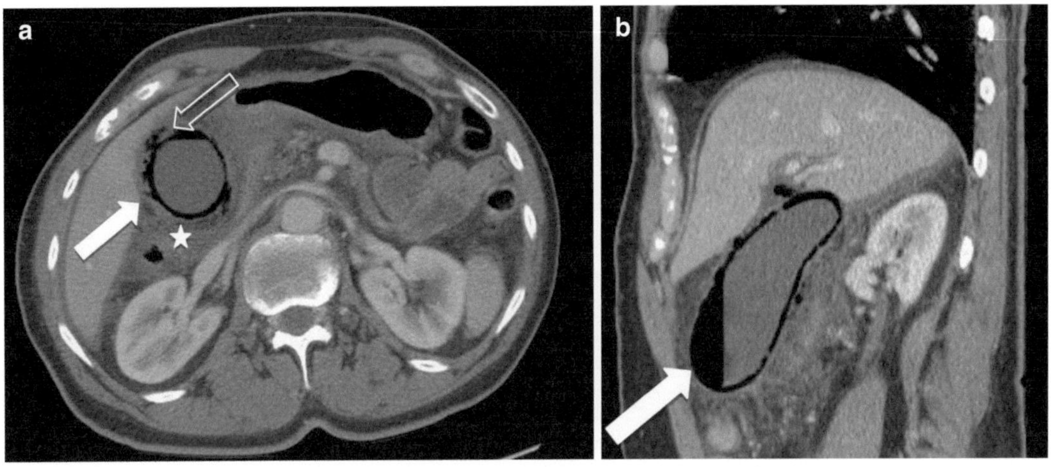

Fig. 4.18 Emphysematous cholecystitis. 74-year-old man with a history of metastatic non-small-cell lung cancer who presented to the emergency department with abdominal pain and vomiting. Axial (**a**) and sagittal (**b**) IV contrast-enhanced CT images reveal a distended gallbladder with a large amount of gas within its irregular wall and lumen (arrows). Multiple foci of discontinuity are seen in the gallbladder wall (open arrow, **a**), with dissection of free gas into the portocaval region (not shown). There was moderate perihepatic free fluid (star). There was a small amount of pneumobilia in the left hepatic lobe (not shown)

the gallbladder. Imaging findings in perforation include discontinuity of the gallbladder wall, bulging of the wall suggesting an underlying defect, and a pericholecystic fluid collection. MR imaging with T1-weighted post-gadolinium images and T2-weighted fat-suppressed images may be particularly useful when the perforation is discrete. Hemorrhage may be seen in CT as hyperattenuating blood, or in MR as T1 hyperintense signal as a result of the T1-shortening effect of methemoglobin [33].

4.4 Biliary Ducts

4.4.1 Choledocholithiasis

Choledocholithiasis is the most common cause of biliary obstruction, and may result in pancreatitis, jaundice, biliary colic, or cholangitis. Calculi lodged in the common bile duct most commonly form in the gallbladder and migrate to the CBD, are dislodged during cholecystectomy, or, rarely, may form in intrahepatic bile ducts and travel to the CBD (5%) [34]. Clinical presentation of choledocholithiasis ranges from mild to severe depending on the degree of obstruction and the presence of concomitant superinfection leading to cholangitis, which requires emergent drainage. Common symptoms include acute right upper quadrant pain, pruritus, and jaundice, with increased serum alkaline phosphatase and direct bilirubin levels. Common complications other than cholangitis include pancreatitis and secondary biliary cirrhosis.

The sensitivity of US for calculi in the central bile ducts ranges from 55 to 91% [35], with particular limitations due to duodenal gas artifact adjacent to the pancreatic head. A calculus is seen as an echogenic focus with posterior acoustic shadowing (Fig. 4.19). Ten percent of calculi may produce no acoustic shadowing. Associated US findings include biliary duct dilation, >6 mm for the common bile duct (age-appropriate adjustments must be taken into account), and >2 mm for the intrahepatic bile ducts. CT sensitivities range from 70 to 80%, and may show an intraductal calculus (usually calcified in up to 80%), with a rim of surrounding bile (meniscus

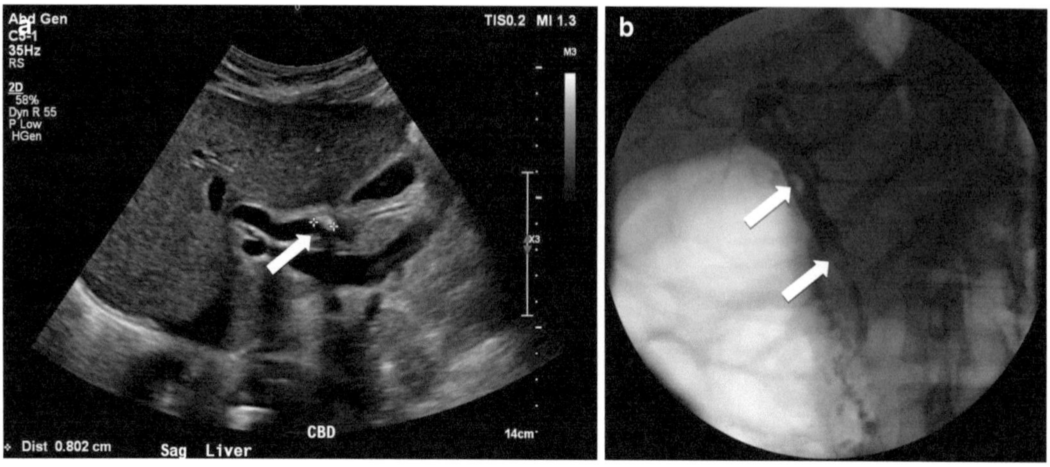

Fig. 4.19 Choledocholithiasis. 34-year-old woman with abnormal liver function tests. Longitudinal ultrasound image (**a**) demonstrates a shadowing calculus in the dilated common bile duct (arrow). Therapeutic ERCP (**b**) performed the next day shows two calculi in the common bile duct (arrows)

or bull's eye sign). Pure cholesterol calculi may not be seen, as they have the same density as bile. Indirect signs include biliary duct dilation, with abrupt termination of the CBD.

MRCP is commonly performed when only indirect signs are seen on ultrasound and/or CT where other diagnoses cannot be excluded, including CBD obstruction from pancreatic or ampullary malignancy, chronic pancreatitis, cholangiocarcinoma, stenosis or stricture from a variety of causes, and primary sclerosing cholangitis. MRCP has a sensitivity and specificity approaching 100%. Signs on MRCP include a low signal-dependent filling defect in the CBD (Fig. 4.20). It is imperative to review the source images, to avoid potential pitfalls including motion artifact, cholecystectomy clip susceptibility, and vascular compression, among others. The location of the filling defect is essential, as nondependent filling defects are seen in the setting of pneumobilia. When the diagnosis is not definitive on US, CT, or MRCP, ERCP is commonly performed, as it provides both diagnostic and therapeutic options, and is the imaging reference standard.

4.4.2 Acute (Ascending) Cholangitis

Acute cholangitis is characterized by the triad of right upper quadrant pain, fever, and jaundice, and is caused by gram-negative bacteria superinfecting bile in the common bile duct. It is most commonly seen in the setting of biliary tract obstruction, for which CT is most readily used to determine the cause. Eighty percent of biliary obstructions are due to choledocholithiasis, while the remaining are usually due to malignancy, sclerosing cholangitis, or biliary procedures including ERCP. US shows thickening of wall of bile duct with debris (usually pus) in the common bile duct and associated intra- and/or extrahepatic biliary duct dilation. Urgent antibiotics with gram-negative coverage and biliary decompression are potentially lifesaving. If severe, mortality rates have been reported up to 50–90%. CT and MR are useful to determine the cause of cholangitis when a calculus is not readily seen on US, and when the diagnosis is not clinically evident. Early, inhomogeneous arterial enhancement of the liver is seen in CT, although this finding is nonspecific. T1-weighted fat-suppressed post-gadolinium MR images show thickened bile duct walls with increased enhancement. T2-weighted MR images may show ill-defined periportal hyperintense signal from inflammation, and wedge-shaped hyperintense regions of infection (Fig. 4.21). These findings also help in distinguishing primary sclerosing cholangitis.

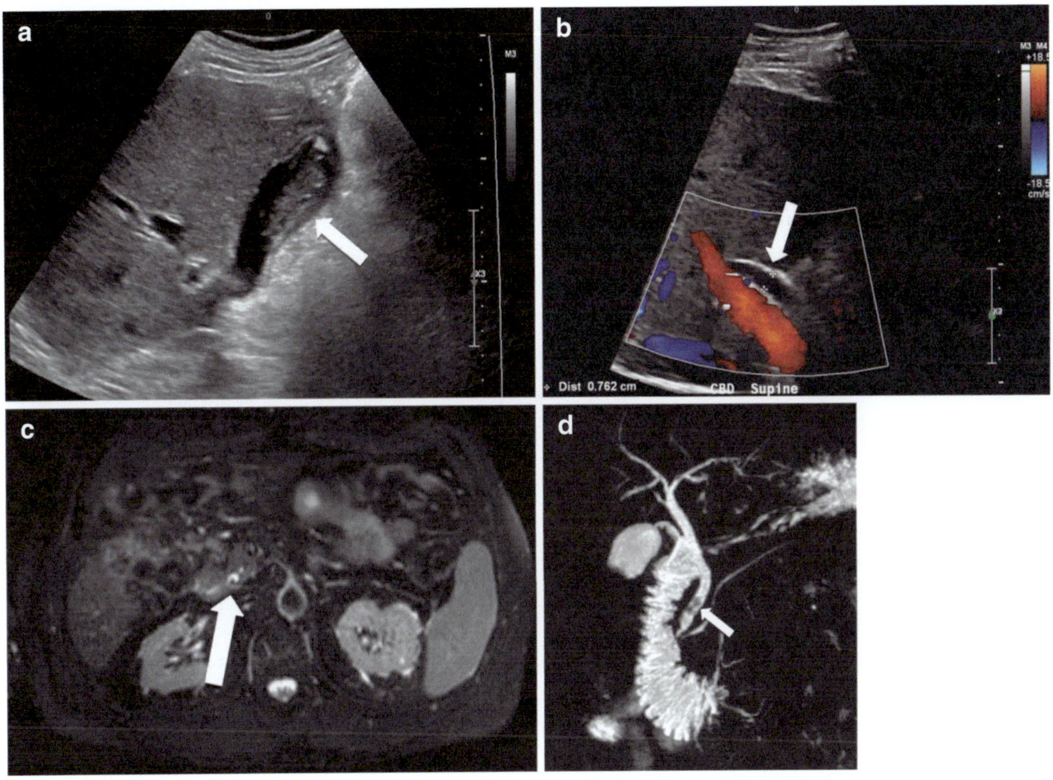

Fig. 4.20 Cholelithiasis and choledocholithiasis. 62-year-old man with right upper quadrant pain. Initial ultrasound performed shows cholelithiasis without cholecystitis (arrow, **a**), and a dilated common bile duct (arrow, **b**). The patient underwent an MRCP given his biliary colic and dilated common bile duct. Axial T2-weighted fat-saturated (**c**) and 3D MRCP images (**d**) reveal calculi in the distal common bile duct (arrows)

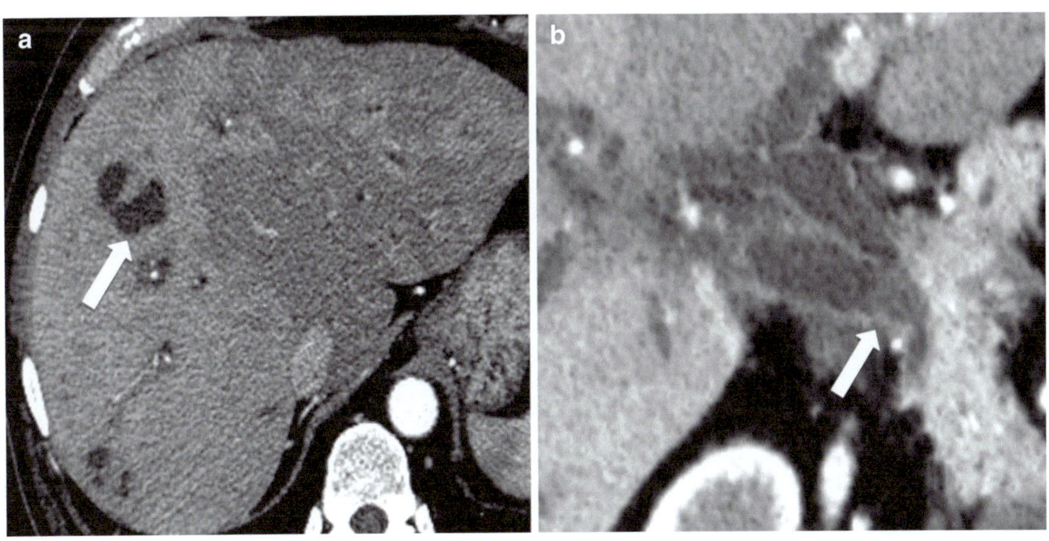

Fig. 4.21 Ascending cholangitis caused by Mirizzi's syndrome. 38-year-old man presents with right upper quadrant pain and fever. Axial (**a**) IV contrast-enhanced CT image show heterogeneous enhancement of the liver parenchyma, dilated intrahepatic bile ducts, and multiple liver abscesses (arrow). Coronal (**b**) IV contrast-enhanced CT image reveals dilatation of the cystic duct and common hepatic duct caused by obstruction by a noncalcified calculus (arrow) located at the junction of both ducts. Also note thickening and hyperenhancement of the biliary duct walls

4.4.3 Recurrent Pyogenic Cholangitis

Recurrent pyogenic cholangitis is caused by pigment calculus formation in the biliary tract, which is thought to be related to parasite infection with *Ascaris lumbricoides* or *Clonorchis sinensis* [36]. The proposed pathophysiology is that parasitic organisms are infesting the biliary tract, and inducing inflammatory and fibrotic changes in the bile duct walls, leading to strictures, bile stasis, disproportional dilation of the extrahepatic bile ducts, intrahepatic calculi, and progressive biliary obstruction with recurrent infection, leading to multiple cholangitic hepatic abscesses, and even cirrhosis (Figs. 4.22 and 4.23) [36]. Parasitic biliary infections are an established risk factor for cholangiocarcinoma [37].

4.5 Acute Traumatic and Iatrogenic Injury to the Biliary Tract

4.5.1 Traumatic Injury

In the setting of trauma, biliary injury is intimately associated with multiple organ injuries: 91% in hepatic injuries, 54% in splenic injuries, and 54% in duodenal injuries [38]. As such, when these injuries are identified, the radiologist must actively search for signs of gallbladder, common bile duct, and intrahepatic bile duct injury, and make recommendations for additional imaging accordingly. Identification of biliary tract injuries in the setting of trauma poses a diagnostic challenge, as these injuries are easily overlooked if there is multi-organ injury. Mechanisms of injury include torsion, shearing, compression, blunt injury, acute deceleration, and penetrating trauma. Although bile duct injuries are rare, occurring in approximately 0.1% of trauma patients, and usually do not pose an imminent threat to life, delayed diagnosis results in high morbidity and mortality from complications including bile leak and superinfection. In the setting of missed diagnosis, symptoms are usually not present until bile is superinfected, resulting in delayed, vague symptoms including abdominal pain, nausea, and vomiting. Laboratory findings may demonstrate rising or persistently elevated bilirubin.

Bile duct injury may involve the intra- or extrahepatic bile ducts, and can be seen as tear or transection, with a frequency of 0.5–21% after hepatic trauma [39]. Injury to the intrahepatic ducts is commonly seen with liver injuries, and usually affects small, subsegmental ducts. Extrahepatic injuries (which include the common hepatic duct and common bile duct) are less frequent, but require treatment with percutaneous, endoscopic, or surgical interventions. Major ducts are usually injured extrahepatically near the hilum due to anatomic fixation due to shear from deceleration or blunt trauma. Many intrahepatic injuries are self-limiting, as they are contained by surrounding liver parenchyma. In a study conducted at our institution, 28% of patients who sustained liver injuries were found to have contained and/or free bile leaks, so the incidence of hepatobiliary injury may be higher than previously thought [40].

In the era of increasing nonoperative management of trauma patients and damage-control surgery with perihepatic packing for liver injuries, open abdomen with subsequent staged surgeries, and decreased use of resection with closing laparotomy and drain placement, identification of a bile leak may be delayed or even go unrecognized for months to years [41]. Patients may present with signs or symptoms of bile leak or bile duct transection or ligation, including jaundice, biliary peritonitis, and cholangitis. However, diagnosis is frequently delayed due to nonspecific symptoms, including abdominal pain, malaise, nausea, and anorexia, which may be attributed to other more frequent postoperative complications [42]. Late manifestations include recurrent cholangitis and secondary biliary cirrhosis due to strictures. Early diagnosis of bile leaks after trauma has been shown to result in a shorter hospital length of stay, with imaging playing an integral role in decreasing morbidity and mortality [43].

A multimodality approach is often warranted to care for these complex patients. There is absence of consensus both in the literature and in

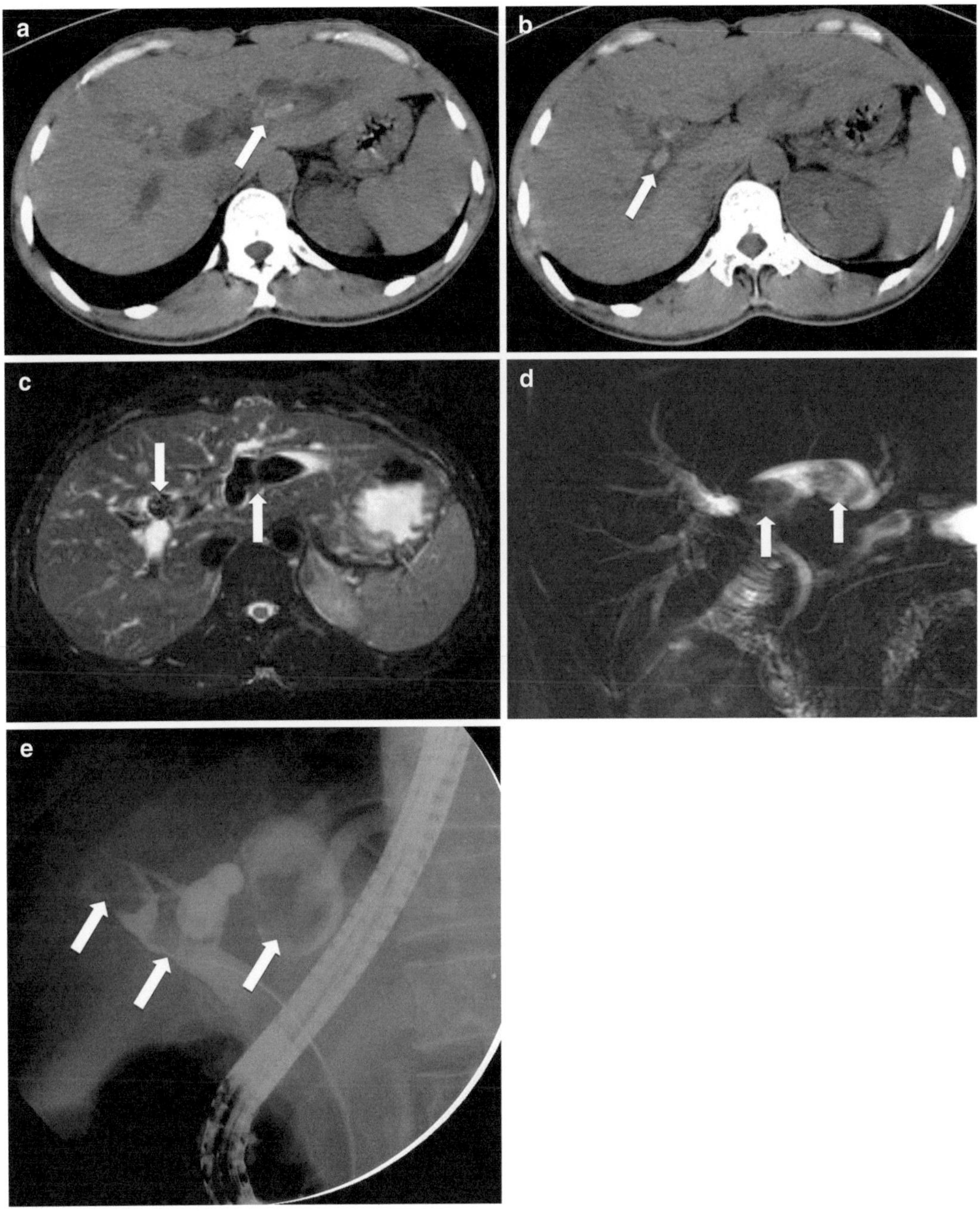

Fig. 4.22 Recurrent pyogenic cholangitis. 46-year-old Asian man who presented with abdominal pain radiating to the back. A non-contrast urinary calculus protocol CT was obtained. Axial images (**a**, **b**) from this examination reveal diffuse, relatively marked intrahepatic bile duct dilation with numerous large intraductal calculi (arrows). Axial T2-weighted fat-saturated (**c**) and 3D MRCP (**d**) images show the same findings (arrows). The patient underwent ERCP (**e**) for calculus extraction and sphincterotomy. Again seen is extensive bile duct dilation, greater in the left hepatic lobe, with multiple bile duct calculi (arrows). These findings are characteristic of recurrent pyogenic cholangitis

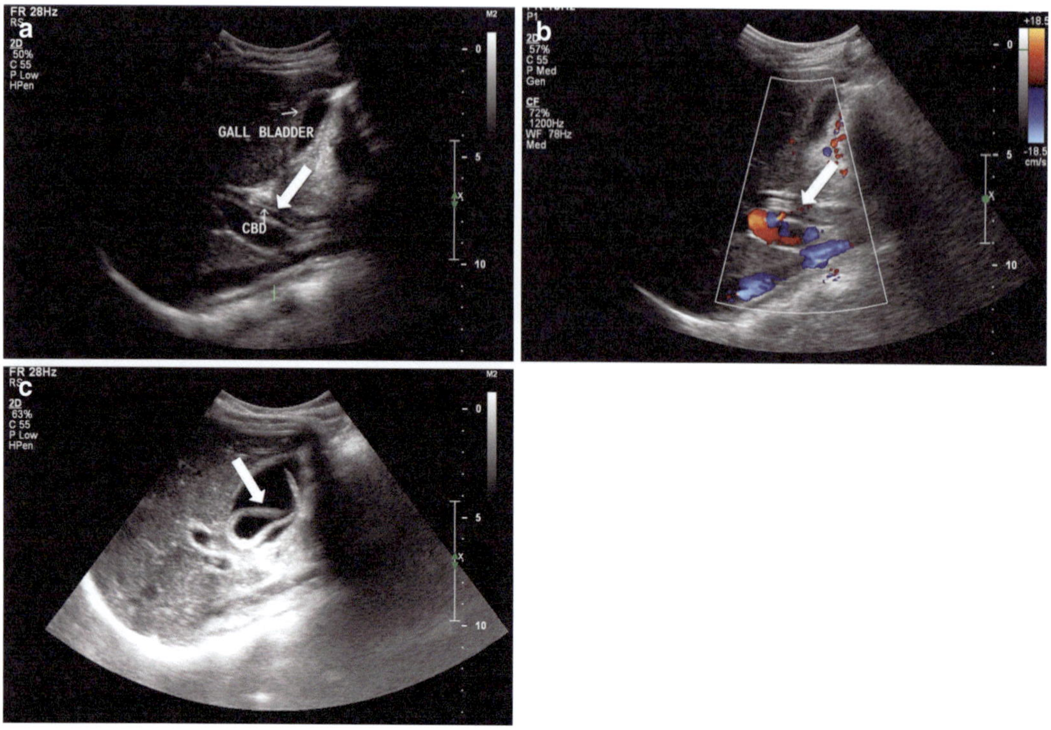

Fig. 4.23 Biliary ascariasis. 22-year-old man from India with right upper quadrant pain. Grayscale (**a**, **c**) and color Doppler (**b**) longitudinal ultrasound images reveal linear and curvilinear echogenic, non-shadowing structures within the common bile duct (arrows in **a**, **b**) and gallbladder (arrow, **c**). Biliary ascariasis was confirmed at ERCP (not shown) (images courtesy of Dr. Tharakeswara Bathala)

practice for an algorithmic approach to the diagnosis of posttraumatic bile leaks. To our knowledge, decisions are often based on the extent of the biliary injury, associated organ injuries, and local expertise. Hemodynamically stable patients who have sustained blunt trauma often undergo CT at the time of admission to delineate their injuries and triage their management. If there is a low suspicion for a bile leak and anatomic detail of the biliary tract is not necessary, hepatobiliary scintigraphy is appropriate for excluding a bile leak. At our institution, our surgical colleagues routinely order hepatobiliary scintigraphy 3–4 days after liver injury. Conversely, if there is a high clinical suspicion for biliary injury including rising serum albumin levels, increasing ascites, enlarging perihepatic fluid collections, or central liver lacerations, MRCP with hepatobiliary contrast material is obtained to provide both anatomic and functional information, which helps guide treatment.

4.6 Iatrogenic Injury

Due to advances in both open and laparoscopic techniques in the last few decades, there has been an increase in the number of hepatobiliary surgeries, including open and laparoscopic cholecystectomy, hepatic resection, and hepatic transplantation, as well as liver biopsy. As a result, there has been a rise in the number of biliary injuries, including bile leak, transection, stricture (Fig. 4.24), and obstruction by surgical clips, which can lead to the development of bilomas, biliary peritonitis, cholangitis, sepsis, biliary cirrhosis, portal hypertension, and hepatic or multi-organ failure.

Detection of biliary injury in the iatrogenic setting is difficult as the patients' clinical symptoms are often nonspecific, including abdominal pain, malaise, nausea, and anorexia, which are frequently seen in association with other more

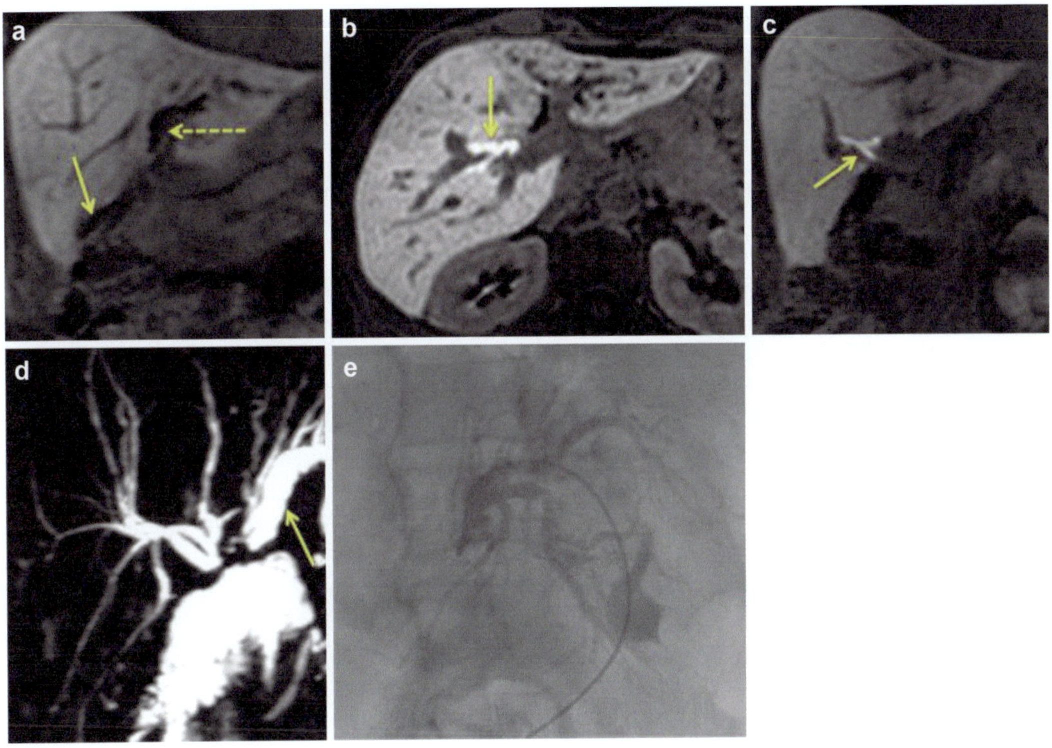

Fig. 4.24 Hepatico-jejunostomy anastomotic stricture. 46-year-old woman with a history of hepatico-jejunostomy now presents with abdominal pain and hyperbilirubinemia. 3D fast spin-echo (3DFSE) MR images demonstrate dilated intrahepatic bile ducts with independent anastomoses of the right (arrow, **a**) and left hepatic ducts (**a**; dashed arrow). On the post-contrast delayed-phase images following the administration of a hepatobiliary contrast agent, the right hepatic duct is shown to be patent (arrow, **b** and c), while the left is obstructed (arrow, **d**). The patient subsequently underwent drainage of the left system via percutaneous transhepatic cholangiography (**e**). Abdom Radiol, Iatrogenic, blunt, and penetrating trauma to the biliary tract, vol 42, 2017, 28–45, LeBedis CA, Bates DDB, Soto JA. ©Springer Science + Business Media New York 2016. With permission of Springer

commonly encountered postoperative complications [42, 44]. The reported rates of bile duct injury are 0.3–0.72% for laparoscopic cholecystectomy, 0.1–0.2% for open cholecystectomy, and 2–25% for orthotopic liver transplantation or hepatic resection, particularly in nonanatomic hepatic resections. Only approximately 25% of bile duct injuries are identified intraoperatively [45, 46]. In addition, intraoperative cholangiography is no longer commonly performed due to risk of a tear at the confluence of the cystic and common bile duct at the site of ligation, increased operative time, and increased procedural cost [47]. Thus, a high index of suspicion must be maintained postoperatively for biliary injury.

4.7 Biliary Tract Injury Imaging

Imaging plays a crucial role in the diagnosis of bile duct injury, as well as assessment of its location and severity. A multimodality imaging approach to biliary injury is often necessary, as each modality has its own strengths and limitations. Options include US, CT, MRCP, hepatobiliary scintigraphy, percutaneous transhepatic cholangiography (PTC), and fluoroscopy with a contrast agent injected through a surgically or percutaneously placed biliary drainage catheter [48]. CT is routinely used as the first-line imaging modality in the setting of trauma and the ill postoperative patient, often showing subtle and nonspecific findings associated with posttraumatic or iatrogenic biliary injury. Liver lacerations, focal perihepatic or intrahepatic fluid collections, and ascites may be the only indicators of bile duct injury. A high level of suspicion is required in the presence of these findings, particularly when other organ injuries (liver, spleen, and duodenum) are noted in the trauma patient, or in the persistently ill postsurgical patient. In these patients, recommending follow-up imaging is essential for the diagnosis of potential late biliary leaks. For example, persistent or increasing low-attenuation intraperitoneal fluid in the setting of recent trauma (Figs. 4.25 and 4.26) or surgery is concerning for bile leakage. Additional findings of peritoneal thickening and hyperenhancement are suggestive of bile peritonitis, and a site of leak should be searched for with advanced imaging modalities [49].

US may be useful in follow-up of known complication to show increasing or decreasing perihepatic fluid, and as a quick and convenient imaging modality for routine follow-up assessment in nonoperative management of hepatic trauma, to detect or confirm the absence of bile leak-related complications [50]. Possible findings in the setting of biliary injury include gallbladder wall thickening, collapsed gallbladder in the setting of perforation, perihepatic and intrahepatic fluid collections, and ascites. More advanced imaging modalities are increasingly recommended and used, as a normal MRCP essentially excludes bile duct injury. When results are indeterminate

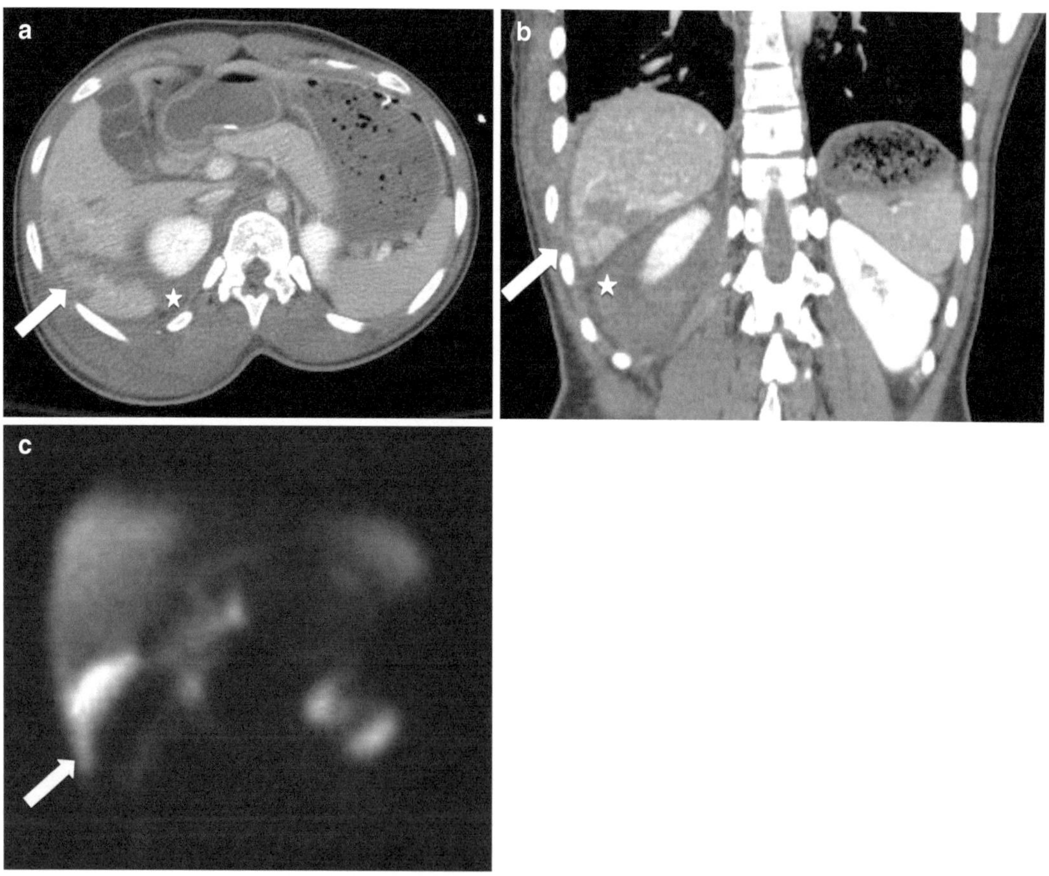

Fig. 4.25 Bile leak due to liver laceration from blunt trauma. 21-year-old woman following a motor vehicle collision who was ejected from her vehicle. Axial (**a**) and coronal (**b**) IV contrast-enhanced CT images reveal an AAST grade 3 laceration (arrows) of segments six and seven with associated perihepatic hemoperitoneum (star). Hepatobiliary scintigraphy (**c**) performed due to concern for a bile leak shows radiotracer extravasating from the liver into the peritoneum (arrow)

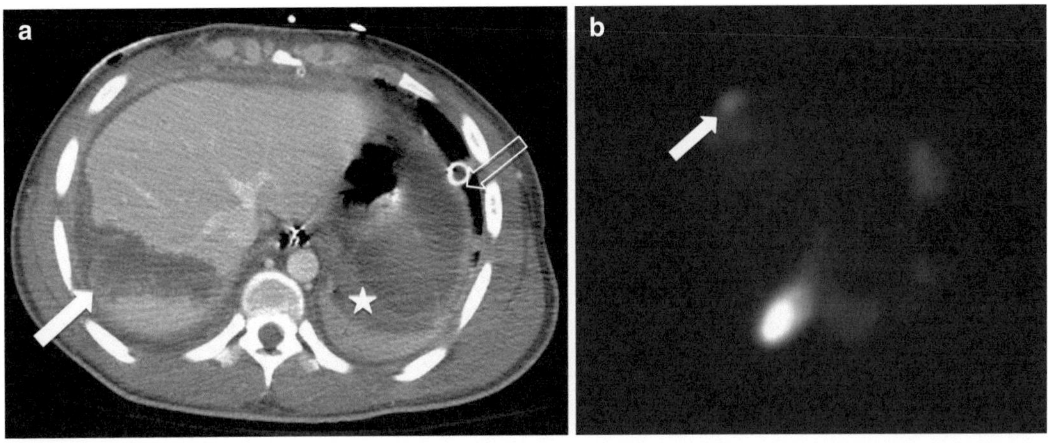

Fig. 4.26 Bile leak due to liver laceration from penetrating trauma. 27-year-man who sustained multiple gunshot wounds to the abdomen and thorax. Axial IV contrast-enhanced CT images show an AAST grade 4 liver laceration at the dome of the liver (**a**, arrow), hemoperitoneum extending into the left upper quadrant (star), and a left chest tube (open arrow). Hepatobiliary scintigraphy (**b**) was subsequently performed, revealing a contained biloma at the site of the laceration at the dome of the liver (arrow)

due to artifacts from peritoneal fluid or tissue edema, hepatobiliary scintigraphy or ERCP may prove definitive in diagnosis.

MRCP with hepatocellular contrast agents provides detailed anatomic information, as well as functional information, with the added advantage of potentially showing the exact site of bile leak and safely permitting differentiation between fluid of biliary and non-biliary origin. MRCP with hepatocyte-selective agents, including gadoxetic acid, can be performed as the initial imaging examination, as it can be used to guide subsequent management, whether it be endoscopic, percutaneous, or surgical [51]. Gadoxetic acid causes T1 shortening of bile, and in conjunction with an MRCP may help in revealing biliary anatomy and bile leaks (Fig. 4.27).

Hepatobiliary scintigraphy provides physiologic information, and is sensitive for demonstrating a bile leak, but delayed 4-h imaging is essential. However, decreased spatial resolution limits the ability to accurately reveal the site of leak, information which governs treatment decisions; thus, evaluation with additional modalities including MRCP and ERCP is commonly needed.

Endoscopic retrograde cholangiopancreatography (ERCP) has both diagnostic and therapeutic capabilities, and remained the reference of imaging standard for decades for biliary tract imaging and intervention. In recent years, ERCP has been commonly reserved solely for patients requiring therapeutic intervention, as imaging modalities have substantially advanced to become the standard diagnostic option for accurate diagnosis [52]. ERCP is more invasive, and is usually pursued after noninvasive imaging examinations have shown or revealed findings suspicious of or definitive for a bile duct injury. Treatment options during the procedure include stenting to bypass and secondarily heal the injury by diverting bile flow with or without sphincterotomy. Another consideration with sphincterotomy is the inherent short-term risk of pancreatitis and a long-term risk of stricture, especially in young patients [53]. The optimal duration of biliary stenting remains to be elucidated to our knowledge, and has been reported to vary from 3 to 16 weeks in prior reports [39, 54].

Percutaneous transhepatic cholangiogram (PTC) and fluoroscopy via an indwelling catheter are useful techniques to guide percutaneous transhepatic biliary drain (PTBD) placement, which can provide biliary drainage and/or diversion in the setting of biliary injury [46]. Compared with ERCP, PTC has the advantage of being able to demonstrate the proximal biliary tract, common bile duct, and, if present, an aberrant right hepatic duct [46].

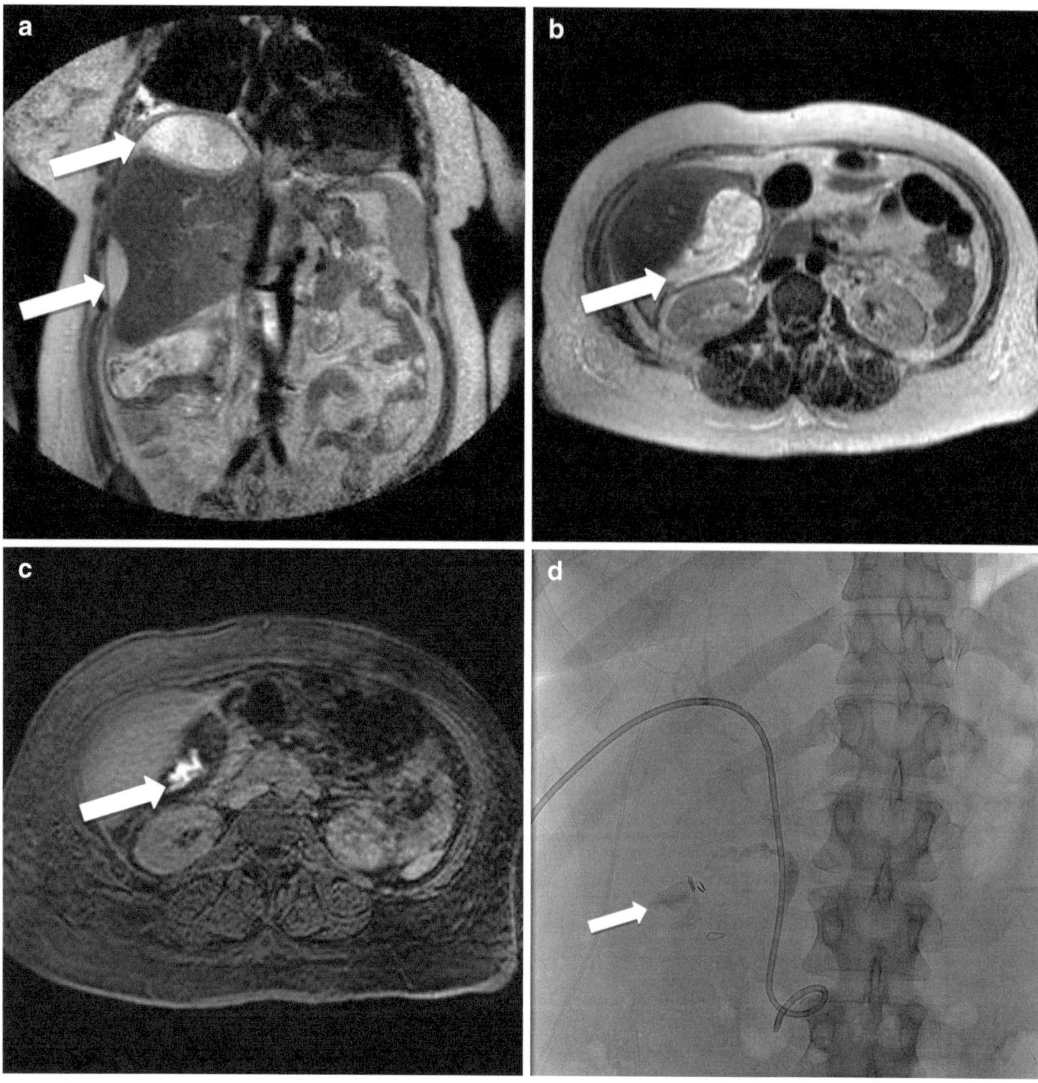

Fig. 4.27 Bile leak after cholecystectomy. 32-year-old woman with worsening abdominal pain 10 days after cholecystectomy. Coronal (**a**) and axial (**b**) T2-weighted MR images demonstrate large perihepatic fluid collection (arrow). Axial T1-weighted gadoxetate disodium-enhanced 20-min delayed MR image (**c**) demonstrates direct leakage of biliary contrast from the cystic duct into the perihepatic fluid collection (arrow). The patient underwent placement of a percutaneous transhepatic biliary drain placement. During this procedure, contrast extravasation confirmed a leak from the cystic duct remnant (arrow, **d**)

4.8 Biloma

A bile leak occasionally results in a biloma which may be intra- or extrahepatic. Since bile is sterile and is absorbed by the peritoneum, patients may not experience any symptoms for weeks after the initial trauma. If the bile becomes superinfected, patients may present with systemic inflammatory response syndrome (SIRS) and respiratory distress [55]. If the biloma results in extrahepatic biliary duct compression, laboratory evaluation may show signs of cholestasis (i.e., elevation of serum alkaline phosphatase, total and direct bilirubin) [55].

In the setting of abdominal trauma, studies report up to a 20% incidence of biliary ascites or bilomas in patients treated conservatively [43, 56]. Bilomas are most commonly described post-iatrogenic injury from cholecystectomy or partial hepatectomy, with an incidence of <0.1% [55]. Other less common causes of biloma include cholangiocarcinoma, acute cholecystitis, tuberculosis, hepatic abscess, infarction, and, rarely, choledocholithiasis in the setting of spontaneous rupture of the biliary tree.

US may have a role in patients with a history of recent trauma or hepatobiliary surgery who present with right upper quadrant pain, chills, and fever, and shows a well-circumscribed, anechoic fluid collection increased through transmission, debris, or septations, in a subphrenic, subhepatic, or intrahepatic location [55]. Loculated ascites or other postoperative collections may appear identical to a biloma, and the need for more advanced imaging or fluid sampling is usually warranted. CT reveals progressive growth of a well-circumscribed, low-attenuation perihepatic or intraparenchymal fluid collection. There should be no identifiable capsule or peripheral enhancement which would indicate a nontraumatic liver mass such as a liver abscess or hemangioma. A hepatic hematoma would also be higher attenuation (as that of blood between 30 and 60 HU, depending on acuity).

Hepatobiliary scintigraphy, MR with hepatobiliary contrast agents, or aspiration may be used for differentiation. MR shows a well-defined fluid collection, which is hyperintense on T2-weighted images and hypointense on T1-weighted images. Hepatobiliary contrast agents are excreted into the biliary tract, and may reveal the site of a bile leak in the hepatobiliary phase. Standard MRCP without hepatobiliary contrast cannot definitively reveal the site of bile leak or be used to distinguish biloma from other fluid collection. Hepatobiliary scintigraphy, if positive, shows focal accumulation of radiotracer outside the biliary tract and bowel. In summary, a loculated low-density collection following hepatic trauma or surgery requires further evaluation.

4.9 Biliary Fistulas

Fistulas are abnormal communications between two epithelial-lined surfaces. Biliary fistulas result from communication of the biliary tract with duodenum, colon, bronchi, skin, or even a vessel. Biliary fistulas most commonly result from gallstone erosion through the gallbladder wall. Trauma and iatrogenic injury may also result in biliary fistulas. The type of fistula will be dictated by the underlying injury and its anatomic relation to surrounding structures.

Biliary-enteric fistula is suggested by pneumobilia, which is detected as gas extending peripherally along the portal triads of the liver within the biliary system. This may be seen on all types of imaging, and must be suggested in the absence of prior sphincterotomy, surgical bypass procedure, recent endoscopic retrograde cholangiopancreatography, or passed common duct calculus [57]. In general, cholecystoduodenal fistulas are the most common type, followed by cholecystocolic and choledochoduodenal fistulas [58]. The clinical manifestation of enterobiliary fistulas is often nonspecific, and most patients are diagnosed on the basis of an incidentally detected imaging finding [58].

Biliary-vascular fistulas are rare, but may be suggested on CT when opacification of the biliary system with iodinated contrast is noted, a finding which is rarely diagnosed prospectively. Diagnosis is most commonly suggested by clinical findings suggesting bleeding, or laboratory evaluation showing excessively high serum levels of direct bilirubin, and only moderately elevated liver enzymes indicating bilhemia (bile mixing with blood). Confirmation is done with selective hepatic arteriography, which shows extravasation of contrast material into the biliary tract, and also serves to exclude hepatic artery aneurysm/pseudoaneurysm as a source of bleeding.

Pleural-biliary fistula may be suspected in nonresolving low-density pleural effusion in the setting of trauma or hepatobiliary surgery (Fig. 4.28). This is typically diagnosed with thoracentesis.

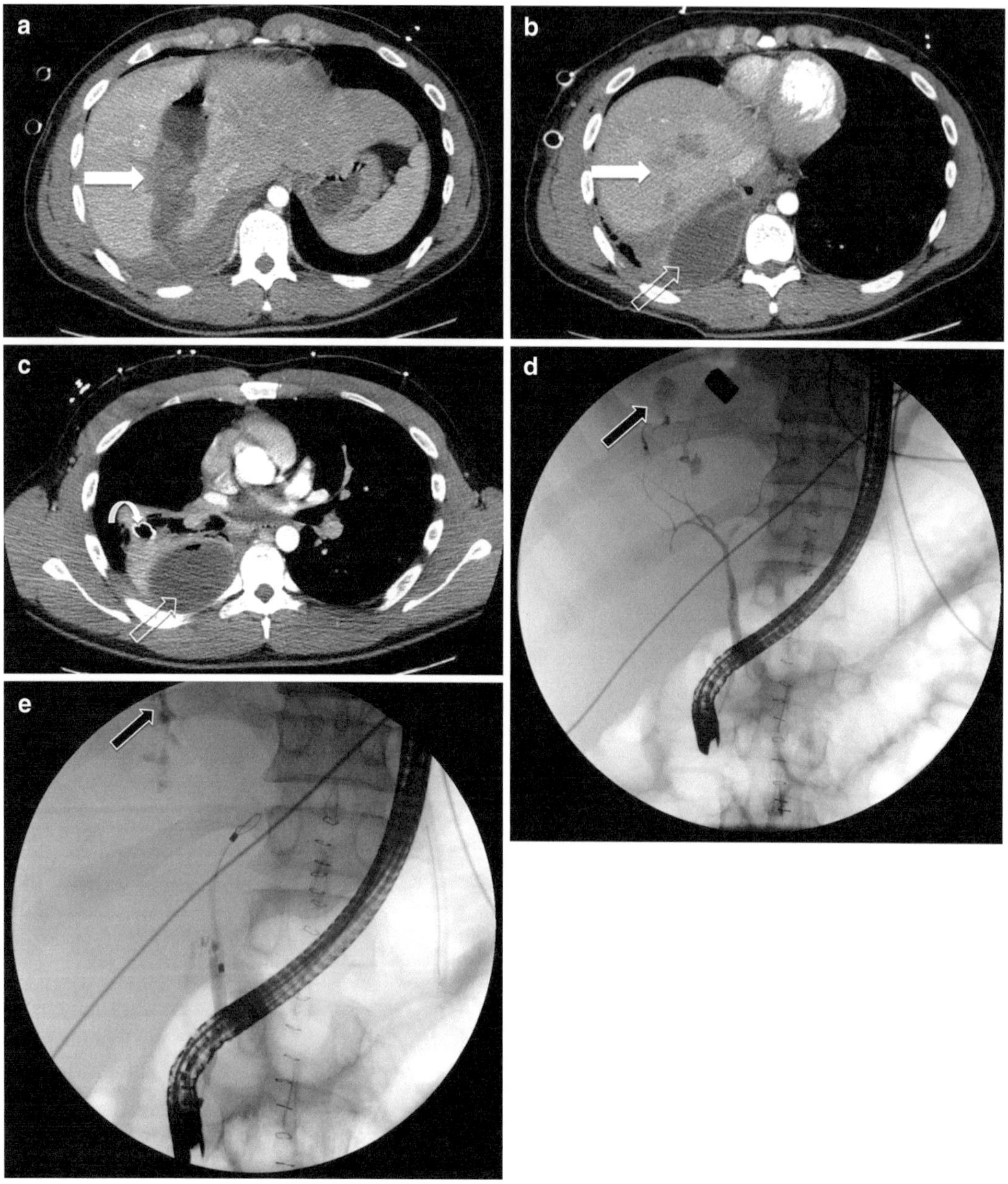

Fig. 4.28 Biliary fistula. 20-year-old man following a gunshot injury, with liver laceration and associated bile leak into the right pleural space. IV contrast-enhanced axial CT images from inferior to superior (**a–b**) reveal an AAST grade 4 liver laceration in the right lobe of the liver along the bullet trajectory (solid arrows), and a right pleural fluid collection (open arrow) with a drainage catheter in place (curved arrow). ERCP images (**d** and **e**) show contrast (arrows) accumulating in the right subphrenic space, and tracking to the right pleural space

4.10 Gallbladder Trauma

Gallbladder injuries include wall contusion, perforation, and avulsion, most of which present as intraluminal or pericholecystic hematoma. Only approximately 2% of patients who undergo laparotomy for traumatic injury are found to have a gallbladder injury [59]. Clinically, a patient with gallbladder injury will develop slowly progressive abdominal complaints, as seen with other traumatic biliary injuries. CT is the first-line

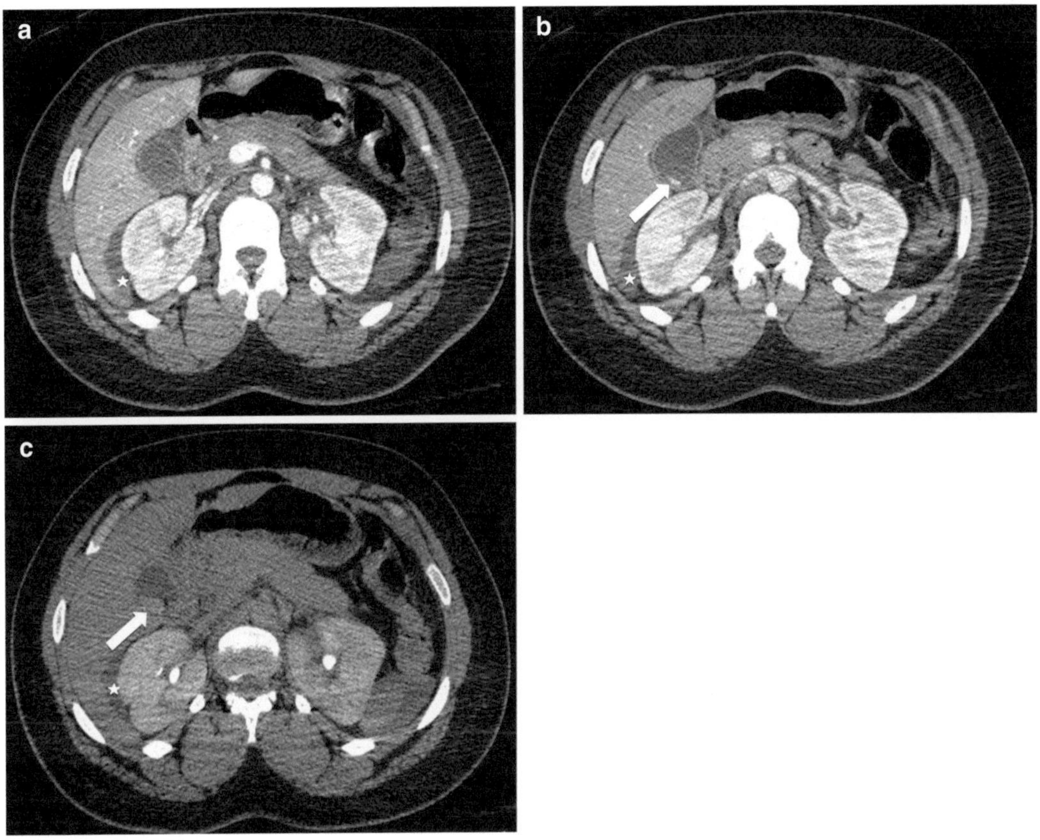

Fig. 4.29 Active gallbladder hemorrhage after blunt trauma. 31-year-old man following rollover motor vehicle collision. Axial IV contrast-enhanced CT images in the arterial (**a**), portal venous (**b**), and 5-min delayed phases demonstrate a focus of hyperattenuation within the gallbladder lumen (arrows in **b** and **c**), which first appears on the portal venous phase, and which expands on the 5-min delayed phase, representing active intraluminal hemorrhage. Perihepatic fluid is also noted (stars)

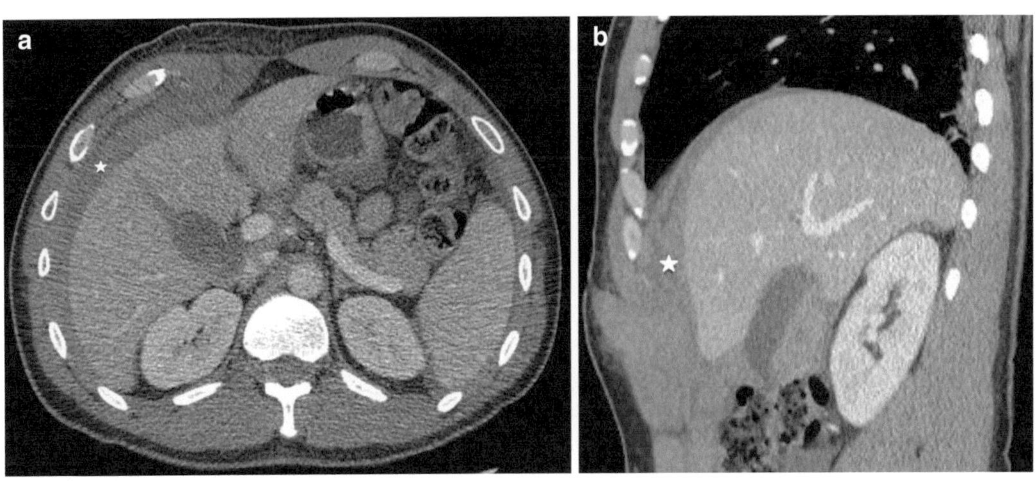

Fig. 4.30 Gallbladder laceration from penetrating trauma. 36-year-old man following stab wound to the right upper quadrant. Axial (**a**) and sagittal (**b**) IV contrast-enhanced CT images show an AAST grade 3 liver laceration extending to the gallbladder wall, and layering hyperattenuating intraluminal material. The patient underwent subsequent cholecystectomy, and a laceration of the gallbladder wall with an associated intraluminal hemorrhage was identified. Perihepatic hematoma was also noted on CT (stars)

imaging modality as it most accurately depicts blood within the gallbladder lumen (Figs. 4.29 and 4.30). Other findings in CT include gallbladder wall thickening, pericholecystic fluid, intramural hematoma or layering blood, indistinct gallbladder wall or discontinuous mucosal enhancement, active bleeding from cystic artery injury, and low-attenuation collections around the liver. An indirect sign of gallbladder wall injury is displacement of the gallbladder from its fossa. US shows echogenic fluid within the gallbladder. Potential mimics of intraluminal blood in the gallbladder on CT include milk of calcium, and vicarious excretion of contrast material from previous CT examinations, which may simulate intraluminal blood [60]. Similar findings are seen with MRI/MRCP. T1-weighted MR images and MRCP aid in identifying intramural hematoma.

Conclusion

A multimodality approach is often warranted to care for patients with hepatobiliary diseases, as they often present as complex diagnostic and therapeutic challenges. In the setting of nontraumatic hepatobiliary injury, as for example with acute cholecystitis, CT and ultrasound remain the imaging examination of choice due to accessibility, low cost, and rapid acquisition. They also serve as useful imaging tools to reveal other causes of acute abdominal pain. High clinical suspicion is often needed to elucidate the more rare presentations of acute abdominal pain, such as a pregnant woman with HELLP syndrome, or a young woman with hemoperitoneum from a ruptured adenoma. In the setting of posttraumatic hepatobiliary injury, there is a lack of consensus, both in the literature and practice, for an algorithmic approach, to our knowledge. Decisions are often based on the extent of biliary injury, associated organ injuries, and local expertise. MRCP often plays an integral role in the diagnosis of posttraumatic complications in stable patients. MRCP is a powerful adjunct imaging tool for equivocal cases, and for showing complications, either from known hepatobiliary disease or in the postoperative setting. It is expected that as MR becomes more advanced in providing accelerated acquisition times, artifact reduction, and cost reduction, it will become a primary imaging modality in emergency hepatobiliary settings where there is a high clinical suspicion for aforementioned diseases and injuries.

References

1. Boll DT, Merkle EM. Diffuse liver disease: strategies for hepatic CT and MR imaging. Radiographics. 2009;29(6):1591–614.
2. Chundru S, Kalb B, Arif-Tiwari H, et al. MRI of diffuse liver disease: characteristics of acute and chronic diseases. Diagn Interv Radiol. 2013;20(3):200–8.
3. Pickhardt PJ, Fleishman MJ, Fisher AJ. Fitz-hugh curtis syndrome: multidetector CT findings of transient hepatic attenuation difference and gallbladder wall thickening. Am J Roentgenol. 2003;180(6):1605–6.
4. Hertzberg B, Middleton W. Ultrasound: the requisites. Philadelphia, PA: Elsevier; 2016. p. 6–68.
5. Semelka R. Abdominal-pelvic MRI. Hoboken, NJ: John Wiley and Sons, Inc.; 2010. p. 418–37.
6. Semelka RC, Kelekis NL, Sallah S, et al. Hepatosplenic fungal disease: diagnostic accuracy and spectrum of appearance on MR imaging. Am J Roentgenol. 1997;169(5):1311–6.
7. Semelka RC, Shoenut JP, Greenberg HM, et al. Detection of acute and treated lesions of hepatosplenic candidiasis: comparison of dynamic contrast-enhanced CT and MR imaging. J Magn Reson Imaging. 1992;2(3):341–5.
8. Oto A, Akhan O, Ozmen M. Focal inflammatory disease of the liver. Eur J Radiol. 1999;32:61–75.
9. Hertzberg B, Middleton W. Ultrasound: the requisites. Philadelphia, PA: Elsevier; 2016. p. 78.
10. Semelka R. Abdominal-pelvic MRI. Hoboken, NJ: John Wiley and Sons, Inc.; 2010. p. 388–98.
11. Brancatelli G, Vilgrain V, Federle MP, et al. Budd-Chiari syndrome: spectrum of imaging findings. Am J Roentgenol. 2007;188(2):W168–76.
12. Torabi M, Hooseinzadeh K, Federle MP. CT of nonneoplastic hepatic vascular and perfusion disorders. Radiographics. 2008;28:1967–82.
13. Valls C, Cos M, Figueras J, et al. Pre-transplantation diagnosis and staging of hepatocellular carcinoma in patients with cirrhosis: value of dual-phase helical CT. Am J Roentgenol. 2004;182(4):1011–7.
14. Mittal S. Epidemiology of HCC: consider the population. J Clin Gastroenterol. 2013;47:s2–6.
15. Semelka R. Abdominal-pelvic MRI. Hoboken, NJ: John Wiley and Sons, Inc.; 2010. p. 189–238.
16. Casillas VJ, Amendola MA, Gascue A, Pinnar N, Levi JU, Perez JM. Imaging of nontraumatic hemorrhagic hepatic lesions. Radiographics. 2000;2:367–78.

17. MacSween R, Anthony P, et al. Pathology of the liver. 3rd ed. London: Churchill Livingston; 1994.
18. Webb WR, Brant WE, Major NM. Fundamentals of body CT. Philadelphia, PA: Elsevier; 2006. p. 225–6.
19. Thomeer MG, Broker M, Verheij J, et al. Hepatocellular adenoma: when and how to treat? Update of current evidence. Ther Adv Gastroenterol. 2016;9(6):898–912.
20. Semelka R. Abdominal-pelvic MRI. Hoboken, NJ: John Wiley and Sons, Inc.; 2010. p. 107.
21. Pritchard JA, Weisma R Jr, Ratnoff OD, Vosburgh GJ. Intravascular hemolysis, thrombocytopenia and other hematologic abnormalities associated with severe toxemia of pregnancy. NEJM. 1954;250:89–98.
22. Sibai BM, Barton JR. Expectant management of severe preeclampsia remote from term: patient selection, treatment, and delivery indications. Am J Obstet Gynecol. 2007;196:514.e1–9.
23. Benedetto C, Marozio L, Tancredi A, et al. Biochemistry of HELLP syndrome. Adv Clin Chem. 2011;53:85–104.
24. Perronne L, Dohan A, Bazeries P, et al. Hepatic involvement in HELLP syndrome: an update with emphasis on imaging features. Abdom Imaging. 2015;40(7):2839–49.
25. O'Connor OJ, Maher MM. Imaging of cholecystitis. Am J Roentgenol. 2011;196(4):W367–74.
26. Soto JA, Lucey BC. Emergency radiology: the requisites. Philadelphia, PA: Elsevier; 2010. p. 334–44.
27. Mirvi S, Kubal W, Shanmuganathan K, et al. Problem solving in emergency radiology. Philadelphia, PA: Elsevier; 2015. p. 452–3.
28. Yang C, Zhang S, Jia Y, et al. Clinical application of dual-energy spectral computed tomography in detecting cholesterol gallstones from surrounding bile. Acad Radiol. 2017;24(4):478–82.
29. Bilgin M, Shaikh F, Semelka RC, Bilgin SS, Balci NC, Erdogan A. Magnetic resonance imaging of gallbladder and biliary system. Top Magn Reson Imaging. 2009;20(1):31–42.
30. Hjartarson JH, Hannesson P, Sverrisson I, Blondal S, Ivarsson B, Bjornsson ES. The value of magnetic resonance cholangiopancreatography for the exclusion of choledocholithiasis. Scand J Gastroenterol. 2016;51(10):1249–56.
31. Soto JA, Lucey BC. Emergency radiology: the requisites. Radiology. 2010;257(2):334.
32. Genevieve BL. CT findings in acute gangrenous cholecystitis. Am J Roentgenol. 2002;178:275–81.
33. Bates D, et al. Use of MR in pancreaticobiliary emergencies. Magn Reson Imaging Clin N Am. 2016;24(2):422–48.
34. Webb WR, Brant WE, Major NM. Fundamentals of body CT. Philadelphia: Elsevier; 2006. p. 233–46.
35. Liu TH, Consorti ET, Kawashima A, Tamm EP, Kwong KL, Gill BS, Sellin JH, Peden EK, Mercer DW. Patient evaluation and management with selective use of magnetic resonance cholangiography and endoscopic retrograde cholangiopancreatography before laparoscopic cholecystectomy. Ann Surg. 2001;234:33–40.
36. Hffernan EJ, Geoghegan T, Munk PL, Ho SG, Harris AC. Recurrent pyogenic cholangitis: from imaging to intervention. Am J Roentgenol. 2009;192(1):W28–35.
37. Tyson GL, El-Serag H. Risk factors of cholangiocarcinoma. Hepatology. 2011;54(1):173–84.
38. Gupta A, Stuhlfaut JW, Fleming KW, Lucey B, Soto JA. Blunt trauma of the pancreas and biliary tract: a multimodality imaging approach in diagnosis. Radiographics. 2004;24:1381–95.
39. Winick AB, Waybill PN, Venbrux AC. Complications of percutaneous transhepatic biliary interventions. Tech Vasc Interv Radiol. 2001;4:200–6.
40. Melamud K, LeBedis CA, Anderson SW, et al. Biliary imaging: multimodality approach to imaging of biliary injuries and their complications. Radiographics. 2014;34:613–23.
41. Pachter HL, Knudson MM, Esrig B, et al. Status of nonoperative management if blunt hepatic injuries in a multicenter experience with 404 patients. J Trauma. 1996;40:31–8.
42. Vachhani PG, Copelan A, Remer EM, et al. Iatrogenic hepatopancreaticobiliary injuries: a review. Semin Interv Radiol. 2015;32:182–94.
43. Baghdanian AA, Baghdanian AH, Khalid M, et al. Damage control surgery: use of diagnostic CT after life-saving laparotomy. Emerg Radiol. 2016;23(5):483–95.
44. Lee CM, Stewart L, Way LW. Postcholecystectomy abdominal bile collections. Arch Surg. 2000;135:538–44.
45. Stewart L. Iatrogenic biliary injuries. Surg Clin North Am. 2014;94:297–310.
46. Lau WY, Lai EC, Lau SH. Management of bile duct injury after laparoscopic cholecystectomy. ANZ J Surg. 2010;80:75–81.
47. Fletcher DR, Hobbs MS, Tan P, et al. Complications of cholecystectomy: risks of the laparoscopic approach and protective effect of operative cholangiography: a population-based study. Ann Surg. 1999;229:449–57.
48. Thompson CM, Saad NE, Quazi RR, et al. Management of bile duct injuries: role of the interventional radiologist. Radiographics. 2013;33:117–34.
49. Vassiliu P, Touttouzas KG, Velmahos GC. A prospective study of posttraumatic biliary and pancreatic fistuli.The role of expectant management. Injury. 2004;35:223–7.
50. Chiu WC, Wong-You-Cheong JJ, Rodriguez A, et al. Ultrasonography for interval ssessment in the nonoperative management of hepatic trauma. Am Surg. 2005;71:841–6.
51. Aduna M, Larena JA, Martin D, et al. Bile duct leaks after laparoscopic cholecystectomy: value of contrast-enhanced MRCP. Abdom Imaging. 2005;30:480–7.
52. Bor R, Madácsy L, Fábián A, Szepes A, Szepes Z. Endoscopic retrograde pancreatography: when should we do it? World J Gastrointest Endosc. 2015;7(11):1023–31.
53. Walsh RM, Henderson JM, Vogt DP, et al. Long-term outcome of biliary reconstruction from bile duct injuries from laparoscopic cholecystectomies. Surgery. 2007;142:450–6.

54. Stewart L, Way LW. Laparoscopic bile duct injuries: timing of surgical repair does not influence success rate—a multivariate analysis of factors influencing surgical outcomes. HPB (Oxford). 2009;11:516–22.
55. Tana C, D'Alessandro P, Tartaro A, Tana M, Mezzetti A, Schiavone C. Sonographic assessment of a suspected biloma: a case report and review of the literature. World J Radiol. 2013;5(5):220–5.
56. Croce MA, Fabian RC, Menke PG, et al. Nonoperative management of blunt hepatic trauma is the treatment of choice for hemodynamically stable patients: reports of a prospective trial. Ann Surg. 1995;221:744–53.
57. Pickhardt PJ, Bhalla S, Balfe DM. Acquired gastrointestinal fistulas: classification, etiologies, and imaging evaluation. Radiology. 2002;224(1):9–23.
58. Inal M, Oguz M, Aksungur E, Soyupak S, Boruban S, Akgul E. Biliary-enteric fistulas: report of five cases and review of the literature. Eur Radiol. 1999;9:1145–51.
59. Soderstrom CA, Maekawa K. Gallbladder injuries resulting from blunt abdominal trauma: an experience and review. Ann Surg. 1981;193:60–6.
60. Wittenberg A, Minotti A. CT diagnosis of traumatic gallbladder injury. Am J Roentgenol. 2005;185:1573–4.

5 Advances in Acute Pancreatic Imaging

Dan Van Roekel, Stephan Anderson, and Trevor Morrison

Abstract

Emergent imaging of the pancreas falls into two broad categories: nontraumatic and traumatic. Imaging for nontraumatic causes is often performed in the evaluation of nonspecific acute abdominal pain in the ER setting, or to assess for severity and complications in known or suspected patients with pancreatitis. Imaging for injury of the pancreas is usually performed as part of a general evaluation for blunt or penetrating trauma to the abdomen, as trauma to the pancreas most often occurs in the setting of multi-organ injury. While evaluation of the pancreas is critical during a traumatic event, as morbidity and mortality are high if the pancreas is injured, actual. An additional category, beyond these causes, includes evaluating acute and delayed complications after pancreatic surgery, which can necessitate emergent imaging of the pancreas. The radiologist requires a basic understanding of the types of pancreatic surgical and other procedures, as a lack of familiarity with the altered anatomy can be an impediment to accurate and efficient diagnosis. In nearly all cases of pancreatic injury requiring emergent imaging, multi-detector computed tomography is the frontline modality. MRI/MRCP and endoscopic retrograde cholangiopancreatography (ERCP) play vital secondary roles. Ultrasonography has a limited, but specific role in the evaluation of the acute pancreas, and radiography has no role in the evaluation of the acutely injured or inflamed pancreas.

5.1 Introduction

Emergent imaging of the pancreas falls into two broad categories: nontraumatic and traumatic. Imaging for nontraumatic causes is often performed in the evaluation of nonspecific acute abdominal pain in the ER setting, or to assess for severity and complications in known or suspected patients with pancreatitis. Imaging for injury of the pancreas is usually performed as part of a general evaluation for blunt or penetrating trauma to the abdomen, as trauma to the pancreas most often occurs in the setting of multi-organ injury. While evaluation of the pancreas is critical during a traumatic event, as morbidity and mortality are high if the pancreas is injured, actual. An additional category, beyond these causes, includes evaluating acute and delayed complications after pancreatic surgery, which can necessitate emergent imaging of the pancreas. The radiologist requires a basic understanding of the types of pancreatic surgical and other procedures,

D. Van Roekel, M.D. • S. Anderson, M.D. (✉)
T. Morrison, M.D.
Department of Radiology, Boston University Medical Center, Boston, MA, USA
e-mail: Stephan.Anderson@bmc.org

M. Patlas et al. (eds.), *MDCT and MR Imaging of Acute Abdomen*,
https://doi.org/10.1007/978-3-319-70778-5_5

as a lack of familiarity with the altered anatomy can be an impediment to accurate and efficient diagnosis. In nearly all cases of pancreatic injury requiring emergent imaging, multi-detector computed tomography is the frontline modality. MRI/MRCP and endoscopic retrograde cholangiopancreatography (ERCP) play vital secondary roles. Ultrasonography has a limited, but specific role in the evaluation of the acute pancreas, and radiography has no role in the evaluation of the acutely injured or inflamed pancreas.

5.2 Pancreatic Anatomy and Function

The pancreas is a retroperitoneal organ lying in a relatively protected location within the anterior pararenal space of the upper abdomen. The pancreas is bordered by the rigid and relatively immobile spinal column posteriorly. Anteriorly and laterally, solid organs, hollow organs, and fat form a protective arc of soft tissue overlying the pancreas. The intimate relationships between the anatomic portions of the pancreas, including the head, uncinate process, neck, body, and tail with the adjacent organs, vasculature, and spinal column, offer diagnostic clues as to the specific location where pancreatic injury may have occurred, as well as to the expected course and distribution where fluid may spread and collect during an episode of acute pancreatitis.

The uncinate process forms a triangular protuberance which insinuates between the superior mesenteric vessels anteriorly and the inferior vena cava and the aorta posteriorly. The head is in intimate contact with the second portion of the duodenum, with a fixed connection between the ampulla and the pancreatic duct. The neck lies anterior to the superior mesenteric vessels. The splenic vein runs along the posterior border of the pancreatic body. The pancreatic tail typically ends in close proximity to the splenic hilum.

An important differentiating structural quality unique to the pancreas is its lack of a capsule. Therefore, the appearance of a pancreatic hematoma will look quite different than a hematoma of the liver, spleen, or kidney. A central pancreatic hematoma may remain contained within the pancreas; however, a peripheral hematoma will most likely have peripancreatic spread guided by the fascial planes of the retroperitoneum and posterior peritoneum. The fascial planes of the posterior peritoneum and retroperitoneum, if intact, guide the distribution of hemorrhage and pancreatic fluid. In the child, the pancreas may have nearly no surrounding fat, while in adults, even thin adults, the pancreas normally lies within a bed of adipose tissue which separates it from the nearby organs. Deep clefts of fat can penetrate the pancreatic parenchyma, which has a lobulated morphology. As adults age, varying degrees of fatty involution of the pancreas occur.

Functionally, the pancreas is both an exocrine and an endocrine organ. Disruption of the exocrine system, with ductal leakage of enzymes into the adjacent soft tissues, can lead to breakdown of the surrounding fat, connective tissue, and vasculature. Vascular disruption can lead to enzymes entering the bloodstream, triggering a systemic response with distant organ failure. It is primarily the leakage of enzymes that is associated with delayed regional and systemic morbidity.

5.3 Nontraumatic Pancreatic Injury and Complications

5.3.1 Acute Pancreatitis

Acute pancreatitis is a common etiology of acute abdominal pain leading to hospital admission, requiring approximately 274,119 hospitalizations in the United States in 2009 [1]. The average cost for a single hospital admission for acute pancreatitis in the United States was $10,000 per patient in 2008 [2]. Having a working knowledge of the diagnosis and management of acute pancreatitis is paramount for this common and costly disease. The spectrum of disease severity ranges from transient epigastric pain, most commonly, to systemic complications, shock, and death. There are a wide range of etiologies of acute pancreatitis, with the two most common causes in the United States being gallstone pancreatitis (38%) and alcoholic pancreatitis (36%) [3].

Imaging plays a vital role in aiding the diagnosis in ambiguous causes of abdominal pain, as well as in helping to elucidate the cause, and in demonstrating complications of acute pancreatitis.

The most widely accepted and used clinical classification system is the Atlanta Classification of Acute Pancreatitis, which was revised in 2012 to improve understanding, management, and communication of the disease, by addressing deficiencies identified in the original 1992 version, and incorporating new knowledge of the disease. The revised 2012 Atlanta Classification establishes four major areas to aid clinicians and radiologists in diagnosis and management of acute pancreatitis. These include outlining new criteria for the diagnosis of acute pancreatitis, categorizing three distinct levels of severity of acute pancreatitis, differentiating between two types of acute pancreatitis, and defining imaging characteristics of pancreatic and peripancreatic collections which develop as complications of acute pancreatitis [4]. For radiologists to communicate effectively with referring clinicians, it is necessary to have a working awareness of this classification system.

To diagnose acute pancreatitis, two of the following three criteria must be met: abdominal pain consistent with acute pancreatitis, serum lipase or amylase level greater than three times the upper limit of normal, and characteristic imaging findings of acute pancreatitis on intravenous contrast-enhanced computed tomography (CECT), MRI, or ultrasound [4]. Therefore, when acute pancreatitis is diagnosed with clinical and laboratory data, CT of the abdomen and pelvis is not necessary to verify the diagnosis. However, an abdominal ultrasound should generally be performed to evaluate for gallstones as an underlying etiology. In patients for which the diagnosis is ambiguous, if the patient does not improve clinically, or if complications are suspected, then IV contrast-enhanced CT (CECT) and/or MRI can aid in diagnosis and further management [5].

The two types of acute pancreatitis are *interstitial edematous pancreatitis* and *necrotizing pancreatitis*. Interstitial edematous pancreatic accounts for 85% of acute pancreatitis [6]. In the first 4 weeks, an *acute peripancreatic fluid collection* (APFC) may develop as a local complication of interstitial edematous pancreatitis. After 4 weeks, if the fluid collection persists, a thick capsule develops and the fluid collection is defined as a *pancreatic pseudocyst* (PP). A peripancreatic or intrapancreatic collection, which develops as a local complication of necrotizing pancreatitis, is known as an *acute necrotic collection* (ANC) within the first 4 weeks, and as *walled-off necrosis* (WON) after 4 weeks (Table 5.1). Any intraparenchymal collection should be considered necrotic. Additional local complications include gastric outlet dysfunction, vascular complications, and colonic necrosis [4], which are discussed in further detail below.

Under the revised Atlanta Classification, stratification of disease severity is divided into mild, moderately severe, and severe, based on the presence and duration of organ failure (respiratory, cardiovascular, or renal), local complications, and systemic complications. The absence of organ failure, local complications, and systemic complications defines mild disease, when mortality is very rare [7]. When organ failure develops, but resolves within 48 h, the disease is considered moderately severe. Moderately severe disease can also be defined when local or systemic complications manifest in the absence of organ failure, or are persistent after resolution of transient organ failure. Severe acute pancreatitis is defined by persistent organ failure longer than 48 h. The mortality rate ranges from 36 to 50% in cases of severe acute

Table 5.1 Definition of collections complicating acute pancreatitis

Interstitial edematous pancreatitis	Necrotizing pancreatitis
Acute peripancreatic fluid collection • Less than 4 weeks • No discernible wall • No solid component	**Acute necrotic collection** • Less than 4 weeks • Variable amounts of solid component • Any fluid collection within the pancreatic parenchyma
Pancreatic pseudocyst • Longer than 4 weeks • Well-defined wall • No solid component	**Walled-off necrosis** • Longer than 4 weeks • Variable amounts of solid component • Any fluid collection within the pancreatic parenchyma

pancreatitis [8–10]. The modified CT severity index (mCTSI) is a radiologic grading system used to help predict disease severity. Points are assigned based on the presence and extent of pancreatic inflammation, parenchymal necrosis, and extraparenchymal complications [11]. Clinical predictors of disease severity include Ranson's Criteria and APACHE II.

While the Atlanta Classification System defines two phases, an early phase consisting of the first week and a subsequent late phase, which may last weeks to months, the radiologist may be better served by dividing phases into the first 72 h, 72 h to 4 weeks, and longer than 4 weeks, as suggested by Zhao et al. [12]. The progression of imaging findings, when thought of in these time blocks, may be more useful in guiding disease management.

IV contrast-enhanced CT is the frontline imaging tool used during the initial evaluation of acute pancreatitis, as it is readily available in the emergency setting, and it offers rapid image acquisition, which is preferred with acutely ill patients. While cross-sectional imaging is not always warranted in the setting of acute pancreatitis, imaging is often performed even when a patient meets clinical criteria for acute pancreatitis. CECT can readily confirm the diagnosis of acute pancreatitis. If a patient is diagnosed with acute pancreatitis and does not receive a CECT, an ultrasound should be performed to evaluate for gallstones. If the ultrasound shows no gallstones, and no other likely cause for acute pancreatitis is found, an MRCP may be performed to further evaluate for malignancy, pancreatic divisum or other pancreatic anomalies, or occult choledocholithiasis.

Necrotizing pancreatitis has a strong association with moderately severe and severe pancreatitis. Early diagnosis could be beneficial in management decisions regarding critically ill or deteriorating patients. However, frank necrosis may not be visible for the first 24–48 h [5, 13]. Both interstitial edematous pancreatitis and necrotizing pancreatitis can demonstrate heterogeneous enhancement due to edema and ischemia. With CECT, the sensitivity for diagnosing pancreatic necrosis within the first 72 h is 60–70% [14, 15].

5.3.2 Interstitial Edematous Pancreatitis, Acute Peripancreatic Fluid Collections, and Pseudocysts

Interstitial edematous pancreatitis (IEP) represents the milder form of pancreatitis, and is much more commonly encountered. Acute, diffuse inflammation of portions of the pancreas or the entire pancreas, as well as the surrounding tissues, usually resolves within a week. Initial IV contrast-enhanced CT findings typically demonstrate edema and enlargement of the pancreas. In mild IEP, the parenchyma should enhance homogeneously, but with lower overall density compared to normal secondary to edema. The contour of the pancreas may be irregular, and the surrounding fat may demonstrate stranding, with fluid in the anterior pararenal space and between the splenic vein and the pancreatic parenchyma (Fig. 5.1).

While CECT is the frontline imaging modality, MRI is more sensitive for pancreatic edema. The most useful images to assess the pancreatic parenchyma for acute inflammation are obtained from T2-weighted sequences, which will demonstrate a hyperintense and enlarged pancreas. Adjacent fat stranding is best assessed with T2-weighted, fat-suppressed sequences (Fig. 5.2).

In more severe IEP, the parenchyma will appear less dense and acute peripancreatic fluid collections (APFC) can develop as fluid leaks out of the pancreas. Typically, within the first 4 weeks of symptom onset, one or more fluid collections develop in the anterior pararenal space or lesser sac, conforming to the fascial planes with a crescentic or spindle morphology. Rarely, APFCs form in the splenic hilum, pelvis, ligamentum venosum, or mediastinum. APFCs lack a capsule, and are not typically round or ovoid in morphology. The fluid within an APFC should be homogeneously hypodense on CECT, hyperintense on T2-weighted sequences, and hypointense on T1-weighted sequences. Superinfection is uncommon, and 85–95% of APFCs resolve spontaneously within the first 4 weeks following the onset of symptoms (Fig. 5.3).

After 4 weeks, persistent peripancreatic fluid collections develop a fibrous capsule, forming

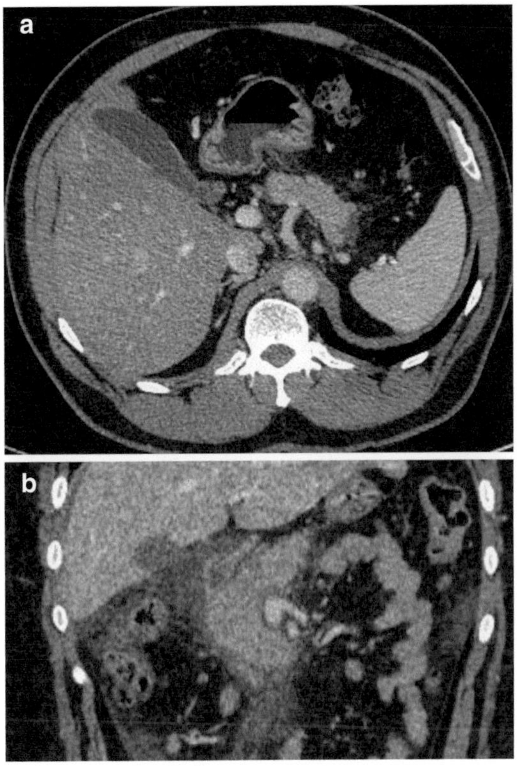

Fig. 5.1 Acute interstitial edematous pancreatitis on CT. (**a**) 51-year-old man presented with acute abdominal pain, nausea, and vomiting. Axial IV contrast-enhanced CT image in the portal venous phase demonstrates mild pancreatic hypodensity, with edema and peripancreatic fat stranding. (**b**) 14-year-old male presented with abdominal pain, nausea, and vomiting. Coronal IV contrast-enhanced CT image demonstrates more severe pancreatic edema with hypodensity involving the head and body, and more severe peripancreatic fat stranding

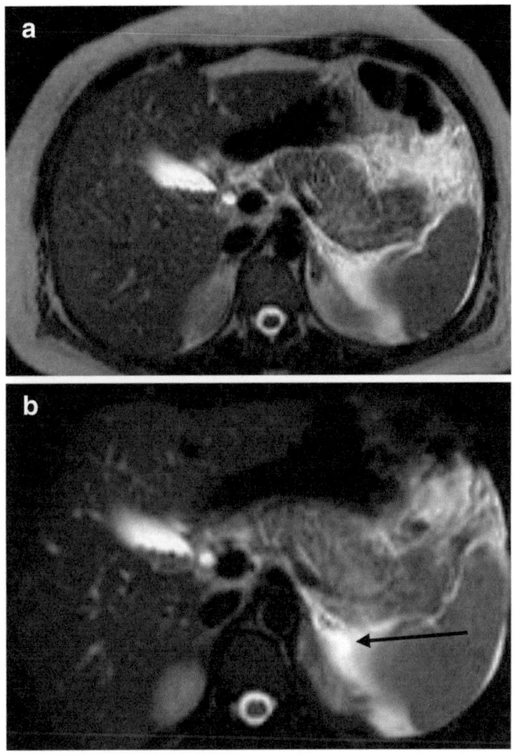

Fig. 5.2 Acute interstitial edematous pancreatitis on MRI. 31-year-old woman presented with abdominal pain. (**a**) T2-weighted and (**b**) T2-weighted fat-suppressed axial MR images demonstrate hyperintensity within the pancreatic body and tail representing edema. Additionally noted is a hyperintense acute peripancreatic collection, better seen on the fat-suppressed image (arrow). Calculi are noted in the gallbladder, and the visualized common bile duct is prominent in this patient with presumed recently passed calculus, leading to gallstone pancreatitis

a pseudocyst. Pseudocysts lack an epithelial layer and, therefore, do not represent true cysts. Pseudocysts are rounded and encapsulated, with homogeneous internal components which demonstrate fluid attenuation of less than 15 HU and an absence of internal solid components. On CECT, the appearance of the fibrous capsule of a pseudocyst is variable in thickness, but should be smooth and may enhance. Debris may lie dependently within the pseudocyst. On MRI, the pseudocyst is typically hyperintense on T2-weighted images and hypointense on T1-weighted images, and visualized debris is specific for a pseudocyst [16] (Fig. 5.4).

Pseudocysts complicate a considerable percentage of patients with acute pancreatitis, with recent studies finding the incidence of pseudocysts to be between 6 and 15% [17–19]. Spontaneous resolution occurs in 40% of pseudocysts. The capability of imaging to be used to predict which pseudocysts will become symptomatic and require treatment is limited, as size and duration have not been shown to be reliable predictors. Numerous complications related to pseudocysts can occur, including erosion of adjacent vessels causing pseudoaneurysm formation, intramural vessels hemorrhaging into the pseudocyst, and large pseudocysts inducing mass effect on local structures causing gastric outlet dysfunction, nausea, and early satiety. Intervention on pseudocysts is avoided unless they are symptomatic or infected. Transgastric or transduodenal/jejunal endoscopic drainage is the stan-

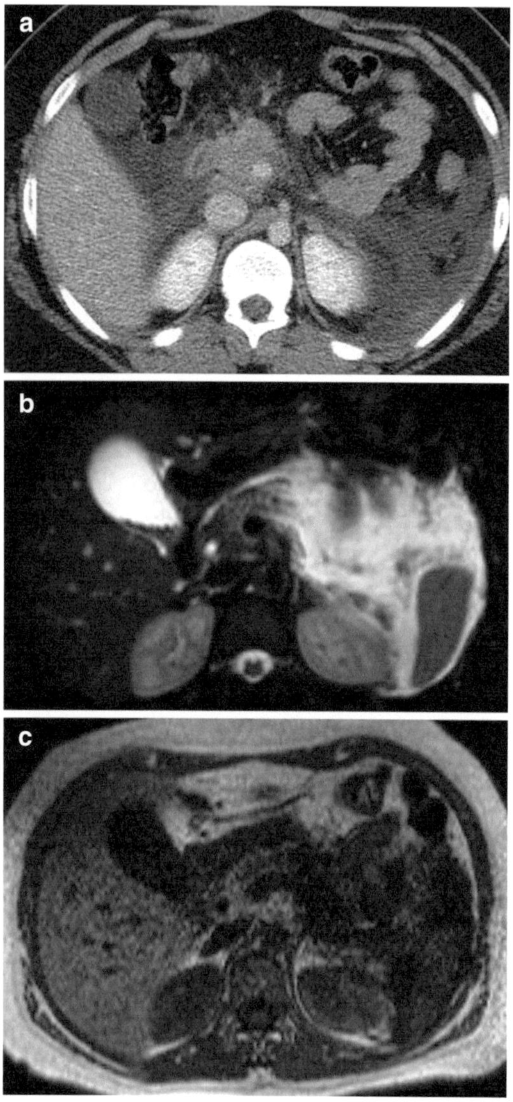

Fig. 5.3 Acute peripancreatic fluid collection on CT and MRI. (**a**) 41-year-old man presented with abdominal pain, emesis, and leukocytosis. Axial IV contrast-enhanced CT image in the portal venous phase demonstrates a large homogeneously hypodense peripancreatic fluid collection. 31-year-old woman presented with abdominal pain. (**b**) Axial T2-weighted fat-suppressed MR image shows a large homogeneously hyperintense peripancreatic fluid collection. (**c**) Axial T1-weighted in-phase MR image demonstrates a homogeneously T1 hypointense peripancreatic fluid collection. Note the absence of a pancreatic capsule on these images

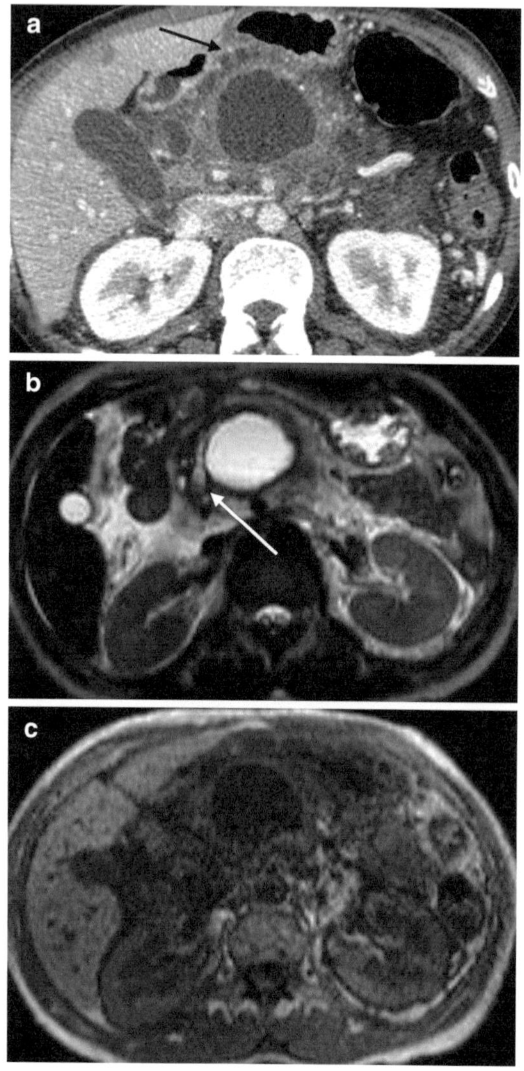

Fig. 5.4 Pseudocyst on CT and MRI. 45-year-old woman with a history of chronic pancreatitis secondary to alcohol abuse, presented with abdominal pain for 1.5 weeks. (**a**) Axial IV contrast-enhanced CT image in the portal venous phase demonstrates an encapsulated hypodense fluid collection posterior to the pancreatic body consistent with a pseudocyst. The pseudocyst was unchanged in size from a prior CT, and was more than 4 weeks old. Note significant mass effect, with anterior displacement of the pancreatic parenchyma. (**b**) T2-weighted and (**c**) T1-weighted axial MR images demonstrate an encapsulated homogeneously T2 hyperintense and T1 hypointense fluid collection posterior to the pancreatic body. Note the characteristic T2 hypointense capsule. Additionally noted are findings of chronic pancreatitis, with pancreatic ductal dilation on the T2-weighted MR image (white arrow), and calcifications within the pancreatic body on CT (black arrow)

dard procedure for draining pseudocysts, during which a fistula is created between the pseudocyst and gastric or duodenal lumen, and a transluminal stent is placed [20, 21].

5.3.3 Necrotizing Pancreatitis, Acute Necrotic Collection, and Walled-Off Necrosis

Acute necrotizing pancreatitis is the more severe local form of pancreatitis, occurring in fewer than 20% of patients with acute pancreatitis. Necrotizing pancreatitis is divided into three morphological subtypes depending on which tissue necroses: pancreatic parenchyma only (less than 5%), pancreatic parenchyma and peripancreatic soft tissue (75–80%), or peripancreatic soft tissue alone (less than 20%) [4, 22]. In addition to the imaging findings seen with IEP, non-enhancing areas are seen within the pancreas and/or heterogeneous regions are seen within the peripancreatic fat. CECT is limited in the evaluation of peripancreatic fat necrosis and, therefore, any heterogeneous peripancreatic collection is presumed to be necrotic. Necrotic parenchyma and peripancreatic fat on MRI will be hypointense on T1-weighted sequences and will not enhance. Necrotic tissue and debris will be hypointense on T2-weighted sequences unless it is liquefied, thereby leading to hyperintense signal [23] (Fig. 5.5). When the peripancreatic fat

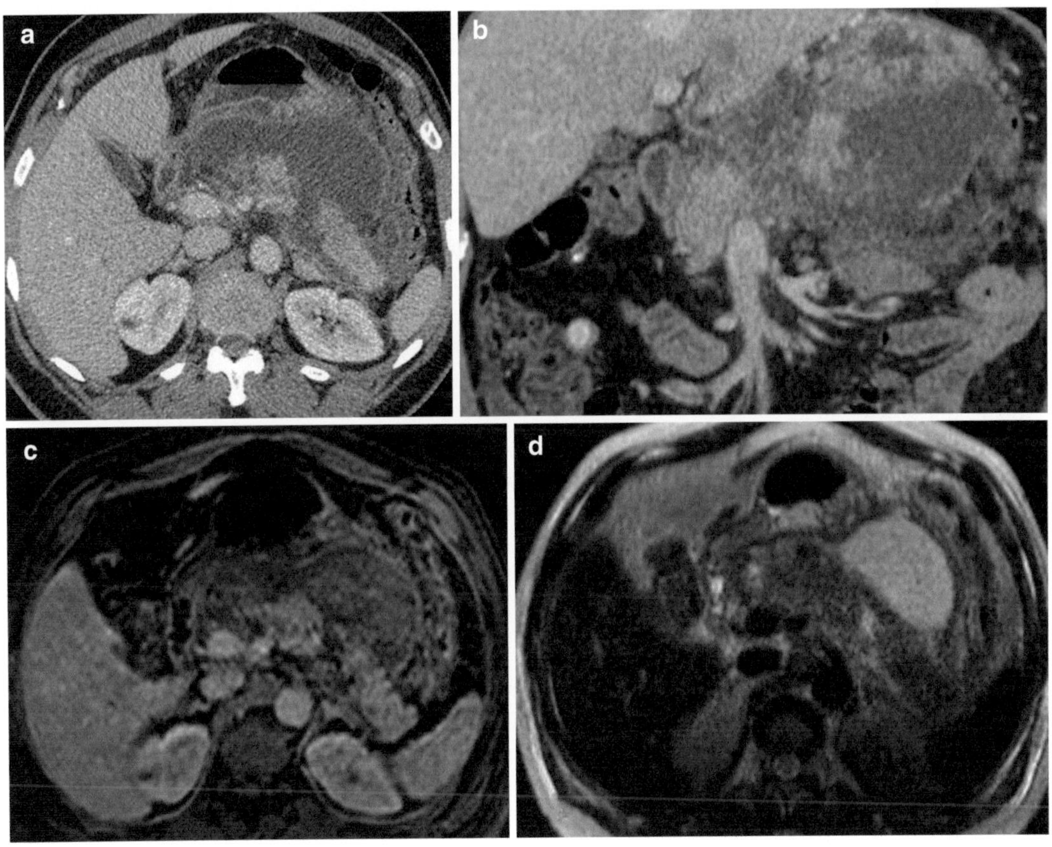

Fig. 5.5 Acute necrotizing pancreatitis on CT and MRI. 64-year-old man presented with abdominal pain and vomiting. (**a**) Axial and (**b**) coronal IV contrast-enhanced CT images demonstrate a non-enhancing portion of pancreas at the body-tail junction with a peripancreatic fluid collection. (**c**) Contrast-enhanced T1-weighted fat-suppressed MR image shows similar findings to CT, with non-enhancement of the body-tail junction. (**d**) T2-weighted MR image demonstrates hyperintensity within the pancreas, and within the peripancreatic collection, indicative of liquefied necrosis

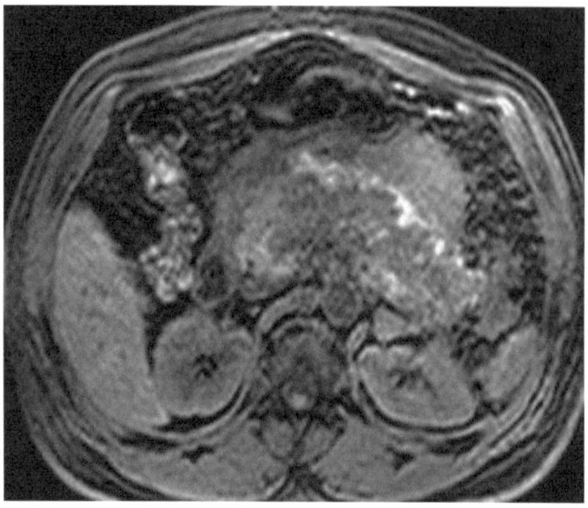

Fig. 5.6 Hemorrhagic fat necrosis. 64-year-old man presented with abdominal pain and vomiting. T1-weighted fat-suppressed axial MR image demonstrates hyperintensity surrounding the pancreas, consistent with hemorrhagic fat necrosis

is hyperintense on fat-suppressed T1-weighted sequences, the fat necrosis is hemorrhagic, which portends a poor prognosis [24] (Fig. 5.6). MRI can be used to better differentiate between fluid collections and necrotic tissue, while CECT is much more limited for distinguishing between the two. Acute necrotic collections are a combination of necrotic soft tissue and the adjacent fluid, and to avoid confusion the word "fluid" is omitted from the terminology in the revised 2012 Atlanta Classification.

Within the first 4 weeks after onset of symptoms, a collection of necrotic pancreatic parenchyma and/or peripancreatic soft tissue with adjacent inflammatory fluid is termed an acute necrotic collection (ANC). Similar to an APFC, a capsule has yet to form around the acute necrotic collection, which may be singular or multiple in nature. Unlike APFCs, ANCs can be intraparenchymal, and may cause main pancreatic duct necrosis and disruption. To distinguish between an ANC and an APFC, solid material within the collection must be identified. On CT, an ANC will have a heterogeneous pattern of hypodense fluid and irregular, intermediate-density, necrotic tissue. On T2-weighted MR sequences, the necrotic tissue will be hypointense, and the liquefied portion will be hyperintense [25, 26].

In up to 9% of patients with pancreatitis, walled-off necrosis (WON) develops after approximately 4 weeks, when a fibrous rim encapsulates the ANC in a similar fashion to the formation of a pseudocyst. Complications from walled-off necrosis include infection, obstruction of adjacent structures, erosion into the adjacent vasculature, and fistula formation [27, 28]. Imaging follow-up is recommended for both symptomatic and asymptomatic WON. WON is most often found in the pancreatic body and tail, but can extend into the paracolic gutters.

The imaging characteristics of WON are similar to pseudocysts. However, walled-off necrosis has a much higher possibility of becoming infected and, therefore, distinguishing between the two entities is important for clinical management. Comparison with prior imaging examinations is helpful, as a region of WON will develop where previously necrotic tissue was seen. CT findings that favor WON over pseudocyst include debris with fat attenuation, involvement of both the pancreas and peripancreatic tissue, extension into the paracolic gutters, irregular capsule margin, growth of the collection, and any collection within the pancreas. Pancreatic duct dilation greater than 3 mm, likely from a compressive effect, favors a pseudocyst [29]. On CT, the hyperdense solid component within the walled-off necrosis may be visualized approximately 45% of the time. MRI can better differentiate the necrotic debris in a similar fashion as with acute necrotic collections (Fig. 5.7). MRCP is recommended in this situation, as walled-off necrosis is complicated by disconnected pancreatic duct syndrome 50–70% of the time [30] (Fig. 5.8). The non-liquefied components are typically removed by laparoscopic, endoscopic, or percutaneous image-guided procedures, or by surgery. Currently, a step-up approach is often employed, starting with the least invasive method, and progressing towards more invasive treatments such as surgical necrosectomy for patients who do not improve or who worsen [31].

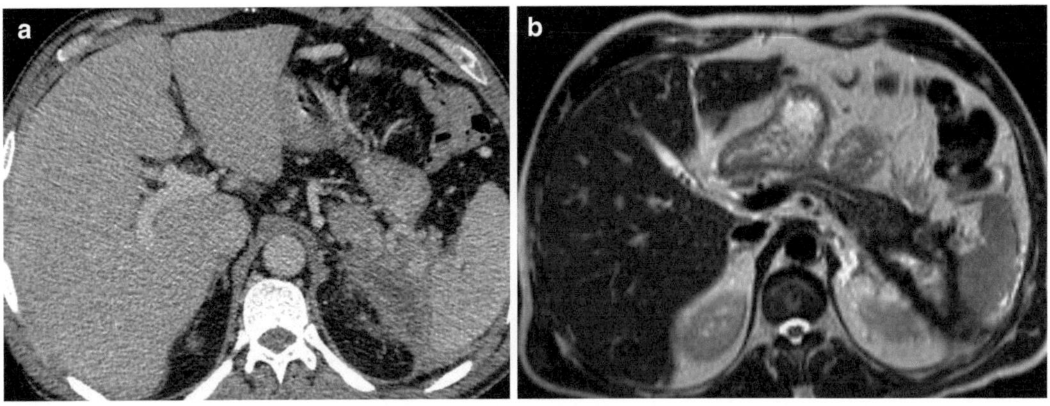

Fig. 5.7 Walled-off necrosis on CT and MRI. 40-year-old man, history of alcohol abuse, prior diagnosis of necrotizing pancreatitis. (**a**) IV contrast-enhanced axial CT image in the portal venous phase demonstrates a thick-walled collection within and surrounding the pancreatic tail, with an irregular margin, in a patient who had presented with pancreatitis months before. (**b**) T2-weighted axial MR image shows thick-walled collection with heterogeneous internal debris, consistent with walled-off necrosis

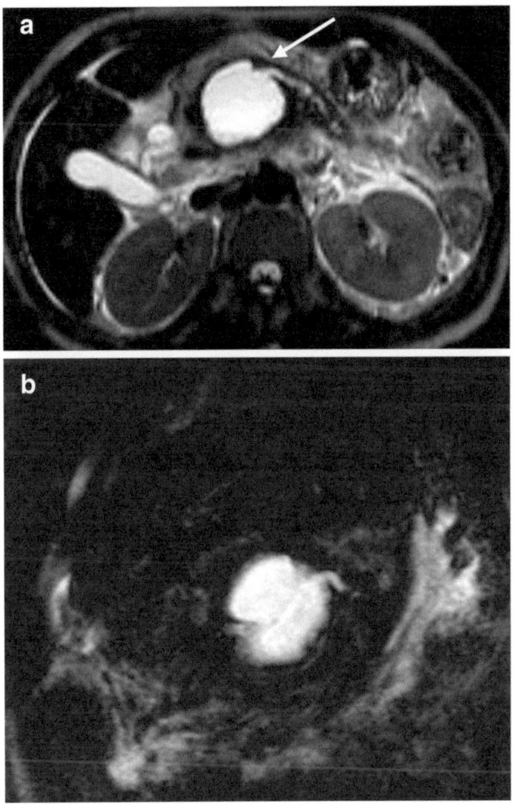

Fig. 5.8 Walled-off necrosis with disconnected duct on MRI. 65-year-old woman with persistent abdominal pain several months after the episode of pancreatitis. (**a**) T2-weighted axial MR image demonstrates walled-off necrosis within the pancreatic body, with communication with the main pancreatic duct (arrow). (**b**) Coronal MRCP image in the same patient shows the collection to be continuous with the main duct

5.3.4 Complications: Infection, Hemorrhage, Disconnected Pancreatic Duct Syndrome

All four types of collections related to acute pancreatitis can become secondarily infected. The non-liquefied component is much more likely to become infected. Infection is typically diagnosed 2–4 weeks after acute pancreatitis onset [29, 32]. The mortality rate of infected pancreatic necrosis approximates 30%, and requires intervention or surgery, whereas noninfected pancreatic necrosis has a reported mortality rate in excess of 10% [33]. On CECT, foci of gas within the collection are suggestive of infection. In the absence of gas but with a clinically suspected infection, fine-needle aspiration can definitively prove infection. CT can more reliably detect small foci of gas compared to MRI (Fig. 5.9).

The most common vascular complication of acute pancreatitis is splenic vein thrombosis, which is non-enhancing on CECT (Fig. 5.10). In the early phase, pancreatic enzymes can erode the wall of the splenic artery, as well as the hepatic artery or gastroduodenal artery, leading to the much rarer development of a pseudoaneurysm. In the late phase, pseudocysts and wall-off necrosis can erode the adjacent vasculature with pseudoaneurysm development. Pseudoaneurysms have the potential to rupture as they increase in size, and are associated with a mortality rate of 40%

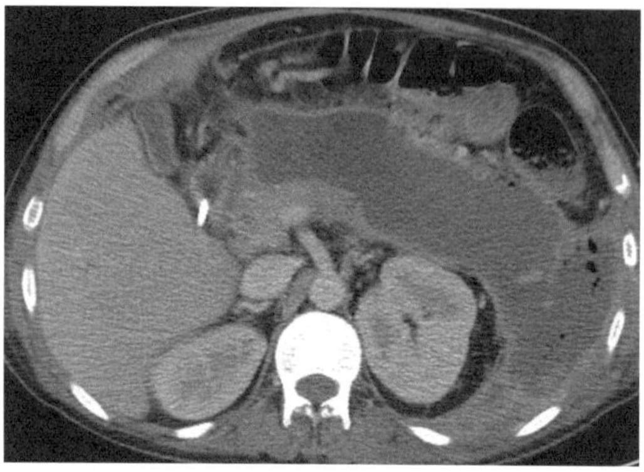

Fig. 5.9 Infected pancreatic necrosis on CT. 31-year-old man presented with abdominal pain. IV contrast-enhanced axial CT image in the portal venous phase demonstrates a large area of peripancreatic walled-off necrosis, extending into the left posterolateral retroperitoneum, which developed foci of air, consistent with infected necrosis. Note the cholecystectomy clip

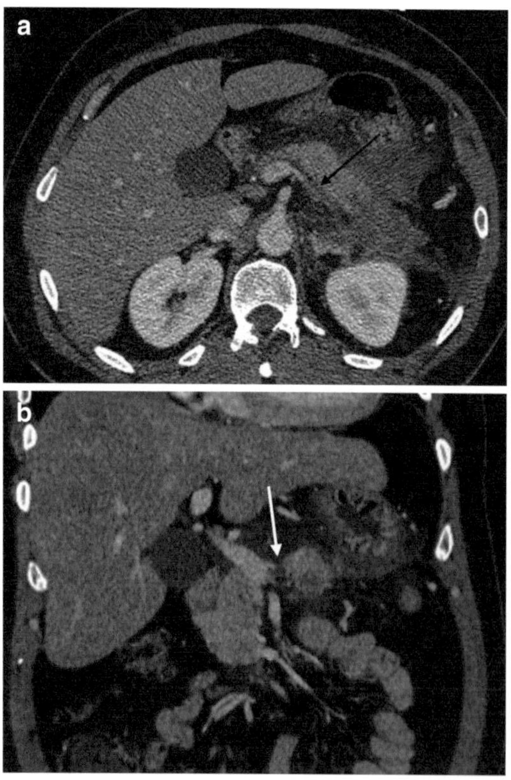

Fig. 5.10 Splenic vein thrombosis on CT. 45-year-old man presented with abdominal pain. (**a**) IV contrast-enhanced axial CT image in the portal venous phase shows attenuation of the splenic vein, with intermediate-density thrombus (black arrow). (**b**) IV contrast-enhanced coronal CT image in the portal venous phase demonstrates acute hypodense clot (white arrow) at the portosplenic confluence

[34]. On IV contrast-enhanced CT and MRI, the pseudoaneurysm and donor artery demonstrate similar enhancement with the rounded pseudoaneurysm arising from the donor artery.

Disconnected pancreatic duct syndrome develops as a complication of acute necrotizing pancreatitis. Pancreatic enzymes continuously leak out at the disruption site, which is often at the pancreatic neck since this is a vascular watershed territory. The enzymes digest the pancreatic and peripancreatic tissue, causing necrosis. MRCP can be used to evaluate ductal integrity, with ERCP used to confirm pancreatic duct disruption, during which pancreatic duct stents and drainage catheters may be placed.

5.3.5 Chronic Pancreatitis

Chronic pancreatitis is a progressive inflammatory disorder during which the pancreatic parenchyma undergoes fibrotic scarring leading to failure of both exocrine and endocrine functions. This most often results from a mixture of environmental and lifestyle factors, including alcohol, cigarettes, and occupational exposure, as well as genetic factors. Alcoholic or idiopathic disease accounts for approximately 90% of chronic pancreatitis. Less commonly, patients develop a hereditary or autoimmune form of chronic pancreatitis. Pain from recurrent bouts of pancreatitis, or constant, disabling pain, is the most common presenting symptom. Chronic pancreatitis is relatively uncommon, with an estimated incidence of 4 per 100,000 and an estimated prevalence of 42 per 100,000 in the United States from 1997 to 2006 [35].

The natural history of chronic pancreatitis can be divided into early, middle, and late phases. The early phase, approximately the first 5 years, is characterized by recurrent episodes of acute pancreatitis, pain, multiple hospitalizations, and interventions. During the middle phase, acute pancreatitis occurs less frequently, but intraductal calcifications, pancreatic duct strictures, and chronic pseudocysts develop (Fig. 5.11). Loss of exocrine and endocrine function manifesting as malnutrition, and diabetes, characterizes the late phase [36].

The unique imaging findings of chronic pancreatitis occur during the middle phase, as the imaging findings in the early phase are similar to those in acute pancreatitis, and emergency imaging is rarely needed in the late phase as the pancreas is no longer functioning. MRI/MRCP has become the standard imaging examination to evaluate chronic pancreatitis, as ERCP precipitates pancreatitis following approximately 4% of procedures, though this is not commonly performed in the acute setting [37]. MRCP demonstrates the main pancreatic duct wall, and when augmented by secretin injection prior to imaging side-duct disease can also be identified.

Pancreaticoduodenal pancreatitis, previously referred to as groove pancreatitis, is a relatively rare form of chronic pancreatitis. In the acute setting, inflammatory changes secondary to biliary or duodenal obstruction are seen in the pancreaticoduodenal groove, which is the potential triangular space bordered by the second portion of the duodenum, the pancreatic head, and the common bile duct. In the chronic phase, scar tissue forms within this space in the pure form and can also involve the pancreatic head in the segmental form [37]. When the pancreatic head is involved, findings can mimic pancreatic adenocarcinoma. Cystic changes and wall thickening of the medial duodenal wall near the ampulla can develop. On CECT, soft tissue within the groove is seen, and may enhance on delayed images (Fig. 5.12a). On MRI, the scar tissue will appear hypointense on T1-weighted sequences compared to the normal pancreatic parenchyma, and iso- to hyperintense on T2-weighted sequences, and demonstrates delayed enhancement (Fig. 5.12b). If small periampullary cysts are seen, their presence, as well as smooth narrowing of the main pancreatic duct by scar tissue, can help differentiate pancreaticoduodenal pancreatitis from pancreatic adenocarcinoma, which irregularly narrows the duct and lacks the cystic changes in the duodenum [38].

Autoimmune pancreatitis may also present acutely. Patients typically present with jaundice, diabetes, weight loss, or pain, but typically do not have the acute, severe pain seen with acute pancreatitis. Imaging will commonly demonstrate a diffusely enlarged pancreas, classically described as sausage shaped. There is typically a loss of the lobular architecture and, sometimes, a peripheral rind or halo of hypoattenuation (Fig. 5.13). The main pancreatic duct is typically not dilated, and may actually be narrowed. A pitfall in diagnosing autoimmune pancreatitis is that only a portion of

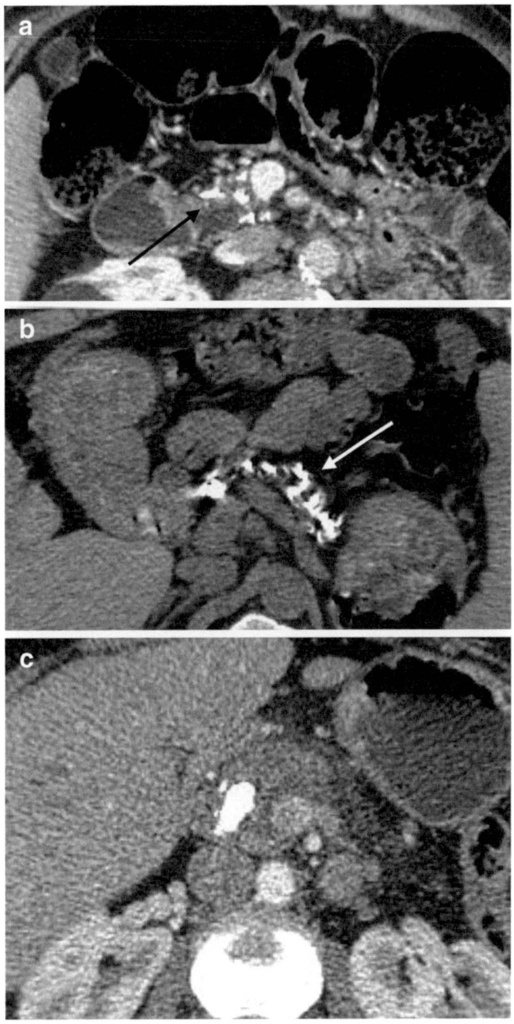

Fig. 5.11 Chronic pancreatitis on CT. CT images from three separate patients with known chronic pancreatitis who presented with acute abdominal pain. (**a**) IV contrast-enhanced axial CT image in the portal venous phase and (**b**) non-contrast axial CT image through the pancreas demonstrate multifocal calcifications in the pancreatic head (black arrow) and body (white arrow), which are related to the patients' histories of chronic pancreatitis. A large ductal calcification is seen in (**c**) with associated distal pancreatic and peripancreatic edema, in this patient with acute-on-chronic pancreatitis

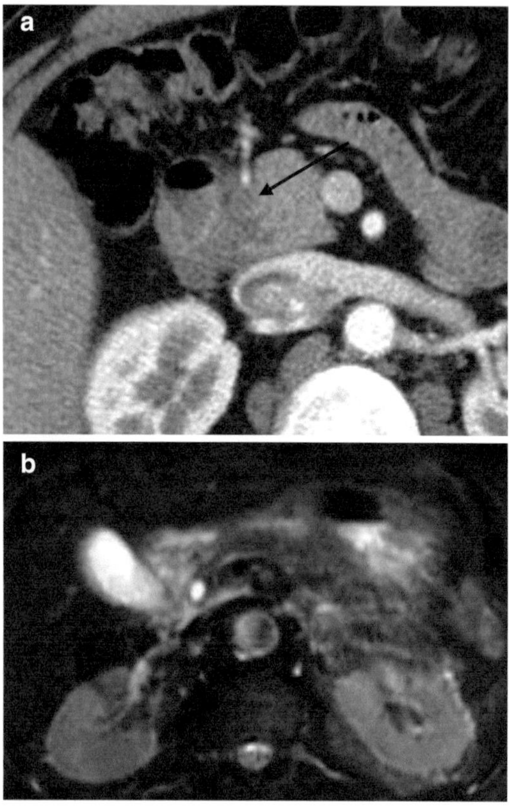

Fig. 5.12 Pancreaticoduodenal pancreatitis on CT and MR. 58-year-old man, with a history of recurrent pancreatitis, presented with acute abdominal pain. (**a**) IV contrast-enhanced axial CT image in the portal venous phase demonstrates hypodense fluid within the pancreaticoduodenal groove (arrow) in a patient presenting with acute abdominal pain. (**b**) Axial T2-weighted MR image demonstrates hyperintensity in and surrounding the pancreaticoduodenal groove, consistent with an acute episode of pancreatitis

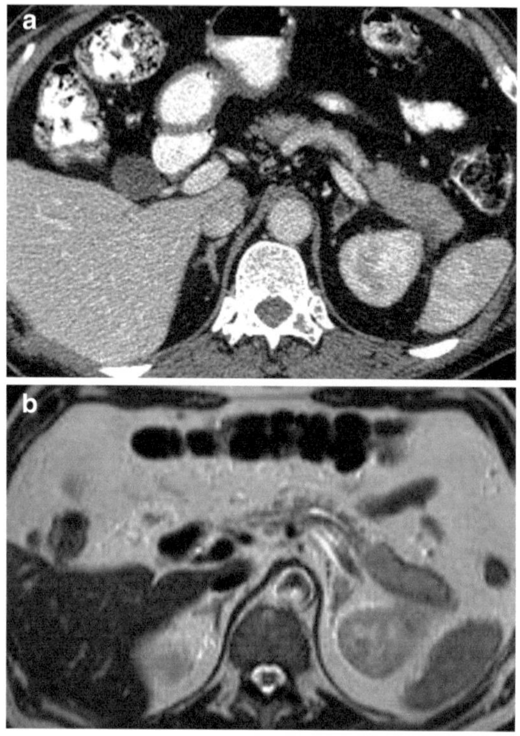

Fig. 5.13 Autoimmune pancreatitis on CT and MRI. 69-year-old man presented with abdominal pain, and elevated IgG4. (**a**) IV contrast-enhanced axial CT image in the portal venous phase and (**b**) T2-weighted axial MR image demonstrate focal mass-like enlargement of the pancreatic tail. Note the contrast to the atrophic pancreatic body

the pancreas can be affected, potentially mimicking pancreatic adenocarcinoma.

Pancreatic congenital malformations can also lead to recurrent episodes of acute pancreatitis and, eventually, chronic pancreatitis. The most common malformation is pancreatic divisum, which is seen in 5–10% of the population [39], which in some patients can lead to recurrent acute pancreatitis. Pancreatic divisum should be suspected in young people who suffer from recurrent episodes of acute pancreatitis, as a reported 12–50% of idiopathic pancreatitis in young people is associated with pancreatic divisum. MRCP should be performed to demonstrate whether the main pancreatic duct connects only to the dorsal duct of Santorini and empties through the minor papilla into the duodenum, or if the main duct communicates anteriorly with the duct of Wirsung and predominantly empties through the major ampulla. In the case of pancreatic divisum, MRCP will demonstrate two distinct non-communicating ducts (Fig. 5.14). Annular pancreas is a rare congenital malformation occurring in 5–15 in 100,000 people [40–42]. On CT or MR, pancreatic tissue surrounds the duodenum, and the pancreatic duct can be seen encircling the second portion of the duodenum. Acute pancreatitis can develop in patients with annular pancreas, and is typically encountered in children, or in adults in their fifth or sixth decade [43] (Fig. 5.15).

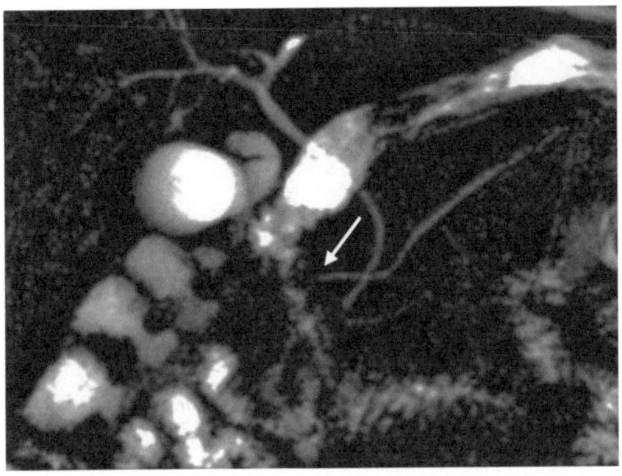

Fig. 5.14 Pancreatic divisum on MRCP. 37-year-old man presented with RUQ pain, and elevated pancreatic enzymes. 2D maximal intensity projection MRCP image shows the main pancreatic duct (white arrow) entering the duodenum, separate from the common bile duct

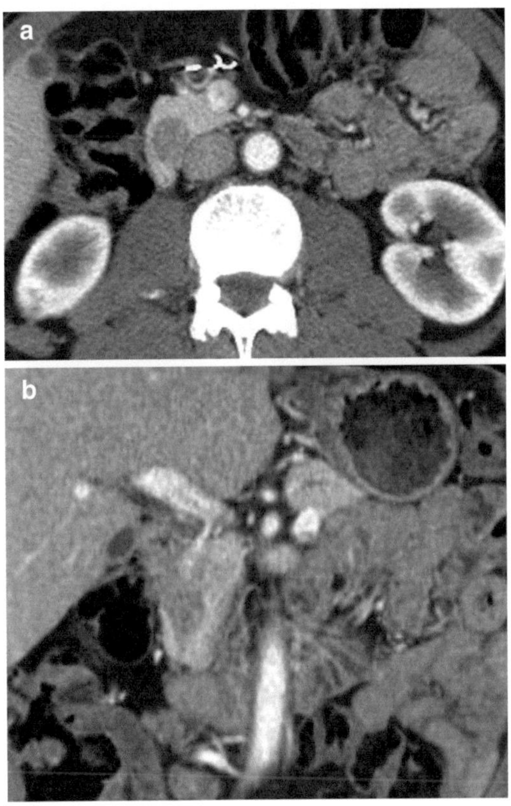

Fig. 5.15 CT of annular pancreas. 57-year-old man with a history of Diffuse large B-cell lymphoma, and surgical clips from prior gastric ulcer repair; an annular pancreas was incidentally discovered on lymph node dissection. IV contrast-enhanced CT images during the portal venous phase in axial (**a**) and coronal (**b**) planes demonstrate pancreatic tissue encircling the second portion of the duodenum

5.4 Traumatic Pancreatic Injury

Penetrating and blunt abdominal trauma represent two common reasons for imaging in the emergency department. In cases of abdominal trauma, pancreatic injury nearly always occurs as part of multi-organ injury. While injury to other abdominal organs is more immediately apparent and life threatening, pancreatic injury is unique in that while it may be apparent immediately after the traumatic event, it may also develop over hours, days, or weeks after the initial event, due to the release of pancreatic enzymes. Regardless of the injury mechanism or evolution, CECT is the primary imaging modality for initial evaluation, with MRI/MRCP and ERCP serving as critical secondary techniques. Knowledge of the most common imaging findings, their anatomic location, and when specific injuries are likely to manifest after the traumatic event will help the radiologist make a rapid and accurate diagnosis. Awareness of imaging pitfalls and mimics is also critical for accurate diagnosis. In patients with the ability to communicate pancreatic injury findings and severity with the trauma surgeons and intensive care physicians, and to advise on the need for any further imaging examinations, is critical to injury management.

Penetrating trauma from gunshots or stab wounds more frequently leads to pancreatic injury than blunt trauma [44]. Isolated injury of the pancreas rarely occurs, as it typically requires a bullet or knife violating multiple layers of soft tissue and adjacent organs before it reaches the pancreas in penetrating trauma. In blunt trauma, the severe anteroposterior forces requisite for pancreatic trauma inevitably lead to concurrent multi-organ injury. In blunt trauma, concurrent injuries to the liver, stomach, major vasculature, spleen, kidneys, and duodenum are most frequently seen [44].

While pancreatic injury is rare, accounting for less than 1% of blunt abdominal trauma [45], delay in diagnosis can have severe consequences, with mortality reported to be up to 16–30% in patients who sustain blunt pancreatic trauma. However, mortality is directly attributable to the pancreatic injury in a small percentage of these patients, ranging from 5 to 15% [45, 46].

The main predictive factors of patient outcomes include the ductal injury, time to diagnosis and/or treatment, and mechanism of injury. A risk factor for mortality in up to 40% of patients with pancreatic injury is delayed diagnosis. Posttraumatic complications occur in 30% of patients with pancreatic injury [47–49].

Pancreatic injury from blunt trauma typically occurs when severe anterior-to-posterior forces compress the pancreas against the spine, injuring the pancreatic neck. Pancreatic neck injury is seen in approximately 60% of patients with blunt pancreatic trauma, with pancreatic head and body/tail injury evenly divided amongst the rest [50]. Shearing and rapid rotation are also significant forces leading to pancreatic injury. Typical scenarios leading to blunt traumatic injury include a motor vehicle driver colliding with the steering wheel, resulting in compression of the upper abdomen, or a passenger slamming against the seatbelt during deceleration. In the pediatric population, a bicyclist falling into/over their handlebars is a more typical scenario. Due to lesser degrees of peripancreatic fat, children are at greater risk for pancreatic injury from blunt trauma. Less common situations include assault or sports injury with direct blows to the abdomen.

Knowledge of the traumatic mechanism, such as those previously described, and an awareness of adjacent organ damage, can give the radiologist significant insight into where a pancreatic injury may have occurred, spurring the radiologist into more detailed interrogation. Injury to the duodenum and liver is more likely to be associated with a concomitant pancreatic head injury. Damage to the superior mesenteric artery and/or vein is likely to have an associated injury to the pancreatic neck and/or the uncinate process. Damage to the stomach may be associated with a pancreatic body and neck injury. When an injury to the left kidney, spleen, or splenic vasculature occurs, concurrent injury to the pancreatic tail is more likely. Gunshot and stab wounds are the most frequent mechanism of penetrating trauma. When evaluating penetrating trauma, injury to the duodenum or stomach should alert the radiologist to search for concomitant injury to the pancreas.

While injury to adjacent organs can clue in the radiologist to a pancreatic injury, these injuries can also obscure a pancreatic injury on CT. Several other unique factors pose a challenge to the radiologist in the initial survey for traumatic pancreatic injury. These include imaging techniques and protocols that prioritize more commonly injured organs, the overall rarity of pancreatic injury, and the often normal appearance of the pancreas on initial imaging.

During the immediate posttraumatic clinical assessment, findings are usually nonspecific, and differentiating pancreatic injury from more commonly or concomitantly injured abdominal organs is limited. On physical examination, ecchymosis or abrasions along the upper abdomen are nonspecific physical examination signs, but increase the likelihood that internal abdominal injury may have occurred. A reliable history from patients may be difficult to obtain as patients typically have other severe injuries requiring intubation or causing them to be altered. Findings that normally present during acute pancreatitis, such as elevated amylase and lipase, leukocytosis, and burning upper abdominal pain, may not develop until a couple of days after the pancreatic injury. Within the first 24 h, serum amylase or lipase may be within normal limits up to 40% of the time [51–53]. When serial serum markers continue to rise, a pancreatic injury should be assumed in the setting of abdominal trauma.

The early phase, approximately the first 48 h, after traumatic pancreatic injury is most critical for patient outcomes. The most devastating injuries are associated vascular injuries, with hemorrhage of the inferior vena cava, splenic vein, or portal vein [44, 46, 50]. Pancreatic duct disruption leading to severe acute pancreatitis and multi-organ system failure is the primary factor leading to mortality and morbidity after the early phase. The most common reported complications include posttraumatic pancreatitis, walled-off necrosis, and development of pseudocysts. Delayed complications may develop within days, or take weeks to years to present. More uncommon, but significant, complications include fistula formation with adjacent structures caused by leakage of pancreatic enzymes, and pseudoaneurysm formation with hemorrhage. When duct disruption occurs, the risk for development of an abscess is 25% and of a fistula is 50%, while the risk of abscess or fistula development is less than 10% when the main duct integrity is intact. Finally, pancreatic duct strictures can be a late cause of recurrent acute pancreatitis [45].

5.5 Imaging

Multi-detector CT plays the primary role in acute injury assessment in the setting of blunt and penetrating abdominal trauma. The speed and ease of acquisition with computed tomography allow for comprehensive evaluation in a timely manner that is unmatched by other modalities. MDCT provides the ability to create thin slices with multi-planar reconstructions (MPR) and three-dimensional reconstructions which are standard in current imaging and which aid in the diagnosis of pancreatic injury. Upon presentation at the emergency department, a trauma patient will typically undergo MDCT using a general abdominal trauma protocol scan performed during the portal venous phase, 70 s after injection of the contrast bolus. An optional low-dose, delayed phase of up to 5 min can be acquired at the radiologist's discretion if parenchymal injury or free fluid is identified after either a portal venous or a pancreatic parenchymal scan, as this can aid in diagnosis of abnormalities including active bleeding with enlarging hematoma.

Modern CT with improved temporal and spatial resolution has shown significant improvement in the identification of pancreatic injury. As previously stated, the integrity of the main pancreatic duct and the duration from injury to diagnosis are the two most critical predictors of outcome following pancreatic injury; therefore, early and accurate diagnosis of pancreatic injury is critical in limiting morbidity and improving the patient's prognosis. However, CT findings can pose a challenge to the diagnostic radiologist as CT findings of pancreatic injury can develop slowly, and a normal appearance does not exclude pancreatic injury. Findings of pancreatic injuries may be absent during the first 12 h on the initial CT scan in up to 20–40% of patients [45, 54, 55].

While the FAST (focused assessment with sonography for trauma) examination is often employed as part of the trauma workup, ultrasound is limited as an examination for evaluating the pancreas. Peripancreatic fluid may be observed on ultrasound, but is a nonspecific finding. Advances in contrast-enhanced ultrasound are currently being explored as a possible additional imaging modality in the setting of pancreatic trauma, but it is not currently part of common practice and remains impractical. MRCP has limited utility during initial injury surveillance, but is increasingly used as a noninvasive secondary tool for the assessment of ductal injury and complications. ERCP can also be used as a secondary test to evaluate for ductal injury, with the added benefit of intervention to stent an injured duct.

Specific findings of pancreatic trauma include laceration, transection or comminution of the pancreatic tissue, parenchymal edema, parenchymal hematoma, and actively collecting hemorrhage between the splenic vein and pancreatic parenchyma. A laceration can appear as a hypodense line or cleft, with normal parenchyma on either side (Fig. 5.16). Complete disruption or comminution of the pancreas can cause hypoattenuation of the entire pancreas. Heterogeneous enhancement with areas of slight hyperenhancement within the gland itself or in the adjacent soft tissue represents hematoma. Fluid between the pancreatic parenchyma and the splenic vein is seen between 60 and 91% of patients with pancreatic trauma and is the most sensitive imaging finding in pancreatic trauma [56, 57].

Pancreatic injury from penetrating trauma should be considered if a foreign body is retained near the pancreas, even when no laceration or hematoma is seen. If no retained foreign body is seen, such as with a stab wound or a through-and-through gunshot wound, the bullet trajectory or knife wound is extrapolated by considering adjacent injuries or tracts of air. These findings can lead the radiologist to assume a degree of pancreatic injury. The placement of markers on wound entry, and exit sites, can aid in the extrapolation of the line of injury.

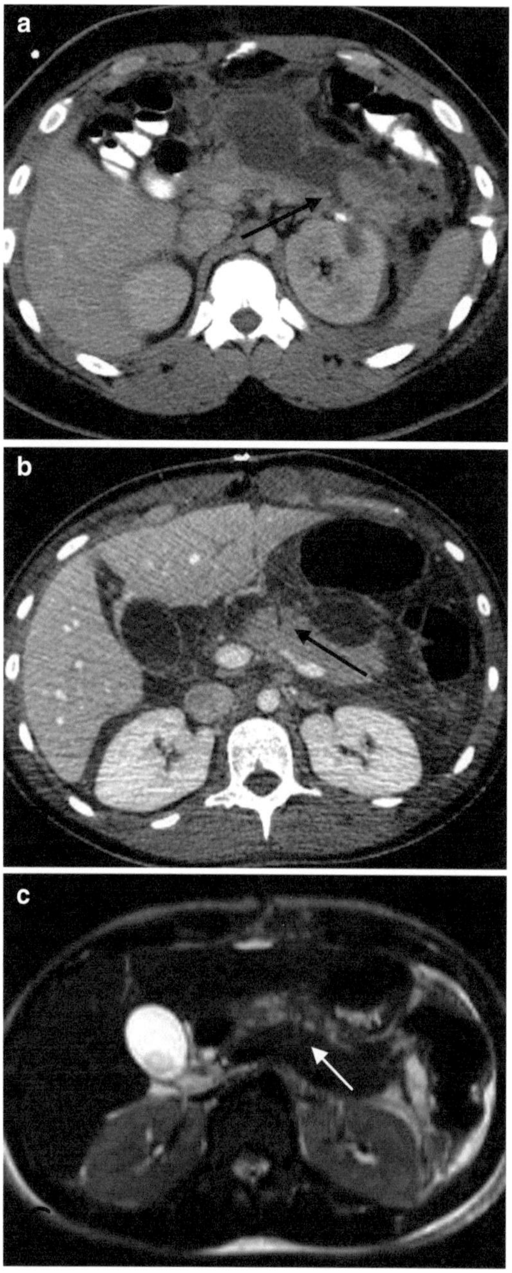

Fig. 5.16 CT and MRI of pancreatic laceration. (**a**) 24-year-old man with gunshot wound. IV contrast-enhanced axial CT image in the portal venous phase demonstrates transection of the pancreatic body-tail junction (black arrow), with a surrounding hypodense fluid collection. (**b**) 20-year-old woman with multiple stab wounds to abdomen. IV contrast-enhanced axial CT image in the portal venous phase demonstrates a partial laceration in the anterior pancreatic body (black arrow). (**c**) T2-weighted MR image from same patient as in (**b**) shows a subtle hyperintense laceration of the pancreatic body (white arrow)

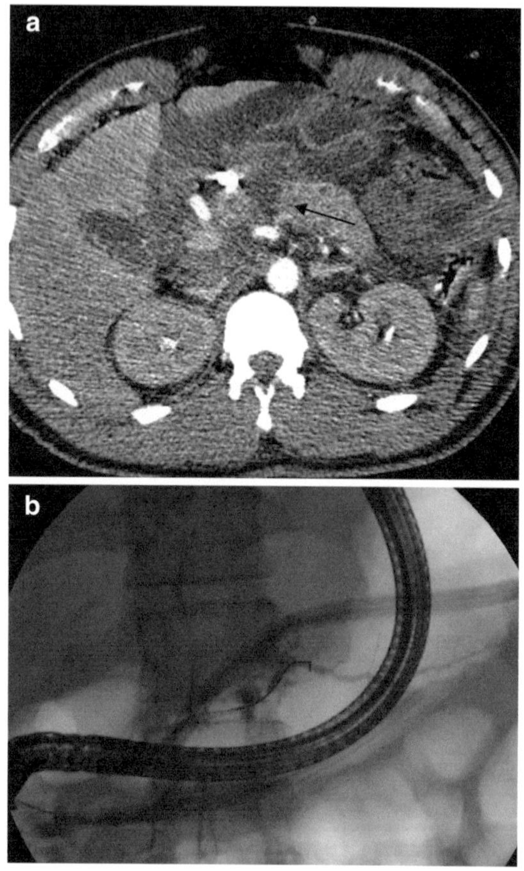

Fig. 5.17 CT and fluoroscopy of pancreatic laceration. 30-year-old man, gunshot wound. (**a**) IV contrast-enhanced CT image in the late arterial phase demonstrates pancreatic transection (arrow) involving the pancreatic body, with a surrounding peripancreatic fluid collection. (**b**) Frontal ERCP image demonstrates a stent being placed across the transected segment

Information acquired from the initial CT can guide further management, including the need for surgical intervention or additional imaging with MRI/MRCP or ERCP. Main duct disruption is usually treated surgically or with stenting, while an intact duct is usually treated medically (Fig. 5.17). For unstable patients who skip initial imaging and undergo immediate exploratory laparotomy, a 24-h follow-up CT scan can be used to identify delayed or initially missed pancreatic injury. The retroperitoneal location of the pancreas limits evaluation during exploratory laparotomy, and injury may not be adequately addressed during surgery.

The most critical finding to determine whether a patient should go to surgery is main pancreatic ductal injury. If a pancreatic laceration extends through the anteroposterior dimension of the pancreas by greater than 50%, loss of ductal integrity is assumed [58]. A post-processing technique termed minimum intensity projection (MinIP), in which thick-slab images are produced by recording the lowest pixel value, can be used to accentuate the main pancreatic duct, and has the potential to improve diagnostic accuracy. In patients where the diagnosis of ductal injury is uncertain and the patient is hemodynamically stable, MRCP can serve as an effective problem-solving test for evaluating the integrity of the pancreatic duct, and should be performed within 24 h of presentation. The sensitivity of MDCT and MRCP for the detection of pancreatic duct injuries was compared in a prospective study by Panda and colleagues, which showed that the two modalities performed similarly, and can complement each other by increasing diagnostic confidence for identification of a pancreatic duct laceration [59].

MRCP sequences are produced with heavily T2-weighted two-dimensional and three-dimensional acquisitions. The pancreatic ductal anatomy along with the biliary tract and fluid-containing structures is readily shown as hyperintense, while surrounding soft tissues remain hypointense. The spatial relationships are more explicit with 3D reconstructions. The pancreatic duct can be visualized from the tail to the pancreatic head, demonstrating ductal anomalies, and allowing for presurgical or pre-ERCP planning. Prior to the acquisition of MRI/MRCP imaging, secretin, a hormone which stimulates pancreatic exocrine secretion, can be given to patients to temporary dilate the pancreatic ducts, increasing the likelihood of laceration detection.

ERCP is now more commonly performed after MRCP in patients who remain equivocal. ERCP is the imaging reference standard in the evaluation of duct integrity, and allows for the therapeutic intervention with ductal stent placement if there is ductal injury. Additionally, a post-ERCP MDCT scan using curved-planar reconstruction along the pancreatic duct can demonstrate extravasation of contrast. While ERCP offers the advantage for therapeutic intervention, there is a risk of complications, particularly acute pancreatitis. For the hemodynamically stable patient, MRCP holds the advantages of being noninvasive and capable of elucidating additional pancreatic parenchymal and bile duct injuries.

Imaging pitfalls may obscure pancreatic trauma or cause the false appearance of pancreatic trauma. Importantly, shortly after trauma, CT findings may be entirely absent. Thin patients and children may have very little peripancreatic fat, which hinders the detection of peripancreatic fluid and injury. Normal clefts of fat, extending deep into the pancreatic parenchyma, may be mistaken for lacerations. After aggressive resuscitation, which is common in the post-trauma patient, fluid can be third-spaced within the fat adjacent to the pancreas, which can mimic abnormal fluid or fat stranding. Additionally, hemoretroperitoneum from adjacent organs such as the kidney may mimic pathologic peripancreatic fluid. When assessing a pancreatic laceration for ductal injury, the 50% rule is limited when considering the pancreatic head as the duct courses more posteriorly with the head.

The American Association for the Surgery of Trauma (AAST) classification system for the grading of pancreatic trauma is the most widely accepted (Table 5.2). This system defines five

Table 5.2 AAST grading of traumatic pancreatic injuries

Grade	Injury	Description
I	Hematoma	Minor contusion without duct injury
	Laceration	Superficial laceration without duct injury
II	Hematoma	Major contusion without duct injury
	Laceration	Major laceration without ductal injury or tissue loss
III	Laceration	Distal transection or parenchymal injury with duct injury
IV	Laceration	Proximal transection or parenchymal injury involving the ampulla
V	Laceration	Massive disruption of the pancreatic head

grades (I–V) for assessing severity. The key components used for evaluating severity are (1) depth of laceration, (2) size of hematoma or contusion, (3) integrity of the main duct, (4) complete disruption of the pancreas, and (5) specific anatomic sections of the pancreas which are involved. Injuries closer to the head receive a higher grade. Mortality for grade I and II injuries is approximately 7%, while grade III and IV injuries have a 29% mortality rate [44, 60].

5.6 The Postsurgical Pancreas

Both acute and chronic complications from pancreatic surgery or procedures can necessitate emergent abdominal imaging. Surgical procedures for resection of pancreatic or periampullary masses or for trauma include pancreaticoduodenectomy, commonly known as a Whipple procedure, central pancreatectomy, distal pancreatectomy, and total pancreatectomy. Drainage procedures used to treat chronic pancreatitis, which has become unamenable to medical management, include the Frey and Puestow procedures. Creation of anastomosis is part of nearly all of these procedures, while resection of adjacent organs is also common. Familiarity with the surgical techniques and postsurgical anatomy is critical in the evaluation of postsurgical complications.

During the Whipple procedure, the pancreatic head, distal common bile duct, duodenum, gastric antrum, and a short segment of the proximal jejunum are resected. The surgery is completed by creation of three anastomoses: pancreaticojejunostomy, hepaticojejunostomy, and gastrojejunostomy. When a modified version with preservation of the pylorus and first 2 cm of the duodenum is performed, a duodenojejunostomy is created instead of a gastrojejunostomy. Shortly after surgery, expected findings include pneumobilia and air within the main pancreatic duct, as well as edema of the gastrojejunostomy, fluid collections, and reactive lymphadenopathy. Complications occur following approximately 40% of pancreaticoduodenectomies, and mortality is approximately 2% [61, 62]. Delayed gastric emptying is the most common complication, which is more typically seen after the pylorus-preserving method. Pancreatic fistulas occur in 17%, and can develop to adjacent organs or spaces [63]. Anastomotic leakage occurs in up to 30% of patients [62], most often occurring at the pancreaticojejunal anastomosis, with associated acute pancreatitis of the remnant pancreas (Fig. 5.18).

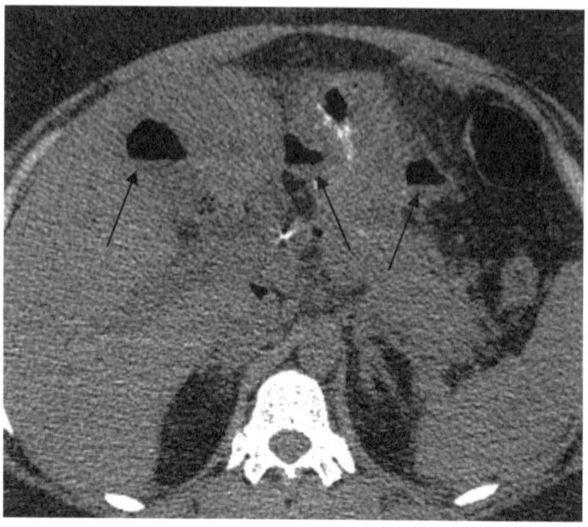

Fig. 5.18 CT of transient anastomotic leak. Non-contrast axial CT image of a patient who underwent a Whipple procedure for a pancreatic head mass. Three air-containing postoperative fluid collections (arrows) were noted 14 days after surgery. The amount of air in the collections suggested origin from the gastrojejunal anastomosis. The patient did well after catheter drainage

The central, distal, and total pancreatectomies are performed much less often than the pancreaticoduodenectomy. The central pancreatectomy involves resection of the pancreatic neck and/or body, with suturing of the cut ends of the pancreatic duct, which is usually followed by anastomosis of the distal pancreatic tail with the jejunum. This procedure is primarily used to treat trauma or chronic pancreatitis. Anastomotic leak is the most common complication, with acute pancreatitis, hemorrhage, and fluid collections occurring less often [64]. Unlike alternative pancreatic resection procedures, the distal pancreatectomy does not involve creation of an anastomosis as the cut end is simply sutured shut. Pancreatic fistulas develop in 5% of patients, with other complications including abscess formation and small-bowel obstruction [65]. During a total pancreatectomy, the entire pancreas is resected, and two anastomoses are created: a hepaticojejunostomy and a duodenojejunostomy.

Drainage procedures, including the Puestow and Frey, are typically indicated for intractable chronic pancreatitis. The pancreatic main duct is usually dilated greater than 6 mm in patients selected to undergo these procedures. A horizontal pancreaticojejunostomy is performed along an 8–10 cm segment of the pancreatic duct to a Roux-en-Y loop of jejunum. The Roux-en-Y loop lies ventral to pancreatic body, and can be mistaken for an abscess on imaging if the surgical history is unknown. The Frey procedure involves excavation of the pancreatic head, while preserving the common bile duct, followed by a similar pancreaticojejunostomy to the Puestow procedure. If the vascular supply to the pancreatic head is damaged during surgery, ischemia can cause necrosis of the common bile duct or duodenum.

IV contrast-enhanced CT is again the initial imaging modality most often employed to assess for postsurgical complications. If enteric contrast is used, it can help differentiate bowel from a fluid collection as well as improve detection of fistulae. An initial non-enhanced CT could be considered to evaluate for hemorrhage and calcifications. Assessment of each anastomosis is critical, and the presence of extraluminal enteric contrast is definitive evidence of a leak, while fluid pooling around the anastomosis or extraluminal air strongly suggests a leak. Foci of air in unexpected locations can also imply a fistulous tract or an abscess. In addition to anastomotic insufficiency, early complications (less than 30 days) include intra-abdominal abscess, pancreaticojejunal fistula, remnant pancreatitis, and hemorrhage. MRI/MRCP represents an important secondary test for the evaluation of the pancreatic duct, as well as for fistulae. In the later phases, chronic complications include gastric outlet obstruction and bowel obstruction from stricture formation of the anastomoses, biliary duct dilation from hepaticojejunostomy structuring, chronic fistula, and peri-anastomotic ulcers [66].

5.7 Summary

Having a working knowledge of emergency pancreatic imaging is critical for anyone who interprets imaging in the emergency department setting. Being able to detect the often subtle findings in pancreatic trauma, knowing how to evaluate for ductal injury, and knowing the complications of acute pancreatitis and what to look for, can potentially significantly improve patient management and outcomes. Knowledge of the etiologies and variants of pancreatitis can also be helpful in order to ensure that patients are directed towards the appropriate treatment. Postoperative pancreatic imaging is always challenging, and having a basic knowledge of the procedures and altered anatomy is crucial in making an accurate diagnosis. Finally, it is important to have a fundamental understanding of the organizational classification systems, particularly the revised Atlanta Classification System and AAST trauma grading, in order to effectively communicate with our colleagues in other fields who work with these systems routinely.

References

1. Peery A, Dellon E, Lund J. Burden of gastrointestinal disease in the United States: 2012 update. Gastroenterology. 2012;143(5):1179–87.
2. Lowenfels AB, Maisonneuve P, Sullivan T. The changing character of acute pancreatitis: epidemiology, etiology, and prognosis. Curr Gastroenterol Rep. 2009;11(2):97–103.
3. Frossard J-L, Steer ML, Pastor CM. Acute pancreatitis. Lancet. 2008;371(9607):143–52.
4. Banks P, Bollen TL, Dervenis C, et al. Classification of acute pancreatitis--2012: revision of the Atlanta classification and definitions by international consensus. Gut. 2013;62:102–11.
5. Tenner S, Baillie J, DeWitt J, Vege SS. American College of Gastroenterology Guideline: management of acute pancreatitis. Am J Gastroenterol. 2013;108(9): 1400–15.
6. Banks PA, Freeman ML. Practice guidelines in acute pancreatitis. Am J Gastroenterol. 2006;101(10): 2379–400.
7. Fagenholz PJ, Ndez-Del Castillo CF, Harris NS, Pelletier AJ, Camargo CJ Jr. Increasing United States hospital admissions for acute pancreatitis, 1988–2003. Ann Epidemiol. 2007;17:491–7.

8. Johnson CD. Persistent organ failure during the first week as a marker of fatal outcome in acute pancreatitis. Gut. 2004;53(9):1340–4.
9. Buter A, Imrie CW, Carter CR, Evans S, McKay CJ. Dynamic nature of early organ dysfunction determines outcome in acute pancreatitis. Br J Surg. 2002;89(3):298–302.
10. Mofidi R, Duff MD, Wigmore SJ, Madhavan KK, Garden OJ, Parks RW. Association between early systemic inflammatory response, severity of multiorgan dysfunction and death in acute pancreatitis. Br J Surg. 2006;93(6):738–44.
11. Balthazar EJ. Acute pancreatitis: assessment of severity with clinical and CT evaluation. Radiology. 2002;223:603–13.
12. Zhao K, Adam SZ, Keswani RN, Horowitz JM, Miller FH. Acute pancreatitis: revised Atlanta classification and the role of cross-sectional imaging. Am J Roentgenol. 2015;205(1):W32–41.
13. Mortele KJ. A modified CT severity index for evaluating acute pancreatitis: improved correlation with patient outcome. Am J Roentgenol. 2004;183(5):1261–5.
14. Tsuji Y, Takahashi N, Fletcher JG, et al. Subtraction color map of contrast-enhanced and unenhanced CT for the prediction of pancreatic necrosis in early stage of acute pancreatitis. Am J Roentgenol. 2014;202(4):W349–56.
15. Casas JD, Díaz R, Valderas G, Mariscal A, Cuadras P. Prognostic value of CT in the early assessment of patients with acute pancreatitis. AJR Am J Roentgenol. 2004;182(3):569–74.
16. Macari M, Finn ME, Bennett GL, et al. Differentiating pancreatic cystic neoplasms from pancreatic pseudocysts at MR imaging: value of perceived internal debris. Radiology. 2009;251(1):77–84.
17. Kim KO, Kim TN. Acute pancreatic pseudocyst. Pancreas. 2012;41(4):577–81.
18. Cui ML, Kim KH, Kim HG, et al. Incidence, risk factors and clinical course of pancreatic fluid collections in acute pancreatitis. Dig Dis Sci. 2014;59(5):1055–62.
19. Lankisch PG, Weber-Dany B, Maisonneuve P, et al. Pancreatic pseudocysts: prognostic factors for their development and their spontaneous resolution in the setting of acute pancreatitis. Pancreatology. 2012;12(2):85–90.
20. Memiş A, Parildar M. Interventional radiological treatment in complications of pancreatitis. Eur J Radiol. 2002;43(3):219–28.
21. Lenhart DK, Balthazar EJ. MDCT of acute mild (nonnecrotizing) pancreatitis: abdominal complications and fate of fluid collections. Am J Roentgenol. 2008;190(3):643–9.
22. Isenmann R, Büchler M, Uhl W, Malfertheiner P, Martini M, Beger HG. Pancreatic necrosis: an early finding in severe acute pancreatitis. Pancreas. 1993;8(3):358–61.
23. Morgan DE, Baron TH, Smith JK, Robbin ML, Kenney PJ. Pancreatic fluid collections prior to intervention: evaluation with MR imaging compared with CT and US. Radiology. 1997;203:773–8.
24. Martin DR, Karabulut N, Yang M, McFadden DW. High signal peripancreatic fat on fat-suppressed spoiled gradient echo imaging in acute pancreatitis: preliminary evaluation of the prognostic significance. J Magn Reson Imaging. 2003;18(1):49–58.
25. Morgan DE. Imaging of acute pancreatitis and its complications. Clin Gastroenterol Hepatol. 2008;6(10):1077–85.
26. Thoeni RF. The revised Atlanta classification of acute pancreatitis: its importance for the radiologist and its effect on treatment. Radiology. 2012;262(3):751–64.
27. Stamatakos M, Stefanaki C, Kontzoglou K, Stergiopoulos S, Giannopoulos G, Safioleas M. Walled-off pancreatic necrosis. World J Gastroenterol. 2010;16(14):1707–12.
28. Boumitri C, Brown E, Kahaleh M. Necrotizing pancreatitis: current management and therapies. Clin Endosc. 2017;50(4):357–65.
29. Takahashi N, Papachristou GI, Schmit GD, et al. CT findings of walled-off pancreatic necrosis (WOPN): differentiation from pseudocyst and prediction of outcome after endoscopic therapy. Eur Radiol. 2008;18(11):2522–9.
30. Gluck M, Ross A, Irani S, et al. Endoscopic and percutaneous drainage of symptomatic walled-off pancreatic necrosis reduces hospital stay and radiographic resources. Clin Gastroenterol Hepatol. 2010;8(12):1083–8.
31. Da Costa DW, Boerma D, Van Santvoort HC, et al. Staged multidisciplinary step-up management for necrotizing pancreatitis. Br J Surg. 2014;101(1):65–79.
32. Besselink MG, Van Santvoort HC, Boermeester MA, et al. Timing and impact of infections in acute pancreatitis. Br J Surg. 2009;96(3):267–73.
33. Petrov MS, Shanbhag S, Chakraborty M, Phillips ARJ, Windsor JA. Organ failure and infection of pancreatic necrosis as determinants of mortality in patients with acute pancreatitis. Gastroenterology. 2010;139(3):813–20.
34. Balachandra S, Siriwardena AK. Systematic appraisal of the management of the major vascular complications of pancreatitis. Am J Surg. 2005;190(3):489–95.
35. Lévy P, Domínguez-Muñoz E, Imrie C, Löhr M, Maisonneuve P. Epidemiology of chronic pancreatitis: burden of the disease and consequences. United European Gastroenterol J. 2014;2(5):345–54.
36. Braganza JM, Lee SH, McCloy RF, McMahon MJ. Chronic pancreatitis. Lancet. 2011;377(9772):1184–97.
37. Mitchell RMS, Byrne MF, Baillie J. Pancreatitis. Lancet. 2003;361(9367):1447–55.
38. Stolte M, Weiss W, Volkholz H, et al. A special form of segmental pancreatitis: "groove pancreatitis". Hepato-Gastroenterology. 1982;29:198–208.
39. Morgan DE, Logan K, Baron TH, Koehler RE, Smith JK. Pancreas divisum: implications for diagnostic

and therapeutic pancreatography. Am J Roentgenol. 1999;173(1):193–8.
40. Ravitch MM, Woods AC Jr. Annular pancreas. Ann Surg. 1950;132:1116–27.
41. Marchese A. Doudenal stenosis by annular pancreas. Arq Cir Clin Exp. 1951;14:201.
42. Vasconcelos E, Sadek HM. Annular pancreas producing duodenal stenosis. Rev Bras Gastroenterol. 1949;1:535.
43. Lloyd-Jones W, Mountain JC. Annular pancreas in the adult. Ann Surg. 1972;176(2):163–70.
44. Linsenmaier U, Wirth S, Reiser M, Körner M. Diagnosis and classification of pancreatic and duodenal injuries in emergency radiology. Radiographics. 2008;28(6):1591–602.
45. Akhrass R, Yaffe MB, Brandt CP, Reigle M, Fallon WF Jr, Malangoni MA. Pancreatic trauma: a ten-year multi-institutional experience. Am Surg. 1997; 63(7):598–604.
46. Bradley EL, Young PR, Chang MC, et al. Diagnosis and initial management of blunt pancreatic trauma guidelines from a multiinstitutional review. Ann Surg. 1998;227(6):861–9.
47. Lucas CE, Ledgerwood AM. Factors influencing outcome after blunt duodenal injury. J Trauma. 1975;15(10):839–46.
48. Heitsch RC, Knutson CO, Fulton RL, Jones CE. Delineation of critical factors in the treatment of pancreatic trauma. Surgery. 1976;80(4):523–9.
49. Smego DR, Richardson JD, Flint LM. Determinants of outcome in pancreatic trauma. J Trauma. 1985; 25(8):771–6.
50. Gupta A, Stuhlfaut JW, Fleming KW, Lucey BC, Soto JA. Blunt trauma of the pancreas and biliary tract: a multimodality imaging approach to diagnosis. Radiographics. 2004;24(5):1381–95.
51. Moretz JA, Campbell DP, Parker DE, Williams GR. Significance of serum amylase level in evaluating pancreatic trauma. Am J Surg. 1975;130(6):739–41.
52. Jobst MA, Canty TG, Lynch FP. Management of pancreatic injury in pediatric blunt abdominal trauma. J Pediatr Surg. 1999;34(5):818–24.
53. Mahajan A, Kadavigere R, Sripathi S, Rodrigues GS, Rao VR, Koteshwar P. Utility of serum pancreatic enzyme levels in diagnosing blunt trauma to the pancreas: a prospective study with systematic review. Injury. 2014;45(9):1384–93.
54. Vasquez M, Cardarelli C, Glaser J, Murthi S, Stein D, Scalea T. The ABC's of pancreatic trauma: airway, breathing, and computerized tomography scan? Mil Med. 2017;182(S1):66–71.
55. Cirillo RL Jr, Koniaris LG. Detecting blunt pancreatic injuries. J Gastrointest Surg. 2002;6(4):587–98.
56. Lane MJ, Mindelzun RE, Sandhu JS, McCormick VD, Jeffrey RB. CT diagnosis of blunt pancreatic trauma: importance of detecting fluid between the pancreas and the splenic vein. AJR. 1994;163: 833–5.
57. Sivit CJ, Eichelberger MR. CT diagnosis of pancreatic injury in children: significance of fluid separating the splenic vein and the pancreas. AJR. 1995;165: 921–4.
58. Gordon RW, Anderson SW, Ozonoff A, Rekhi S, Soto JA. Blunt pancreatic trauma: evaluation with MDCT technology. Emerg Radiol. 2013;20(4):259–66.
59. Panda A, Kumar A, Gamanagatti S, et al. Evaluation of diagnostic utility of multidetector computed tomography and magnetic resonance imaging in blunt pancreatic trauma: a prospective study. Acta Radiol. 2015;56(4):387–96.
60. Venkatesh SK, Wan JMC. CT of blunt pancreatic trauma - a pictorial essay. Eur J Radiol. 2008;67(2): 311–20.
61. Beger HG, Schlosser W, Friess HM, Büchler MW. Duodenum-preserving head resection in chronic pancreatitis changes the natural course of the disease: a single-center 26-year experience. Ann Surg. 1999;230(4):512–9-23.
62. Schafer M, Mullhaupt B, Clavien PA. Evidence-based pancreatic head resection for pancreatic cancer and chronic pancreatitis. Ann Surg. 2002;236(2):137–48.
63. Yeo CJ, Cameron JL, Sohn TA, et al. Six hundred fifty consecutive pancreaticoduodenectomies in the 1990s: pathology, complications, and outcomes. Ann Surg. 1997;226(3):248–57-60.
64. Iacono C, Bortolasi L, Serio G. Central pancreatectomy. Dis Pancreas Curr Surg Ther. 2008;141(2):425–40.
65. Lillemoe KD, Kaushal S, Cameron JL, Sohn TA, Pitt HA, Yeo CJ. Distal pancreatectomy: indications and outcomes in 235 patients. Ann Surg. 1999;229(5):693–8-700.
66. Scialpi M, Scaglione M, Volterrani L, et al. Imaging evaluation of post pancreatic surgery. Eur J Radiol. 2005;53(3 SPEC. ISS):417–24.

MDCT and MRI of Bowel Obstruction and Ischemia

6

Daniel C. Oppenheimer, Constantine A. Raptis, and Vincent M. Mellnick

Abstract

Bowel obstruction and ischemia are common causes of the acute abdomen, with potential for morbidity and mortality if not recognized promptly. Multidetector computed tomography is the current imaging standard for establishing these diagnoses, but emerging techniques including dual-energy computed tomography and magnetic resonance angiography are being utilized with increased frequency. Radiologists must understand the imaging techniques available for evaluating intestinal obstruction and ischemia in order to provide effective and timely care to patients in the emergency and acute inpatient setting.

Keywords

Closed-loop obstruction · Mesenteric ischemia · Ischemic colitis · Dual-energy CT · Magnetic resonance angiography

D. C. Oppenheimer, M.D.
Department of Imaging Sciences, University of Rochester Medical Center, Rochester, NY, USA

C. A. Raptis, M.D. • V. M. Mellnick, M.D. (✉)
Mallinckrodt Institute of Radiology, Washington University in St. Louis School of Medicine, St. Louis, MO, USA
e-mail: mellnickv@wustl.edu

6.1 Bowel Obstruction

6.1.1 Introduction

Intestinal obstruction is a common condition representing either mechanical or functional obstruction of the small or large bowel, resulting in impaired transit of its luminal contents. It is an important cause of morbidity and mortality, accounting for upwards of 15% of emergency department visits for acute abdominal pain [1]. The majority of patients with intestinal obstruction can be adequately treated with conservative nonoperative management, including nasogastric tube decompression, if appropriate [2]. However, if strangulation or ischemia is present, the mortality rises, particularly if surgical management is delayed [3]. Imaging is a critical component in the evaluation of suspected bowel obstruction and its associated complications, and the potential for morbidity and mortality in these patients emphasizes the need for the radiologist to make an accurate and timely diagnosis.

6.1.2 Pathophysiology

A bowel obstruction may be partial or complete. In a partial small bowel obstruction (SBO), some of the luminal contents are able to pass distal to the point of obstruction, whereas in complete SBO, no contents can move distally [4]. The progressive

M. Patlas et al. (eds.), *MDCT and MR Imaging of Acute Abdomen*,
https://doi.org/10.1007/978-3-319-70778-5_6

distension of small bowel loops proximal to the site of obstruction produces several physiologic alterations. Vomiting results in volume depletion and hypokalemic metabolic alkalosis [5]. Stasis of bowel contents leads to overgrowth of intestinal flora, which can result in bacterial translocation across the bowel wall [6, 7]. As the obstructed bowel progressively dilates, the intraluminal pressure may exceed systemic venous pressures, and venous drainage will be impaired. Eventually, arterial flow to the bowel will be compromised, resulting in ischemia, necrosis, and perforation [8].

While patients with SBO usually present with acute onset abdominal pain, nausea, vomiting, and abdominal distension, patients with large bowel obstruction (LBO) typically present with more insidious symptoms of abdominal pain, constipation, and gradual abdominal distension [3]. If the ileocecal valve is competent (approximately 75% of patients), the obstruction cannot decompress into the small bowel, and a LBO will result in a closed-loop obstruction [9]. The cecum is the most capacious portion of the colon and as it progressively dilates, this segment is at greatest risk for ischemia, necrosis, and perforation [10]. If the ileocecal valve is incompetent, however, the LBO will decompress into the small bowel, and the appearance can mimic a distal SBO [11].

6.1.3 Epidemiology and Etiology

Bowel obstruction may be functional in nature, related to dysfunction of the splanchnic innervation or muscular wall, or mechanical due to a physical barrier to the passage of luminal contents. Functional small bowel dilatation is often referred to as "adynamic ileus" or "paralytic ileus," and is frequently seen postoperatively, as a side effect of opioid use, or in the setting of abdominal infection or inflammation including pancreatitis, diverticulitis, or appendicitis [5]. Functional dilatation of the colon is termed subacute chronic pseudo-obstruction (ACPO) or Ogilvie's syndrome [12]. Ogilvie's syndrome, which may apply to either sub-acute or chronic colonic pseudo-obstruction.

In the United States, the most common cause of mechanical SBO is adhesions, followed by hernias and malignancies, which together account for more than 80% of all causes of SBO [4, 13]. Less common etiologies of mechanical SBO include volvulus, stricture, intussusception, foreign bodies, and iatrogenic causes [3]. LBO is four to five times less common than SBO in the United States. Obstructing colonic malignancy is by far the most common cause of LBO (>60%), followed by colonic volvulus and diverticulitis, and less commonly hernias, inflammatory bowel disease, extrinsic compression, and intraluminal contents causing obstruction [14]. While adhesions are a common cause of SBO, they are very rarely the etiology of LBO [11].

In addition to being partial or complete, SBO can be subclassified as simple obstruction or closed-loop obstruction. A simple obstruction occurs when the bowel is obstructed at one or more points along its course, while closed-loop obstruction occurs when two points of intestine are obstructed at a single site, which produces a "C" or "U"-shaped configuration when a short segment is involved, and prone to volvulus, vascular compromise, and ischemia [15].

6.1.4 Bowel Obstruction Imaging

6.1.4.1 Small Bowel Obstruction

While radiography has relatively low accuracy and specificity for bowel obstruction, it may be the first imaging examination obtained in patients with suspected bowel obstruction [8]. Radiographs of the abdomen and pelvis should be obtained with upright or decubitus views if there is clinical concern for bowel obstruction. Upright or decubitus views permit identification of pneumoperitoneum and air-fluid levels, which may not be seen if only supine views are obtained [3]. Dilated small bowel loops containing air-fluid levels wider than 2.5 cm and differing by more than 2 cm in height within the same loop are generally accepted radiographic criteria for SBO [16].

If there is clinical concern for bowel obstruction, most patients will undergo computed tomography (CT). At our institution, in patients with suspected SBO, multidetector CT (MDCT) images are obtained without the use of oral contrast through the abdomen and pelvis. Iodinated

IV contrast is recommended if there are no contraindications to its administration. IV contrast improves detection of ischemia which may be associated with SBO, helps identify extraluminal fluid collections, and also aids in detecting alternative diagnoses which may account for the patient's symptoms.

The radiologist must make several specific observations when presented with a patient with suspected SBO. The first task is to determine if a SBO is present, defined as dilation of small bowel loops proximal to the obstruction measuring greater than 2.5 cm in diameter, often associated with intraluminal air-fluid levels [17] (Fig. 6.1). After confirming the presence of a SBO, the radiologist must make a determination of the severity of obstruction. In high-grade obstruction, there is greater than 50% difference in caliber between the dilated loops proximally and collapsed bowel distally [18]. While positive oral contrast is not typically administered prior to CT at our institution, the presence of oral contrast material beyond the site of obstruction is indicative of a partial obstruction (Fig. 6.2) [19]. The presence of intraluminal particulate material may be identified in the dilated loops of small bowel ("small bowel feces sign"), and can help determine the site of the obstruction, but this finding is not reliable in determining the severity of the obstruction [20] (Fig. 6.3).

Identifying the site of obstruction (transition point) should always be sought when a SBO is suspected. The transition point is identified on CT as the site of focal caliber change between dilated proximal and collapsed distal small bowel loops [18] (Figs. 6.1, 6.4, 6.5, 6.6). Applying a systematic approach of following the entire course of the bowel in an antegrade or retrograde fashion will usually successfully reveal the transition point [21]. The use of multiplanar reconstructions (MPR)—particularly coronal reformatted images—and determining which segments of small bowel contain fecalized material—is useful for determining the site of obstruction [13].

Recognizing closed-loop bowel obstruction is of paramount importance, as this particular configuration of obstruction is at high risk for strangulation and ischemia [3]. The typical appearance of a closed-loop obstruction, as noted above, is a fluid-filled dilated segment of bowel in a "C" or "U"-shaped configuration, with stretched and prominent mesenteric vessels converging in a radial distribution toward the point of fixation [15] (Fig. 6.7). A long-segment closed-loop bowel obstruction may also manifest as a "balloons-on-a-string" appearance, representing several adjacent loops of dilated fluid-filled small bowel radiating from a single point. The narrow pedicle at the point of fixation is prone to torsion, producing a small bowel volvulus which may

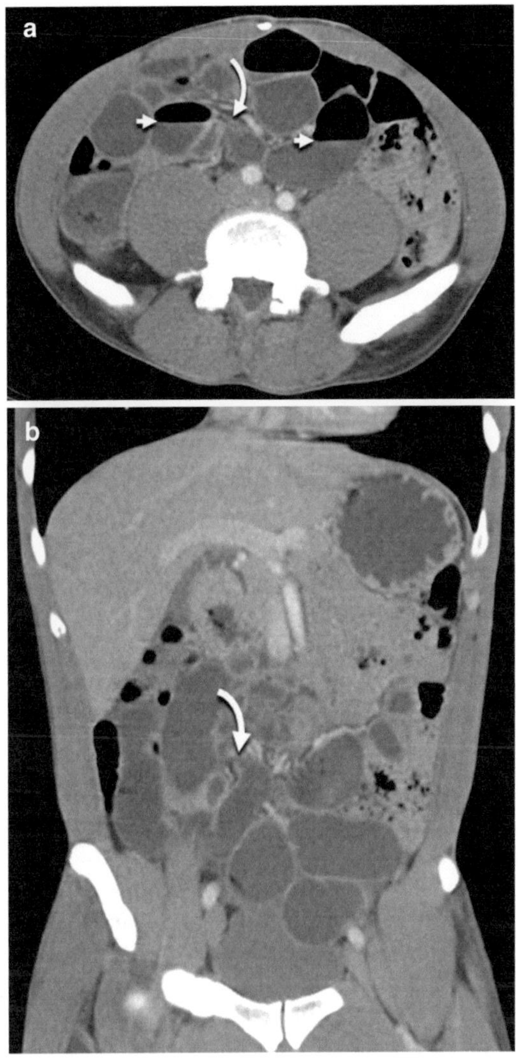

Fig. 6.1 41-year-old male with partial small bowel obstruction. Axial (**a**) and coronal reformatted CECT images (**b**) demonstrate dilated fluid-filled small bowel loops with air-fluid levels (*arrowheads*) compatible with small bowel obstruction, with transition point in the right mid abdomen (*curved arrow*)

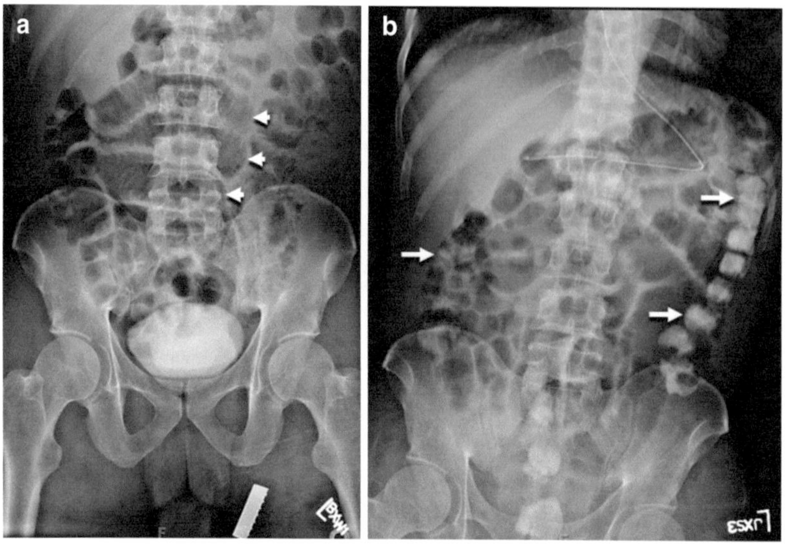

Fig. 6.2 41-year-old male with partial small bowel obstruction. The supine abdominal radiograph obtained on admission (**a**) shows dilated air containing small bowel loops with a stacked appearance (*arrowheads*) and normal caliber colon, compatible with small bowel obstruction. Air-fluid levels are not seen due to the supine positioning of the patient. The follow-up radiograph obtained after placement of a nasogastric tube (**b**) demonstrates persistent air-distended small bowel loops but oral contrast administered previously has reached the colon (*arrows*), indicating a partial small bowel obstruction

produce a "whirl sign," representing the twisted mesentery and vessels [21]. A closed-loop obstruction associated with ischemia is known as a strangulated obstruction, and this condition will be described in detail in the subsequent discussion on intestinal ischemia.

6.1.4.2 Large Bowel Obstruction

Radiographs may be the first imaging examination performed in patients with abdominal pain and LBO [9]. The colon is considered dilated when it is greater than 6 cm in diameter, with the exception of the cecum which can measure up to 9 cm in diameter in normal individuals. LBO is recognized radiographically as dilation of the colon proximal to a site of obstruction, with a paucity of gas distally [11]. Occasionally, air-fluid levels in the colon may be seen with LBO, which may indicate that the LBO is more acute as the intraluminal colonic fluid has not been present for sufficient time to allow absorption [3]. Dilation of the colon may be seen with several other conditions in addition to LBO, including colonic ileus, toxic megacolon, and colonic pseudo-obstruction. Distinguishing between LBO and colonic pseudo-obstruction may be difficult on the basis of radiography alone, and CT should be obtained in patients where the diagnosis is not clear [11].

CT is the imaging examination of choice in the evaluation of suspected or known LBO, with sensitivity and specificity of 96% and 93%, respectively [22]. The findings of LBO on CT are dilated large bowel proximal to a transition point, and collapsed colon distal to the obstruction [23]. CT should be performed with IV contrast if there are no contraindications, as it improves the ability to detect an obstructing colonic mass, as well as signs of inflammation and/or ischemia [11]. The use of oral contrast in the acute setting causes delays in obtaining the CT in patients who may need urgent treatment, distends the bowel which may simulate an obstruction, and can obscure the mucosa, making detection of associated ischemia more difficult [24]. While rectal contrast is not routinely administered and generally not necessary, retrograde rectal administration of water-soluble iodinated contrast can be useful in selected patients for distinguishing between LBO and colonic pseudo-obstruction

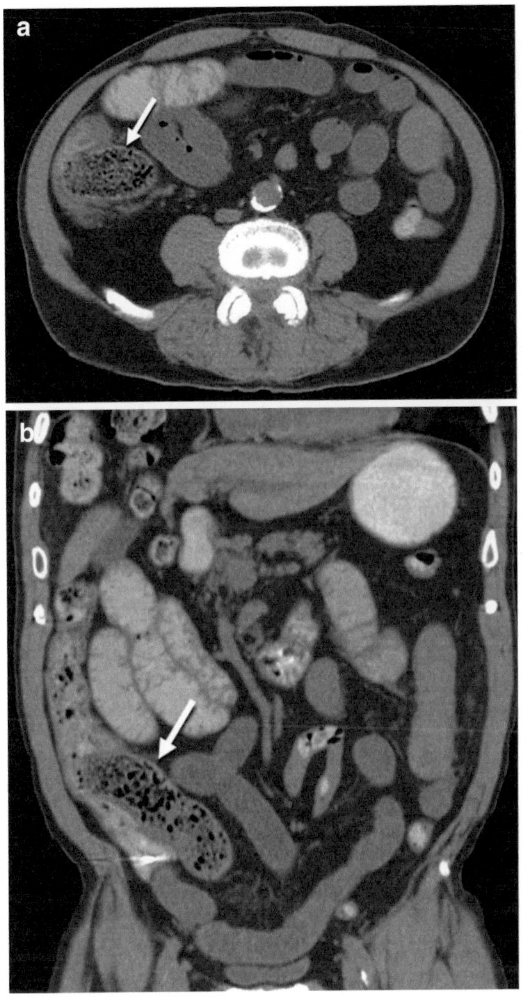

Fig. 6.3 82-year-old male with distal small bowel obstruction secondary to an impacted metallic foreign body. Axial (**a**) and coronal reformatted CECT images (**b**) demonstrate diffusely fluid-filled distended small bowel loops. There is transition at the level of the terminal ileum (*arrows*) where there is a large volume of fecalized intraluminal material

[25], and can also help to confirm or exclude colonic volvulus [3].

Obstructing colon carcinoma is the most common cause of LBO (>60%), and occurs most frequently in the sigmoid colon and at the splenic flexure [26]. CT findings include annular or eccentric short-segment wall thickening, or an enhancing soft-tissue mass which narrows the colonic lumen [27] (Fig. 6.8). Right-sided tumors with an incompetent ileocecal valve can mimic distal SBO, while left-sided tumors cause diffuse colonic distension with transition at the level of the obstruction to smaller caliber more distal colon [11]. Colon cancer may mimic acute diverticulitis if there is pericolonic spread and associated infiltration of the pericolonic fat, and optical colonoscopic follow-up may be indicated in selected patients with what appears to be acute diverticulitis on CT, to evaluate for an underlying mass [28].

Acute colonic volvulus is defined as twisting of the colon upon itself and accounts for approximately 10–15% of LBO [22]. Colonic volvulus, particularly sigmoid volvulus, is most commonly seen in the elderly, who are predisposed to this condition due to a mobile and redundant sigmoid colon. Cecal volvulus is more common in younger patients, particularly those with malrotation or chronic motility disorders. Volvulus of other portions of the colon is very rare [9]. Similar to closed-loop small bowel obstruction, volvulus predisposes to vascular compromise, which will eventually lead to ischemia, necrosis, and perforation. A variety of classic radiographic signs of colonic volvulus have been described, including the "coffee bean" sign and the "bird beak" sign, which represent apposition of the medial walls of a dilated loop of colon simulating a cleft in a coffee bean (Fig. 6.9), and a smooth tapering transition point at the site of obstruction, respectively [29]. CT is superior to radiography in demonstrating distended colon in an abnormal location (classically the right upper abdomen in sigmoid volvulus, and the left upper abdomen in cecal volvulus, although it is variable, especially in cecal volvulus). The "whirl" sign may also be evident—the spiraled appearance of engorged mesenteric vessels radiating from the twisted segment of colon at the site of obstruction [30] (Fig. 6.9). The primary treatment of colonic volvulus is endoscopic detorsion followed by elective resection, although patients with sepsis or peritonitis should be taken directly to the operating room without attempting endoscopic treatment [31].

Acute colonic pseudo-obstruction is an important mimic of LBO. ACPO is defined as acute dilatation of the colon due to interrupted autonomic innervation [32], and is character-

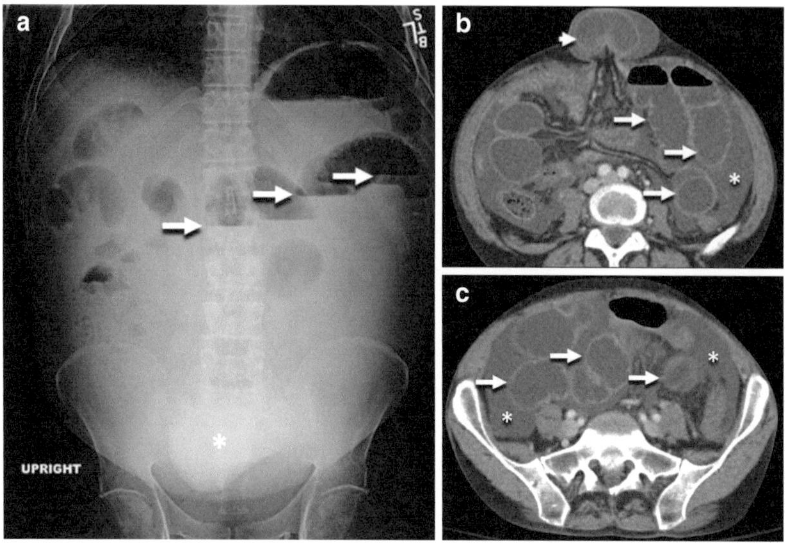

Fig. 6.4 47-year-old male with small bowel obstruction secondary to an incarcerated umbilical hernia. Upright abdominal radiograph (**a**) demonstrates dilated small bowel loops with differential air-fluid levels (*arrows*) compatible with small bowel obstruction. A rounded area of increased opacity is seen overlying the pelvis (*asterisk*), which corresponded to an obvious midline bulge on physical exam. Axial CECT (**b**, **c**) demonstrates a midline umbilical hernia containing dilated small bowel and fluid (arrowhead), and there are dilated small bowel loops with air-fluid levels proximally (*arrows*). Ascites (*asterisk*) was due to underlying cirrhosis, and there was no evidence of ischemia at the time of surgery

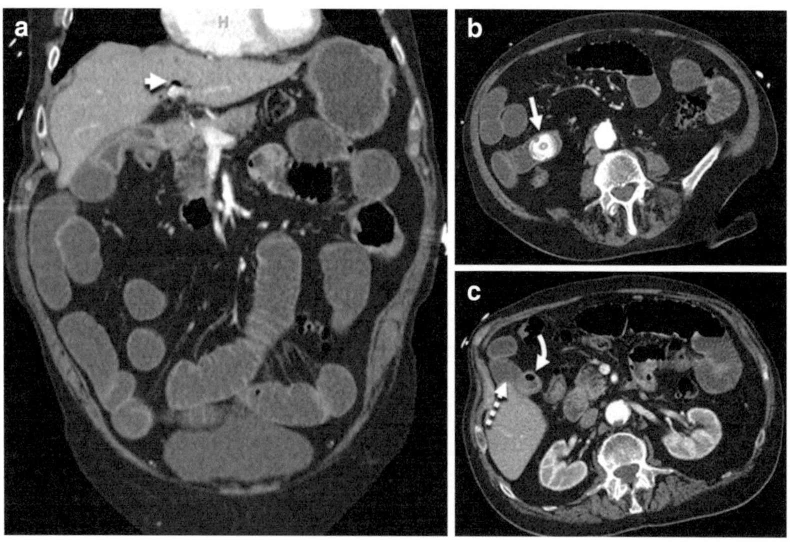

Fig. 6.5 78-year-old male with an impacted gallstone resulting in small bowel obstruction (gallstone ileus). Coronal reformatted image from a CECT (**a**) demonstrates dilated fluid-filled small bowel loops compatible with small bowel obstruction and small amount of pneumobilia (*arrowhead*). Axial CECT (**b**) demonstrates a large round high attenuation intraluminal mass within the distal small bowel (*arrow*) at the transition point of the small bowel obstruction, representing a large gallstone within the small bowel lumen. Axial CECT (**c**) demonstrates the presence of intraluminal gas within the gallbladder (*curved arrow*), which is inseparable from the adjacent small bowel (*dashed arrow*), consistent with cholecystoenteric fistula

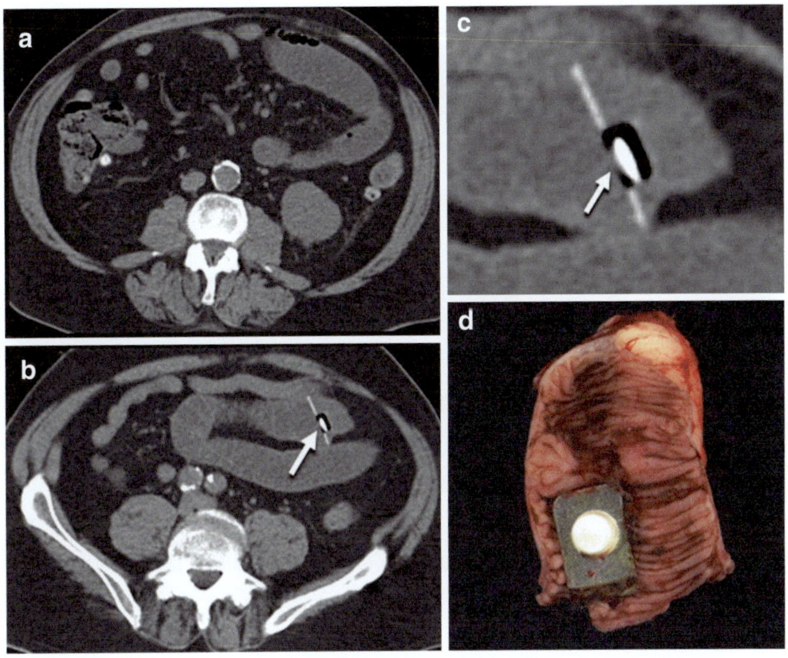

Fig. 6.6 70-year-old male with small bowel obstruction due to ingested foreign body. Axial NECT images (**a**, **b**) demonstrate dilated fluid-filled small bowel loops consistent with small bowel obstruction. The transition point is located at an intraluminal foreign body which contains linear high attenuation and rectangular gas containing components (*arrow*, **b**, **c**). At the time of small bowel resection, the foreign body was identified to be a pill which had not been removed from its outer packaging (**d**)

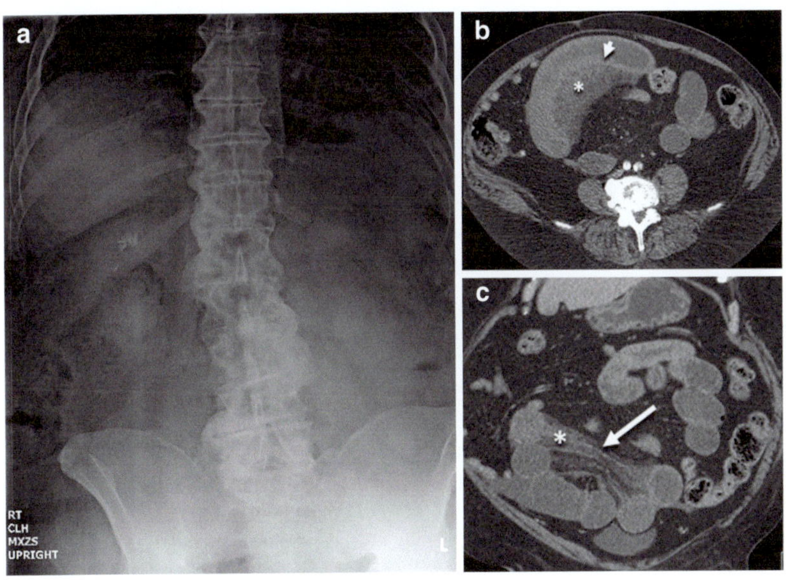

Fig. 6.7 65-year-old male with closed loop bowel obstruction and ischemia. Upright abdominal radiograph (**a**) demonstrates no dilated bowel loops or air-fluid levels and was interpreted as normal. Axial (**b**) and coronal reformatted images from CECT (**c**) show a dilated fluid-filled loop of small bowel in a "U"-shaped configuration with stretched and prominent mesenteric vessels converging in a radial fashion to the point of fixation (*arrow*). There is associated edema within the mesentery (*asterisk*) and high attenuation thickening of the obstructed strangulated small bowel (*arrowhead*) representing intramural hemorrhage. This case exemplifies the increased sensitivity of CT compared to radiography in diagnosing small bowel obstruction

Fig. 6.8 75-year-old male with large bowel obstruction due to colon cancer with perforation. Axial (**a**, **b**) and coronal reformatted images from CECT (**c**) demonstrate distension of proximal large bowel with pseudopneumatosis (*curved arrows*) secondary to a circumferential soft-tissue mass at the hepatic flexure (*arrows*). Scattered foci of extraluminal gas are present in the abdomen (*arrowheads*)

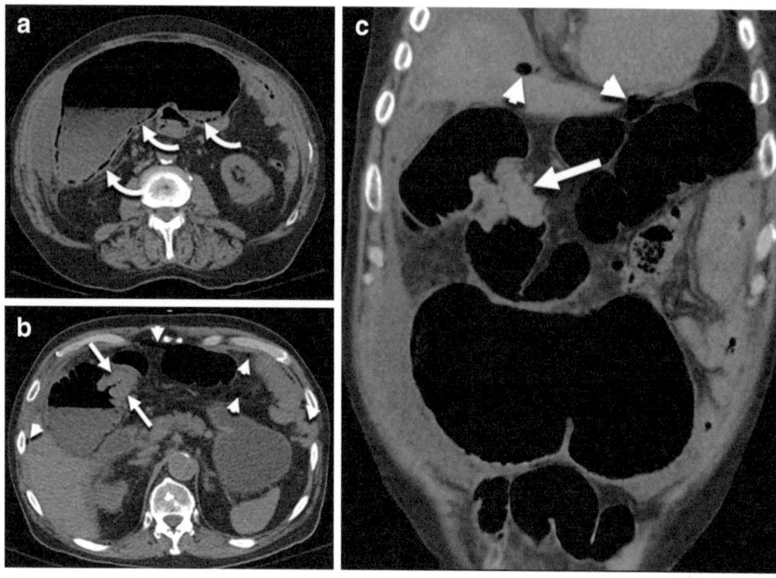

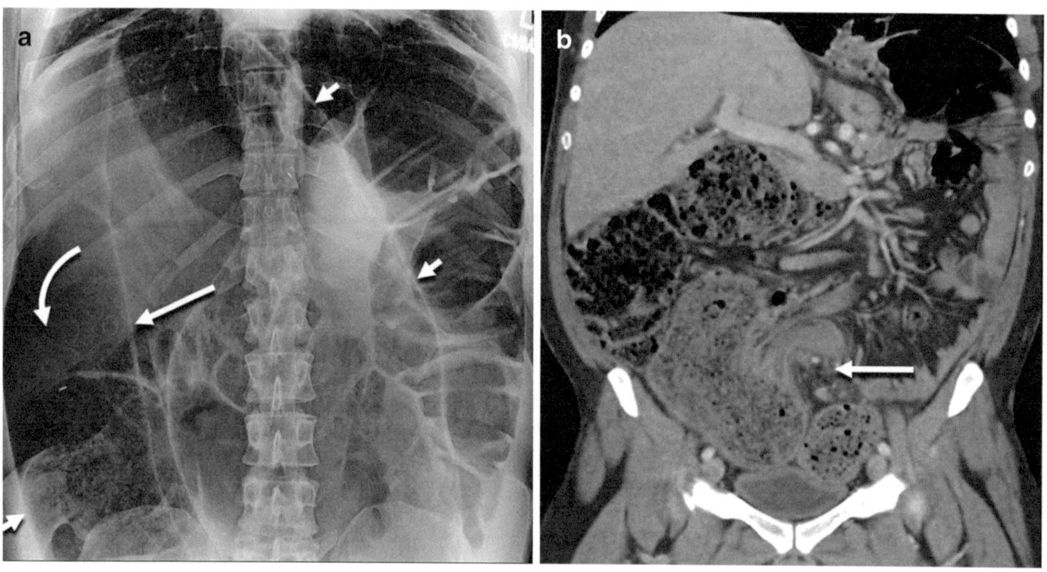

Fig. 6.9 68-year-old male with sigmoid volvulus. Supine abdominal radiograph (**a**) shows markedly dilated large bowel in the right upper quadrant with an inverted "U" configuration. The coffee bean sign is evident, with the medial walls of the dilated sigmoid colon volvulus forming the central cleft (*arrow*) and the lateral walls of the sigmoid colon representing the outer contour of the "bean" (*short arrows*). Gallstones are also visualized in the right hemiabdomen (*curved arrow*). Coronal reformatted image from CECT (**b**) demonstrates the "beak sign" and whirling of the mesentery at the site of volvulus (*arrow*)

ized by colonic dilatation with preserved haustration and normal wall thickness, usually with minimal intraluminal fluid content [33]. It can be challenging to distinguish ACPO from LBO on radiography. Positioning the patient in the right lateral decubitus and/or prone position to demonstrate air filling the distal colon may be successful in differentiating ACPO from LBO [34] (Fig. 6.10). In patients where the diagnosis remains uncertain, contrast enema or CT are use-

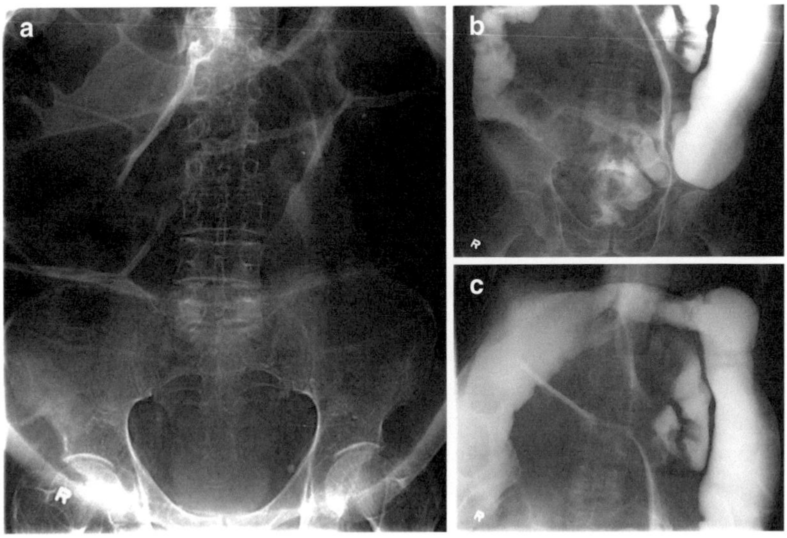

Fig. 6.10 81-year-old male with colonic pseudo-obstruction. Supine abdominal radiograph (**a**) demonstrates markedly dilated air-filled large bowel loops. The differential diagnosis for this appearance includes large bowel obstruction and colonic pseudo-obstruction. Subsequently, the patient underwent contrast enema (**b**, **c**), which shows retrograde opacification of the entire colon and refluxed contrast into the small bowel, without evidence of a transition point. The patient was managed with anticholinergic therapy

ful to exclude the presence of a transition point [35]. While the entire pathophysiology of ACPO remains unclear to our knowledge, the principal treatment is with parasympathomimetic drugs and/or endoscopic decompression [36, 37]. Distension of the colon in the setting of ACPO, particularly the cecum, puts these patients at risk for ischemia and perforation, with a reported incidence of 15%, and a mortality of approximately 50% [38].

6.2 Bowel Ischemia

6.2.1 Introduction

Bowel ischemia refers to hypoxic injury to small and/or large bowel and is estimated to represent approximately 1% of all patients presenting with an acute abdomen [39]. Acute mesenteric ischemia is generally reversible if recognized promptly, but if the diagnosis is delayed, ischemia may progress to infarction, which has a mortality of 60–90% [40, 41]. The widespread availability of CT and magnetic resonance imaging (MRI) and their ability to reveal the severity and extent of ischemic changes has firmly established the role of these imaging modalities in the evaluation of patients with suspected or known bowel ischemia. Recent advancements in imaging technology, including dual-energy CT (DECT), are also being utilized with increasing frequency in evaluating patients with bowel ischemia. Experience and proficiency with emerging imaging techniques will benefit radiologists, surgeons, and clinicians in the years to come.

6.2.2 Pathophysiology

The bowel receives approximately 20% of the total cardiac output under normal circumstances. Splanchnic autoregulation can nearly double perfusion to the bowel postprandially [42]. Conversely, in critical situations such as hypovolemic shock, intestinal perfusion may be reduced to only 10% of the cardiac output [43]. In addition to systemic autoregulation, vasoactive substances including vasopressin and angiotensin play an important role in regulating local intestinal perfusion [44]. The balance of systemic and local autoregulatory mechanisms can generally maintain viability of the bowel at systolic blood pressures greater than 70 mm Hg. Ischemia becomes likely when the systolic blood pressure drops below this level [45, 46].

Hypoxic ischemia of the bowel promotes the release of various substances into the splanchnic circulation, including cytokines and tumor necrosis factor, which potentiate breakdown of the mucosal barrier and damage to the bowel wall, thereby increasing the likelihood of bacterial translocation and sepsis [47]. The presence of intraluminal bacteria and toxins, as well as the production of free radicals during reperfusion of the ischemic segment of bowel, further contributes to the pathogenesis of intestinal ischemia and necrosis [48].

If ischemic damage to the intestinal wall is limited to the mucosa, it is generally reversible and the mucosa will eventually heal completely [49]. When ischemia involves the deeper submucosal and muscular layers, fibrosis and stricture formation may result as a consequence of local reparative changes [50]. Transmural ischemic involvement of all bowel wall layers is most severe, carries a high mortality rate, is frequently associated with perforation, and is a surgical emergency [51].

6.2.3 Epidemiology and Etiology

Acute bowel ischemia comprises two distinct pathologic entities—acute mesenteric ischemia and ischemic colitis. Acute mesenteric ischemia is less common than ischemic colitis, but is associated with greater morbidity and mortality [3]. The incidence of acute mesenteric ischemia has been estimated at 12.9 per 100,000 person-years and affects 2–3 people per 100,000 [52–55].

Acute arterial occlusion related to thrombosis or distal embolization comprises the majority of patients with acute mesenteric ischemia, approximately 60–70% [56]. It is noteworthy, however, that these estimates are based on surgical series and likely underestimate the incidence of nonocclusive mesenteric ischemia. Several conditions may result in occlusion of the mesenteric arterial system, including atrial fibrillation, atherosclerosis, arterial dissection, vasculitis, hypercoagulable states, and iatrogenic causes [57]. Generally, proximal occlusion of only one of the main visceral arteries (celiac, superior mesenteric artery, or inferior mesenteric artery) is compensated by collateral circulation, while distal arterial occlusions and lack of collateralized flow usually lead to the most severe ischemic damage to the bowel [41]. In contrast to acute mesenteric ischemia, ischemic colitis typically occurs with nonocclusive low-flow states and subsequent hypoperfusion to the bowel [58].

Venous occlusion causes 5–10% of acute mesenteric ischemia and is seen in the setting of a variety of causes of a hypercoagulable state, including infection, inflammatory conditions, or neoplasia [59]. Mesenteric venous thrombosis is highly associated with the development of hemorrhagic infarction from disrupted venous outflow and congestion of the bowel wall [4].

Acute nonocclusive mesenteric ischemia comprises the remaining 20–30% of patients and includes low-flow states, including hypovolemic shock, cardiac failure, arrhythmia, and administration or ingestion of various medications and illegal drugs [55, 56]. Ischemic injury may be reversible and localized to watershed areas, or it can be severe and diffuse. An important nonocclusive cause of mesenteric ischemia is mechanical bowel obstruction, either in the setting of strangulated obstruction or distention of bowel loops proximal to an obstruction such that the intraluminal pressure within the dilated loops of bowel results in impaired perfusion [4]. Strangulating obstruction is a form of mechanical bowel obstruction which is associated with bowel ischemia and represents approximately 10% of all patients with small bowel obstruction [60, 61].

6.2.4 Imaging

6.2.4.1 Computed Tomography Angiography Technique

Multidetector computed tomography angiography (CTA) is the most effective noninvasive imaging examination in the evaluation of patients with suspected acute bowel ischemia and has high sensitivity, excellent spatial resolution, widespread availability, rapid acquisition time, and the ability to perform multiplanar reconstructions (MPR), maximum intensity projections (MIP), and three-dimensional rendering post-processing [62]. CTA receives the highest rating from the American College of Radiology Appropriateness Criteria [63] for suspected bowel ischemia and has almost completely replaced conventional angiography for initial diagnosis given its speed, noninvasive nature, and ability to depict pathology associated with bowel ischemia or alternative diagnoses causing the patient's symptoms [64]. A meta-analysis in 2010 showed that CTA had 93.3% sensitivity and 95.9% specificity in the diagnosis of acute mesenteric ischemia [65]. It should be noted that while CTA is the preferred examination, in clinical practice most patients who present with nonspecific symptoms of abdominal pain will undergo standard single-phase portal venous CT of the abdomen and pelvis, rather than a dedicated mesenteric ischemia protocol CTA.

At our institution, the CTA protocol for evaluating suspected acute bowel ischemia includes a triphasic acquisition CT examination, with images obtained from the dome of the liver through the lesser trochanters prior to and following the intravenous administration of iodinated contrast in the arterial and portal venous phases. Nonenhanced computed tomography (NECT) is performed first to evaluate for high attenuation intramural hemorrhage in the bowel wall, a highly specific finding which may be seen with hypoperfusion-reperfusion to the bowel [3, 38]. NECT also has the advantage of depicting vascular calcifications, hyperdense or calcified thrombi, and can aid in the evaluation of bowel wall hypoenhancement by providing a direct comparison with the subsequently obtained IV contrast-enhanced images [66]. In situations where there is known or suspected gastrointestinal hemorrhage, NECT is useful for distinguishing between high attenuation intraluminal contents and extravasated intravenous contrast. While some argue that NECT should always be performed as part of the CTA protocol in suspected bowel ischemia [67], others believe that the inclusion of NECT adds little additional value while contributing additional radiation dose to the patient [68]. Dual-energy CT is an emerging technique with several advantages compared with conventional CTA in the evaluation of acute mesenteric ischemia, including the creation of virtual nonenhanced images and lower radiation dose to the patient. A detailed discussion of dual-energy CT is covered below.

After the rapid (3–5 cc/sec) intravenous administration of iodinated contrast, CT images are then performed through the abdomen and pelvis in the arterial phase and portal venous phase. Bolus tracking or test bolus techniques can be used to maximize opacification of the arterial system and are particularly beneficial in patients with decreased cardiac output where a longer delay after contrast bolus administration may be necessary to achieve peak arterial enhancement. The arterial phase acquisition permits identification of arterial stenosis, embolus, and occlusion. The portal venous phase allows assessment of patency of the mesenteric venous system, detection of bowel wall enhancement, and evaluation of the solid organs. The venous phase also enables detection of perforation, peritonitis, abscess formation, as well as alternative causes of the acute abdomen [41].

At our institution, oral contrast is not used in the evaluation of suspected bowel ischemia. Positive oral contrast adds no value and may even be detrimental, because, as noted above, it can mask potentially subtle high attenuation intramural hemorrhage, bowel wall hypoenhancement, or extravasated intraluminal contrast. To our knowledge, there is no literature supporting its use in the setting of suspected acute mesenteric ischemia. On the other hand, negative or neutral oral contrast may be useful because it permits better visualization of bowel wall enhancement and high attenuation intramural hemorrhage [69]. Despite these potential benefits, negative oral contrast is rarely used in patients at our institution as they are generally too ill, and drinking may increase the risk of aspiration in patients who are vomiting or have altered mental status. It should be noted that protocols remain varied among current radiology practices, and to our knowledge, no consensus has been reached at the time of this writing as to the optimal CT protocol for bowel ischemia.

6.2.4.2 Computed Tomography Angiography Interpretation

Interpretation of CTA in the setting of suspected bowel ischemia should include assessment of bowel wall thickness, attenuation and enhancement, the degree of bowel distension, the presence of mesenteric fat stranding and fluid, and patency/stenosis of the mesenteric arteries and veins. The normal bowel wall measures up to 3–4 mm thick, depending on the degree of luminal distention [70]. While thickening of the bowel wall is a nonspecific finding, it is the most frequently observed CT finding in mesenteric ischemia [4, 38]. However, bowel wall thickening may not always be present with mesenteric ischemia, particularly in severe ischemia, due to arterial occlusion. In that setting, the lack of arterial inflow produces neither mural edema nor hemorrhage, and the bowel wall is thin as a result of loss of tissue vascularity and intestinal muscular tone [41] (Fig. 6.11).

The attenuation of the bowel wall should be carefully observed on both NECT and IV contrast-enhanced CT images. Failure to do so may lead to misinterpretation of high attenuation in the bowel wall on IV contrast-enhanced images as normally enhancing bowel, when in fact the high attenuation is due to intramural hemorrhage (Fig. 6.12). A highly specific but insensitive CT finding of acute mesenteric ischemia is decreased or absent enhancement of the bowel wall [4, 38] (Fig. 6.11). A target/halo appearance or diffuse bowel wall hyperenhancement may be observed with hyperemia due to venous occlusion, reduced venous outflow, or hypoperfusion followed by reperfusion [71] (Figs. 6.13 and 6.14). Pneumatosis intestinalis represents air within the bowel wall, and while it can be seen with a variety of benign conditions, in the setting of suspected bowel ischemia, it is a highly specific finding of transmural infarction [72] (Figs. 6.11 and 6.14). Mesenteric venous and/or portal venous gas may also be observed with pneumatosis due to transmural infarction (Fig. 6.15). While the presence of portomesenteric gas has classically been associated with a poor prognosis [73], more recent studies have suggested that it is not an independent predictor of mortality [74].

Bowel ischemia results in disruption of normal peristalsis, which acutely can cause spastic reflex ileus reflected as diffusely collapsed bowel loops. Subacutely, mesenteric ischemia results in adynamic ileus, which is characterized radiologically as diffuse bowel luminal dilation [38]. When ischemic bowel is distended, it may be either gas- or fluid-filled, although the latter appearance is more commonly seen with venous ischemia and strangulated obstruction [75]. Transudation of fluid into the peritoneal space and mesenteric fat stranding on CT have high sensitivity (85–88%), but are less specific (61–72%) findings of bowel ischemia [41].

Arterial occlusive mesenteric ischemia is diagnosed when a filling defect is seen in the mesenteric arteries or branches, in combination with the other CT findings described above (Fig. 6.11) [70]. When an embolus or thrombus is located in the proximal superior mesenteric artery (SMA), the SMA may be dilated such that its diameter is greater than or similar in caliber compared to the adjacent superior mesenteric vein (SMV) [56]. Infarcts in other organs in the abdomen, such as the spleen and kidneys, may also be observed, classically seen as wedge-shaped peripheral areas of decreased enhancement.

Venous occlusive mesenteric ischemia is diagnosed when a filling defect and dilation of the mesenteric vein is observed on CECT [76] (Fig. 6.13). Unless the venous occlusion is very distal, the severity of ischemia is generally not as substantial as with arterial occlusive mesenteric ischemia. The impaired venous drainage results in elevated hydrostatic pressure and extravascular leakage of red blood cells and plasma into the bowel wall, mesentery, and peritoneal cavity, which is reflected as intramural hemorrhage, mesenteric stranding, and ascites on CT [3] (Figs. 6.12 and 6.13). Bowel loops are

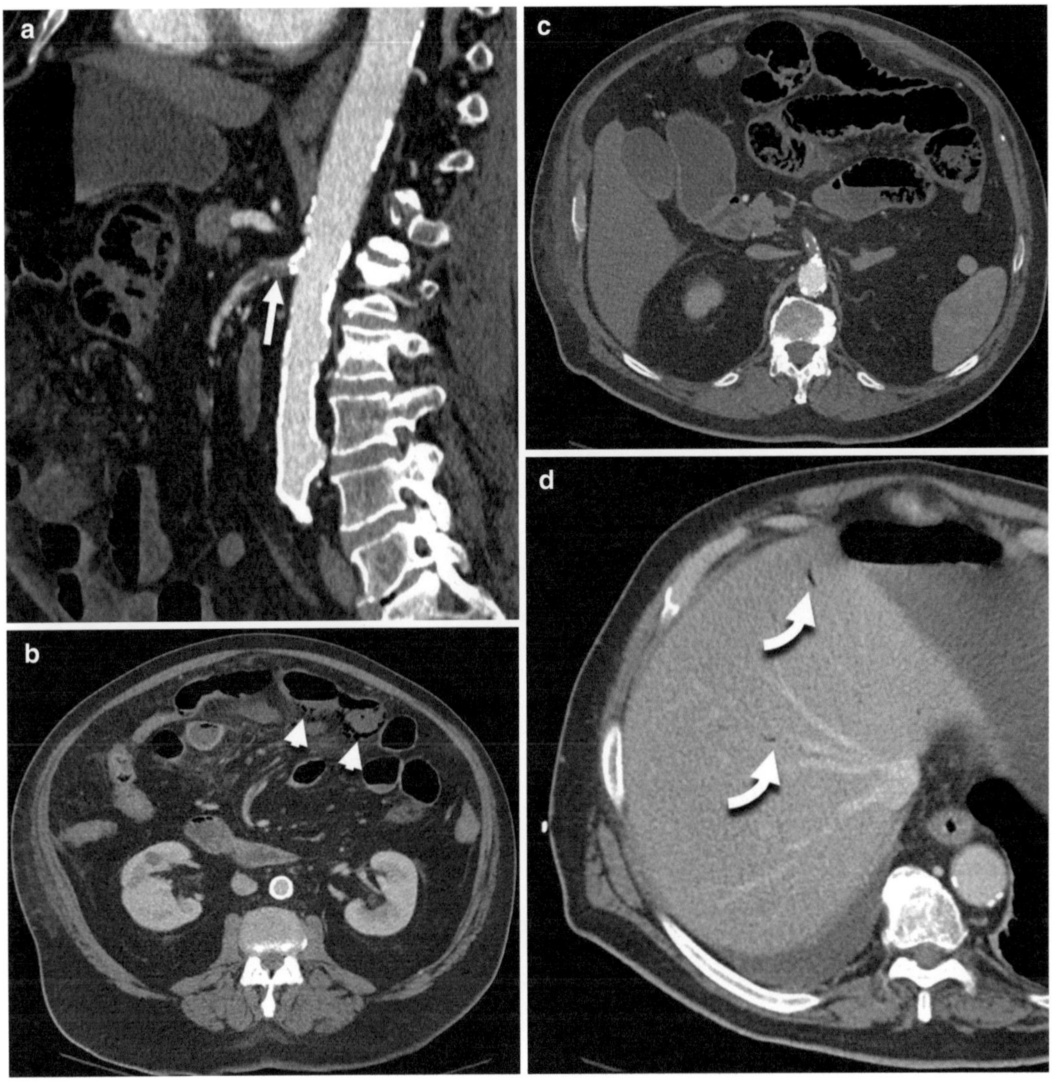

Fig. 6.11 74-year-old male with arterial occlusive mesenteric ischemia. Sagittal reformatted image from CECT (**a**) demonstrates occlusive thrombus at the origin of the SMA (*arrow*) with underlying atherosclerotic disease of the aorta and SMA. Axial CECT (**b–d**) demonstrates pneumatosis of small bowel loops in the left mid abdomen (*arrowheads*) and small volume portal venous gas (*curved arrows*). Note that the ischemic segments of small bowel wall are hypoenhancing and thin rather than thick-walled, due to the arterial occlusive nature of the ischemia in this case

typically dilated, fluid-filled, and thick-walled [4]. The bowel wall of affected segments may be hypoenhancing, nonenhancing, diffusely hyperenhancing, or show a halo/target pattern of enhancement [4, 38].

6.2.4.3 Dual-Energy Computed Tomography

In conventional CT, materials which have different elemental composition may be represented with the same CT attenuation value, which makes differentiation and classification of different tissue types challenging. Dual-energy CT (DECT) is a technique that utilizes CT imaging at two different photon energies, enabling the decomposition of a mixture of materials into its constituents, a principle which was initially described by Godfrey Hounsfield [77], and subsequently investigated by Alvarez and Macovski [78]. DECT can be accomplished in several different ways, includ-

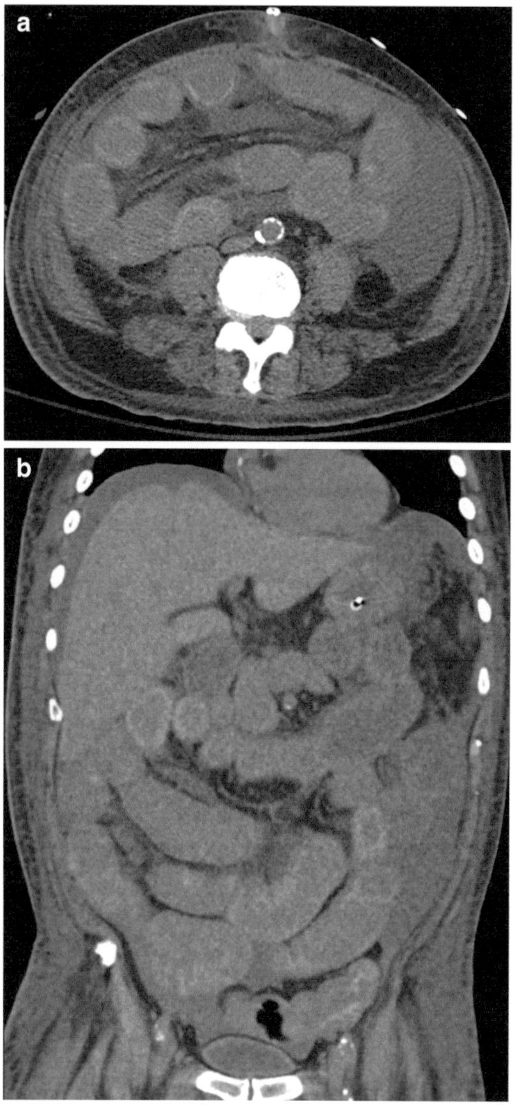

Fig. 6.12 67-year-old male with intramural hemorrhage secondary to mesenteric ischemia. Axial (**a**) and coronal reformatted NECT images (**b**) demonstrate dilated fluid-filled small bowel loops with extensive areas of high attenuation in the wall of the majority of the small bowel as well as mesenteric edema and ascites. No IV or oral contrast was administered. The findings are compatible with ischemic ileus with small bowel intramural hemorrhage due to ischemia. Skin staples and NGT are present in this patient who recently underwent subtotal colectomy for clostridium difficile colitis

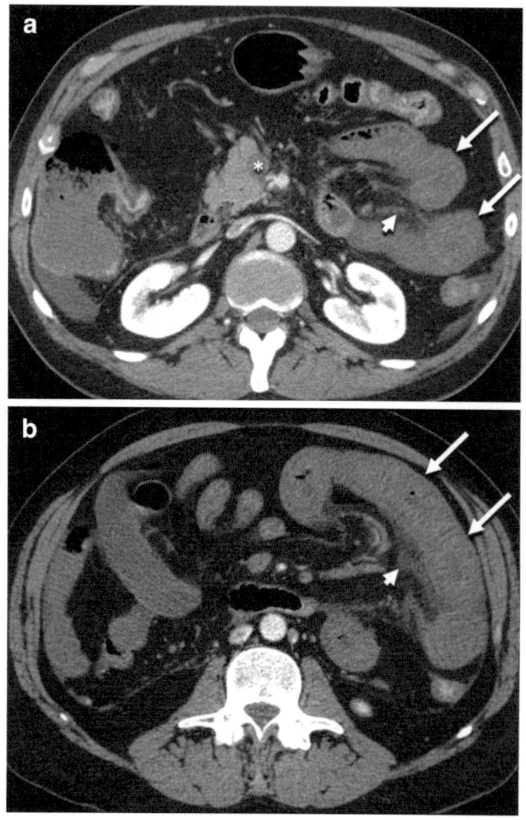

Fig. 6.13 55-year-old male with venous occlusive mesenteric ischemia. Axial CECT (**a**, **b**) demonstrates enlargement and occlusive filling defect in the SMV (*asterisk*) consistent with thrombosis. Small bowel loops in the left hemiabdomen are dilated and thick-walled with mucosal hyperenhancement (*arrows*) and mesenteric edema/stranding (*arrowheads*)

ing the use of rapid kVp switching, multilayer detectors, or dual X-ray sources [79, 80].

As described above, a key and highly specific CT finding of bowel ischemia is detecting decreased enhancement in the wall of ischemic bowel. While the specificity of bowel wall hypoenhancement in bowel ischemia is high, the sensitivity of CTA for this finding is poor [38]. Utilizing DECT, the degree of hypoenhancement between ischemic and normal bowel can be made more conspicuous by post-processing the images and creating iodine maps [79] (Fig. 6.16). A recent study by Poetretzke et al. utilized a swine model, and confirmed two important findings with respect to DECT of bowel ischemia [81]. First, the attenuation difference between perfused and ischemic segments of bowel at 51-keV was nearly double that of conventional 120-kVp images, and second, the creation of iodine material density maps enabled accurate quantification

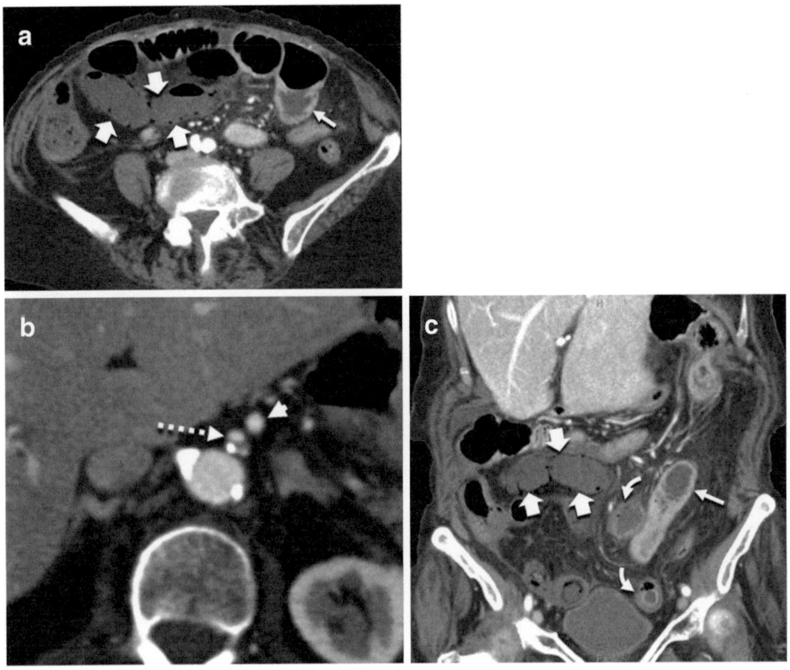

Fig. 6.14 79-year-old female with nonocclusive mesenteric ischemia. Axial (**a**, **b**) and coronal reformatted CECT images (**c**) demonstrate pneumatosis of distal small bowel loops which are thin-walled and hypoenhancing (*fat arrows*) relative to more proximal normal nonischemic small bowel in the left hemiabdomen (*arrows*). Loops of ileum in the pelvis which are less severely ischemic demonstrate mucosal hyperenhancement and wall thickening (*curved arrows*, **c**). There is atherosclerotic luminal narrowing at the SMA origin (*dashed arrow*, **b**). The normal celiac trunk (*arrowhead*, **b**) is seen adjacent to the SMA

of iodine content within the bowel wall, which significantly improved conspicuity of ischemic segments of bowel compared with conventional CT. An additional benefit of DECT is the ability to differentiate between hemorrhage and iodine in the bowel wall, the former being a highly specific sign of bowel ischemia [4, 82]. Lastly, DECT enables the creation of virtual nonenhanced images, obviating the need for a separate precontrast acquisition, thereby saving radiation dose to the patient, but still providing the benefits of NECT images [78]. A variety of other emerging applications of DECT in abdominal imaging continue to be explored, some of which are discussed elsewhere in this book, including the detection of bowel hyperemia in patients with inflammatory bowel disease, and identification of pancreatic adenocarcinoma and the hypovascular liver masses [83–85].

6.2.4.4 Magnetic Resonance Angiography

While CTA receives the highest ACR appropriateness rating in the evaluation of suspected acute mesenteric ischemia, IV contrast-enhanced magnetic resonance angiography (CE-MRA) of the abdomen is assigned a rating of 7, indicating that it is also “usually appropriate” [63]. Advances in MR technology have enabled fast single breath-hold acquisitions in the arterial and portal venous phases, which permit evaluation of the proximal celiac axis and SMA for stenosis or occlusion [86] (Fig. 6.17). Compared to CTA, CE-MRA is less sensitive for distal occlusion of celiac and SMA branches, and only permits evaluation of the inferior mesenteric artery in approximately half of patients [87]. Additionally, MR examination times are significantly longer than with CTA and are not safe for unstable patients.

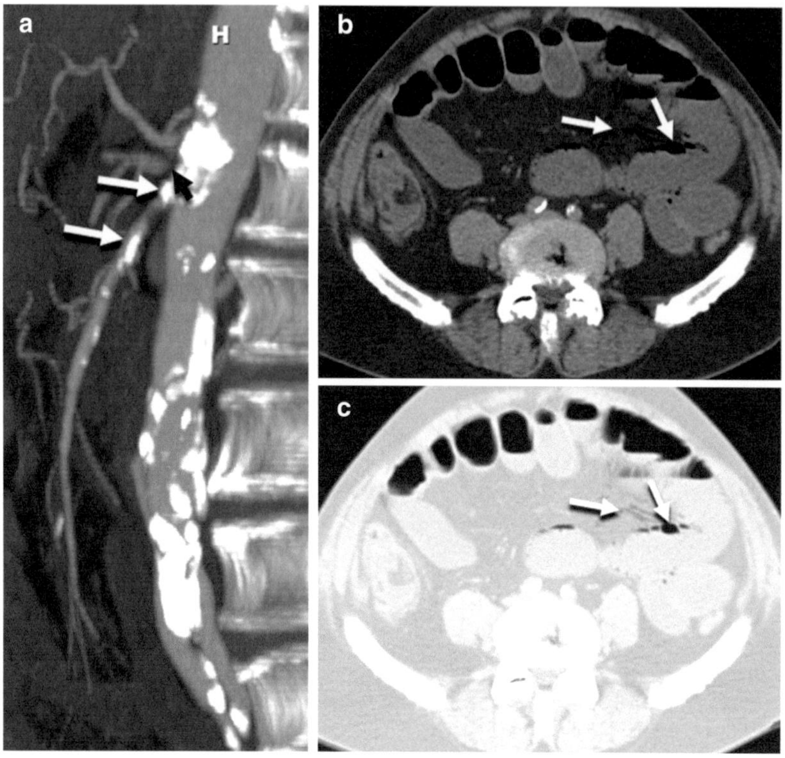

Fig. 6.15 67-year-old male with mesenteric ischemia. Sagittal volume rendered MIP image from CTA of the abdominal aorta and branches (**a**, obtained on an earlier exam before the patient developed acute symptoms) demonstrates dense atherosclerotic calcification of the aorta with severe stenosis at the celiac origin (*arrowhead*) and multifocal high-grade stensoses in the proximal SMA (*arrows*). There is variant anatomy with a separate origin of the left gastric artery arising directly from the aorta just cranial to the celiac trunk. The patient later presented with acute onset abdominal pain. Axial NECT images displayed at soft-tissue window (**b**) and lung window (**c**) demonstrate dilated loops of small bowel with pneumatosis and mesenteric venous gas (*arrows*). Note the absence of wall thickening in the affected segments of small bowel due to the arterial occlusive nature of the ischemia

Acutely ill patients may not be capable of breath-holding, which is necessary to obtain MR images without motion artifacts. A recent study evaluating the utility of CE-MRA in patients who had recently underwent conventional portal venous phase CT showed that there was a high degree of concordance between the two examinations for interpreting vascular findings, and that MRA added little value when obtained subsequent to portal venous CT in assessing bowel ischemia [88]. Therefore, while MRA is capable of revealing findings of mesenteric ischemia, its role at the present time is secondary to CTA, and its use is usually restricted to patients who cannot receive iodinated contrast.

MRA of the abdomen can also be obtained without the use of IV gadolinium-based contrast agents in patients with allergies, decreased renal function, or other contraindications to its use. Time-of-flight, phase contrast, and fresh-blood imaging MRA techniques can be used for vascular imaging, but are time consuming and sensitive to bowel and respiratory motion [86]. Quiescent-interval single-shot (QISS) MRA is a new technique that is less sensitive to patient motion, can be obtained in a single breath-hold, and does not require the use of subtraction [89] (Fig. 6.18).

6.2.4.5 Ischemic Colitis

Ischemic colitis is the most frequent form of intestinal ischemia (70%) [41]. Acute ischemic colitis is most commonly seen in the elderly, with a peak incidence in the seventh decade of life [90]. In contrast to acute mesenteric ischemia,

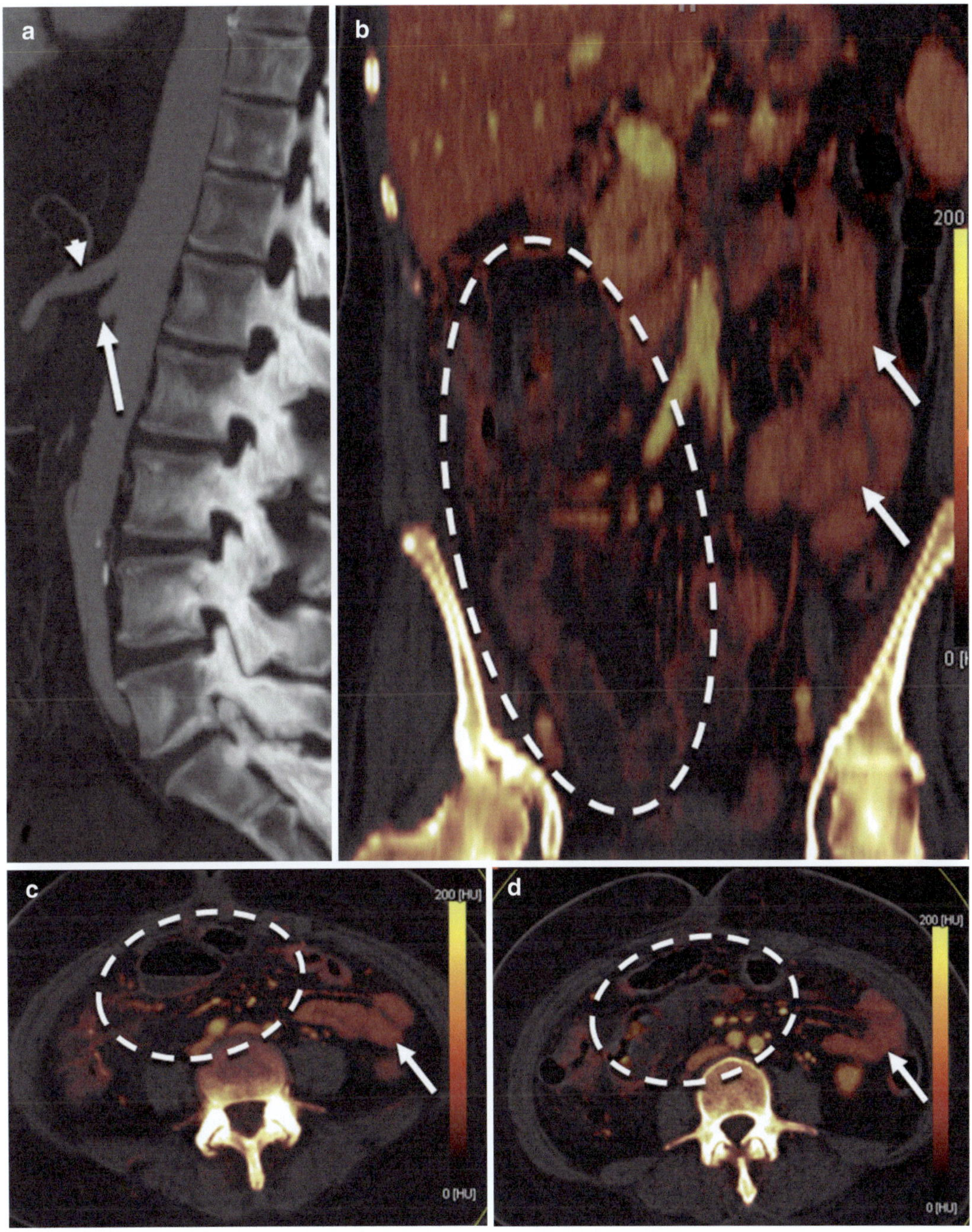

Fig. 6.16 46-year-old female with SMA occlusion and acute on chronic mesenteric ischemia on DECT. Sagittal MIP reformatted CECT image (**a**) from CTA demonstrates occlusion of the SMA just distal to the origin (*arrow*). The celiac is widely patent (*arrowhead*). Coronal (**b**) and axial iodine maps (**c**, **d**) from DECT exam demonstrates decreased iodine concentration within the wall of mid and distal small bowel and proximal colon in the right hemiabdomen (*dashed ovals*) relative to the normal proximal small bowel in the left hemiabdomen (*arrows*), compatible with mesenteric ischemia and ischemic colitis

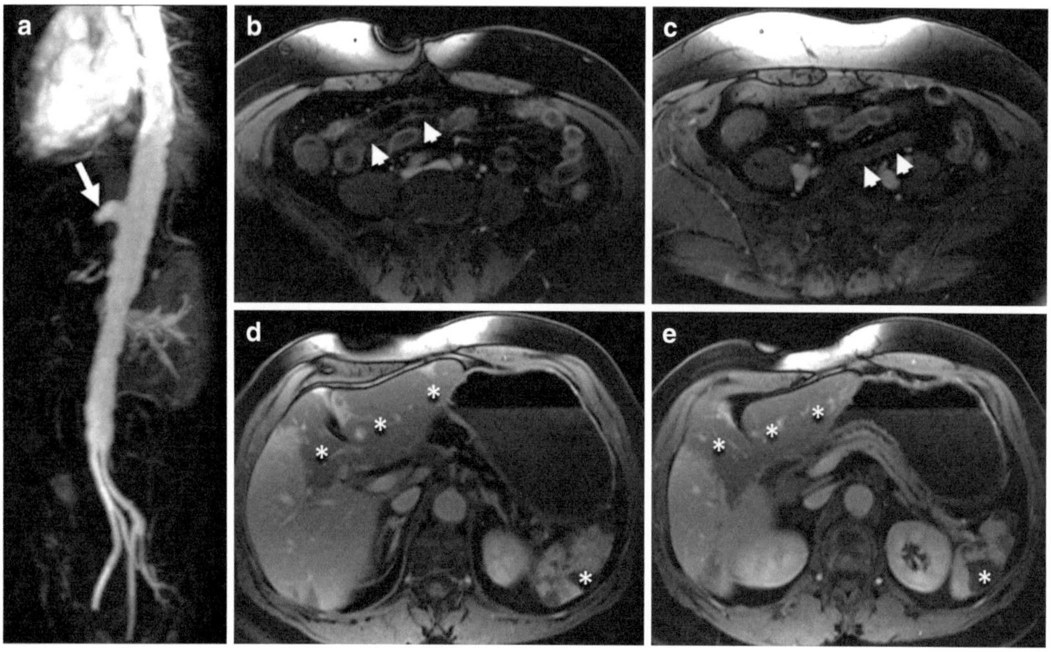

Fig. 6.17 71-year-old female with a history of SMA occlusion status post SMA and hepatic artery jump grafts with mesenteric ischemia on MRA. Sagittal MIP reformatted image from MRA (**a**) demonstrates occlusion of the supraceliac to SMA and hepatic artery graft just beyond its origin (*arrow*). The native celiac and SMA were chronically occluded. Axial fat suppressed T1 weighted post contrast images (**b–e**) demonstrate segments of small bowel which are thin-walled and hypoenhancing (*arrowheads*). Geographic areas of hypoenhancement are present in the liver and spleen (*asterisk*), compatible with infarcts

vascular occlusion is usually not the etiology of acute ischemic colitis [91]. Given the nonocclusive etiology in most patients, ischemic colitis has classically been described to affect the "watershed" regions of vascular supply to the colon, specifically the splenic flexure and rectosigmoid junction [92]. However, more recent studies have not shown there to be preferential involvement for these regions, and the location of ischemic colitis can be variable [54]. Ischemic colitis is usually segmental in distribution rather than diffuse [93]. Ischemic injury limited to the mucosa or submucosa results in mucosal edema, hemorrhage, ulcerations, and/or patchy areas of mucosal necrosis which is generally reversible. Necrosis involving the muscularis may lead to the development of a fibrotic stricture, while transmural necrosis is associated with perforation and sepsis [94].

While the diagnosis of ischemic colitis is confirmed on histopathology, patients are often first evaluated with CT [95]. The most frequently observed findings are colonic wall thickening, mesenteric fat stranding, and abnormal colonic wall enhancement, while the presence of pneumatosis, luminal dilatation, and free fluid are indicative of severe ischemia [90] (Figs. 6.19 and 6.20). Although commonly seen with ischemic colitis, colonic wall thickening is a nonspecific finding which can also be seen with nonischemic conditions including infection, inflammation, and angioedema, although the distribution of colonic wall thickening and presence of bloody diarrhea are strongly suggestive of the diagnosis, especially in an older patient in the appropriate clinical context. Colonic pneumatosis in the setting of ischemia is rare, but can be indicative of bowel necrosis, although other conditions including infectious, inflammatory, and benign causes can also produce pneumatosis [71]. Bowel wall hyperenhancement has been postulated to represent redistribution of blood during early reperfusion and recovery from ischemia [96].

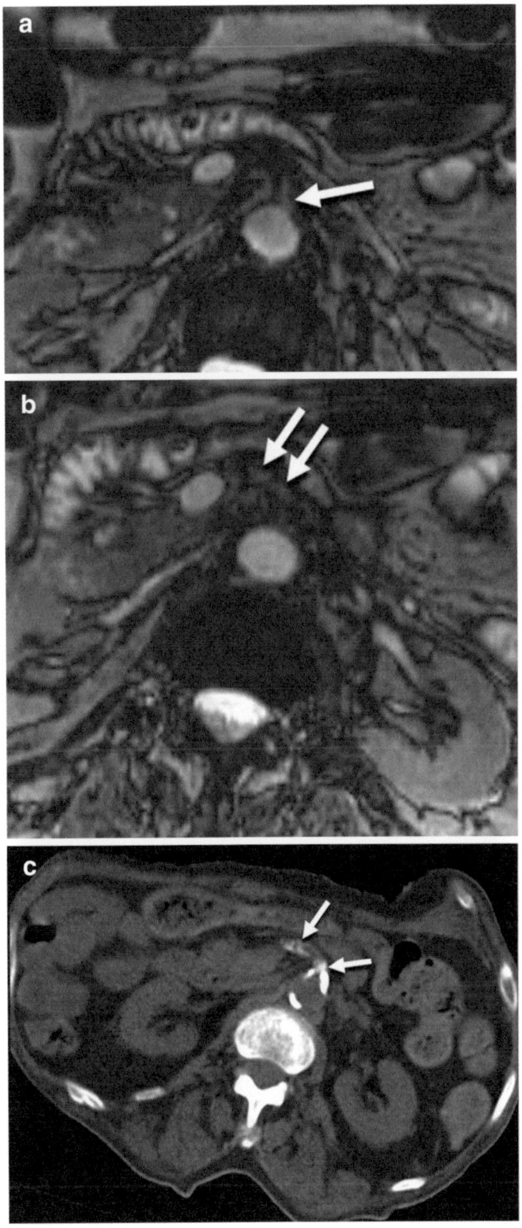

Fig. 6.18 91-year-old male with severe SMA stenosis on non-contrast MRA and NECT. Axial balanced steady-state free precession images (**a**, **b**) demonstrate severe stenosis of the SMA at the origin and proximal aspects (*arrows*). The corresponding axial NECT (**c**) demonstrates the large volume of calcified atherosclerotic plaque narrowing the lumen of the SMA

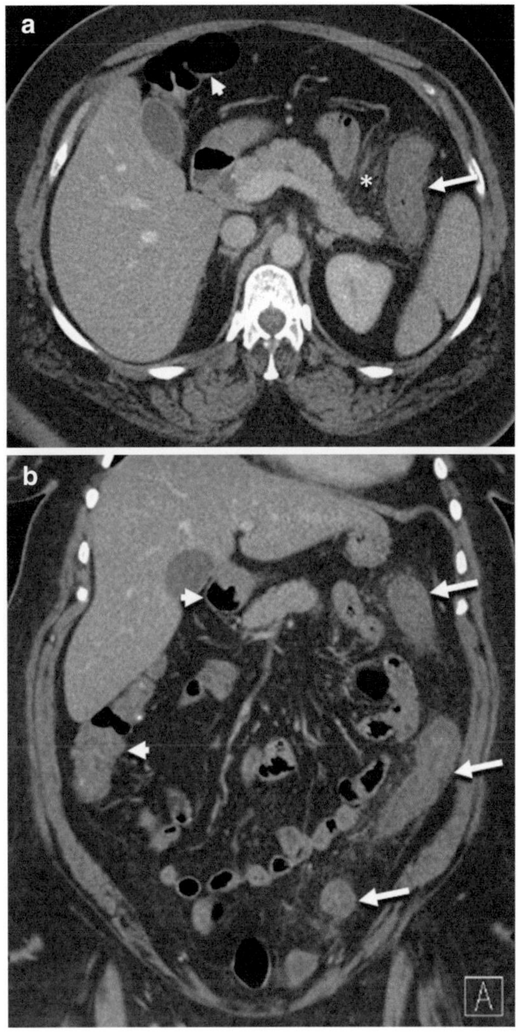

Fig. 6.19 56-year-old female with ischemic colitis. Axial (**a**) and coronal (**b**) reformatted CECT demonstrate circumferential wall thickening and mucosal hyperenhancement of the descending and sigmoid colon (*arrows*), with adjacent fat stranding (*asterisk*). Note the segmental nature of the colitis with sparing of the transverse and ascending colon (*arrowheads*)

6.2.4.6 Chronic Mesenteric Ischemia

Chronic mesenteric ischemia has a different pathophysiology and a more indolent presentation than acute mesenteric ischemia [97]. This condition was first described nearly a century ago by Goodman as “abdominal angina” [98]. The classic clinical history in chronic mesenteric ischemia is recurrent postprandial abdominal pain, weight loss, and “food fear” [99]. Most patients with chronic mesenteric ischemia have atherosclerosis of the mesenteric arteries, result-

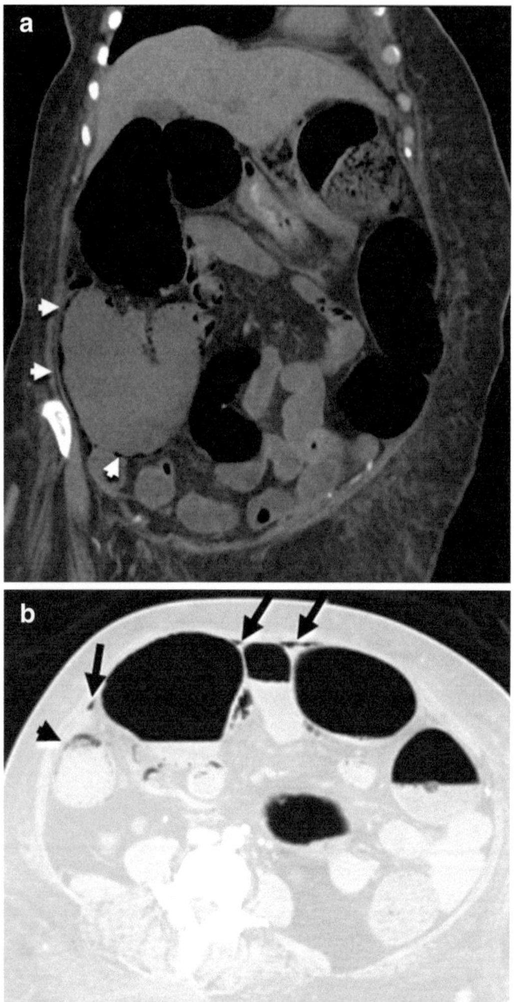

Fig. 6.20 75 woman with ischemic colitis and cecal perforation. Coronal reformatted CECT (**a**) demonstrates cecal distension and pneumatosis (*arrowheads*). Axial CECT displayed at lung windows (**b**) demonstrates small locules of free air adjacent to cecum (*arrows*) as well as cecal pneumatosis (*arrowhead*)

ing in slowly progressive luminal stenosis [100]. Less common causes of chronic mesenteric ischemia include vasculitis, thromboangiitis obliterans, and radiation-induced vasculopathy [101]. The majority of patients are older than 60 years of age, and this condition affects women more frequently than men [102]. The slow process of worsening atherosclerotic narrowing enables the development of collateral pathways of perfusion to the intestine; symptoms develop when collateralization is not adequate to maintain perfusion [103].

CT is useful in depicting calcified and noncalcified atherosclerotic plaque in the aorta and mesenteric arteries, as well as the extent of collateral pathways in patients with chronic mesenteric ischemia [38] (Fig. 6.21). The use of MIP and three-dimensional reformatting techniques are particularly well suited for evaluating collateral vessels. The most common collateral pathways between the celiac trunk and SMA include pancreaticoduodenal arteries running between the gastroduodenal artery and the proximal SMA, while the arch of Riolan and marginal artery of Drummond form the predominant collaterals between the SMA and inferior mesenteric artery [96].

Although the classic teaching is that at least two of the three main mesenteric arteries (celiac, superior mesenteric, and inferior mesenteric) must be diseased before symptoms develop, some patients with a single arterial stenosis have pain, and others with multivessel disease are asymptomatic [104]. Therefore, other more patient-specific factors are likely involved in the symptomatology of chronic mesenteric ischemia, including the location of stenoses, the pace of the development of the stenoses, and the ability to form collaterals [99].

The small bowel is usually normal appearing in patients with chronic mesenteric ischemia, although patients with chronic mesenteric ischemia are at risk for developing acute mesenteric ischemia. Therefore, careful observation for the findings of acute mesenteric ischemia in any patient presenting with abdominal pain is paramount. MRA is capable of demonstrating stenosis and occlusion in the celiac and SMA in patients with chronic mesenteric ischemia, but is less reliable in evaluation of the inferior mesenteric artery [86].

Catheter angiography demonstrates stenosis, and the pressure gradient across a stenosis can be measured to determine its hemodynamic significance [102]. In addition, endovascular treatment of mesenteric arterial stenoses with angioplasty and/or stent placement has been shown to have high technical and clinical success rates, with

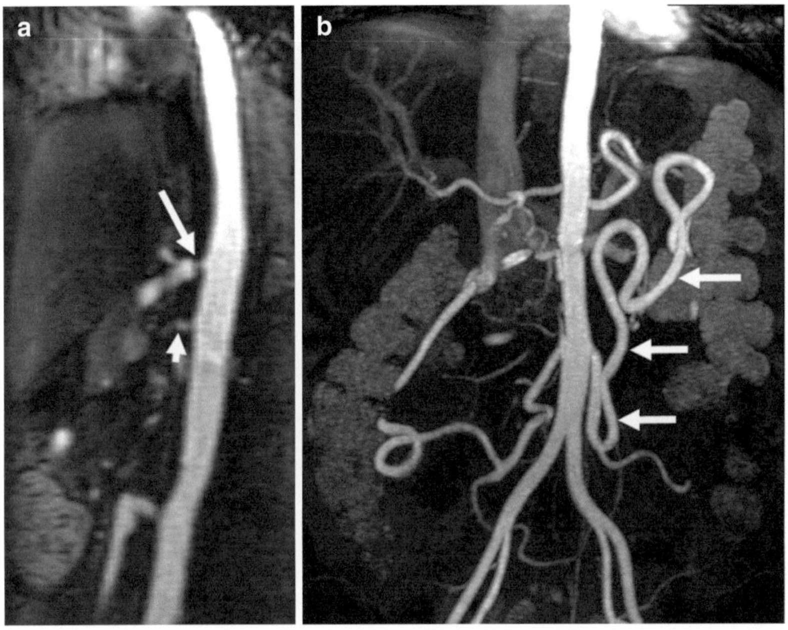

Fig. 6.21 Severe celiac and SMA stenosis with chronic mesenteric ischemia and compensatory hypertrophy of IMA and arc of Riolan. Sagittal MRA (**a**) demonstrates severe stenosis at the origin of the celiac (*arrow*) with post stenotic dilatation and minimal flow through the severely stenotic SMA (*arrowhead*). Coronal MIP MRA (**b**) demonstrates the hypertrophied IMA and prominent arc of Riolan (*arrows*) providing collateral flow to the SMA territory and an additional hypertrophied collateral supplying the ileocolic territory in the right lower quadrant

lower complication rates and 30-day mortality compared to open surgical repair [101]. It should be noted, however, that recurrent symptoms and reintervention rate are higher in patients previously treated endovascularly compared to those initially treated with open surgery [105]. Despite the likelihood of repeat intervention, endovascular treatment of chronic mesenteric ischemia is generally the first-line treatment in these patients due to the other comorbidities frequently seen in this patient population [98]. With respect to endovascular treatment, stenting of the mesenteric arteries, as opposed to angioplasty alone, is associated with a higher patency rate [106].

Conclusion

Bowel obstruction and ischemia are common potentially life-threatening conditions, especially if not recognized promptly. While MDCT is the current imaging standard, emerging techniques including DECT and MRA are being used with increased frequency. Imaging plays an important role in evaluating patients with suspected bowel obstruction or ischemia, and radiologists must carefully interpret these examinations to accurately identify the critical findings.

References

1. Irvin TT. Abdominal pain: a surgical audit of 1190 emergency admissions. Br J Surg. 1989;76(11):1121–5.
2. Peetz DJ Jr, Gamelli RL, Pilcher DB. Intestinal intubation in acute, mechanical small-bowel obstruction. Arch Surg. 1982;117(3):334–6.
3. Rubesin SE, Gore RM. Small bowel obstruction. In: Gore RM, Levine MS, editors. Textbook of gastrointestinal radiology, vol. 1. 3rd ed. Philadelphia, PA: Saunders Elsevier; 2008. p. 871–99.
4. Jeffrey RB. Small bowel obstruction. In: Federle MP, Jeffrey RB, Woodward PJ, Borhani AA, editors. Diagnostic imaging: abdomen. 2nd ed. Salt Lake City, Utah: Amirsys; 2010. p. 44–7.
5. Kulaylat MN, Doerr RJ. Small bowel obstruction. In: Holzheimer RG, Mannick JA, editors. Surgical treatment: evidence-based and problem-oriented. Munich: Zuckschwerdt; 2001.

6. Sagar PM, MacFie J, Sedman P, May J. Intestinal obstruction promotes gut translocation of bacteria. Dis Colon Rectum. 1995;38:640–4.
7. Rana SV, Bhardwaj SB. Small intestinal bacterial overgrowth. Scand J Gastroenterol. 2008;43(9):1030–7.
8. Wangensteen OH. Understanding the bowel obstruction problem. Am J Surg. 1978;135(2):131–49.
9. Welch J. Bowel obstruction: differential diagnosis and clinical management. Philadelphia, PA: Saunders; 1989. p. 59–95.
10. Kottler RE, Lee GK. The threatened caecum in acute large-bowel obstruction. Br J Radiol. 1984;57(683):989–90.
11. Jaffe T, Thompson WM. Large-bowel obstruction in the adult: classic radiographic and CT findings, etiology, and mimics. Radiology. 2015;275(3): 651–63.
12. Eisen GM, Baron TH, Dominitz JA, et al. Acute colonic pseudo-obstruction. Gastrointest Endosc. 2002;56(6):789–92.
13. Miller G, Boman J, Shrier I, Gordon PH. Etiology of small bowel obstruction. Am J Surg. 2000;180(1): 33–6.
14. Biondo S, Parés D, Frago R, et al. Large bowel obstruction: predictive factors for postoperative mortality. Dis Colon Rectum. 2004;47(11):1889–97.
15. Nicolaou S, Kai B, Ho S, Su J, Ahamed K. Imaging of acute small-bowel obstruction. AJR Am J Roentgenol. 2005;185(4):1036–44.
16. Lappas JC, Reyes BL, Maglinte DD. Abdominal radiography findings in small-bowel obstruction: relevance to triage for additional diagnostic imaging. AJR Am J Roentgenol. 2001;176(1):167–74.
17. Fukuya T, Hawes DR, Lu CC, Chang PJ, Barloon TJ. CT diagnosis of small-bowel obstruction: efficacy in 60 patients. AJR Am J Roentgenol. 1992;158(4):765–9.
18. Silva AC, Pimenta M, Guimarães LS. Small bowel obstruction: what to look for. Radiographics. 2009;29(2):423–39.
19. Canon CL. Gastrointestinal tract. In: Lee JKT, Sagel SS, Stanley RJ, Heiken JP, editors. Computed body tomography with MRI correlation. 4th ed. Philadelphia, PA: Lippincott Williams & Wilkins; 2006. p. 771–828.
20. Jacobs SL, Rozenblit A, Ricci Z, et al. Small bowel faeces sign in patients without small bowel obstruction. Clin Radiol. 2007;62(4):353–7.
21. Khurana B, Ledbetter S, McTavish J, Wiesner W, Ros PR. Bowel obstruction revealed by multidetector CT. AJR Am J Roentgenol. 2002;178(5):1139–44.
22. Taourel P, Kessler N, Lesnik A, Pujol J, Morcos L, Bruel JM. Helical CT of large bowel obstruction. Abdom Imaging. 2003;28(2):267–75.
23. Godfrey EM, Addley HC, Shaw AS. The use of computed tomography in the detection and characterization of large bowel obstruction. N Z Med J. 2009;122(1305):57–73.
24. Huynh LN, Coughlin BF, Wolfe J, Blank F, Lee SY, Smithline HA. Patient encounter time intervals in the evaluation of emergency department patients requiring abdominopelvic CT: oral contrast versus no contrast. Emerg Radiol. 2004;10(6):310–3.
25. Chapman AH, McNamara M, Porter G. The acute contrast enema in suspected large bowel obstruction: value and technique. Clin Radiol. 1992;46(4):273–8.
26. Garcia-Valdecasas JC, Llovera JM, deLacy AM, et al. Obstructing colorectal carcinomas: prospective study. Dis Colon Rectum. 1991;34(9):759–62.
27. Horton KM, Abrams RA, Fishman EK. Spiral CT of colon cancer: imaging features and role in management. Radiographics. 2000;20(2):419–30.
28. Chintapalli KN, Chopra S, Ghiatas AA, Esola CC, Fields SF, Dodd GD 3rd. Diverticulitis versus colon cancer: differentiation with helical CT findings. Radiology. 1999;210(2):429–35.
29. Burrell HC, Baker DM, Wardrop P, Evans AJ. Significant plain film findings in sigmoid volvulus. Clin Radiol. 1994;49(5):317–9.
30. Peterson CM, Anderson JS, Hara AK, Carenza JW, Menias CO. Volvulus of the gastrointestinal tract: appearances at multimodality imaging. Radiographics. 2009;29(5):1281–93.
31. Gingold D, Murrell Z. Management of colonic volvulus. Clin Colon Rectal Surg. 2012;25(4):236–44.
32. Ogilvie H. Large-intestine colic due to sympathetic deprivation; a new clinical syndrome. BMJ. 1948;2(4579):671–3.
33. Batke M, Cappell MS. Adynamic ileus and acute colonic pseudo-obstruction. Med Clin North Am. 2008;92(3):649–70, ix
34. Low VH. Colonic pseudo-obstruction: value of prone lateral view of the rectum. Abdom Imaging. 1995;20(6):531–3.
35. Choi JS, Lim JS, Kim H, et al. Colonic pseudoobstruction: CT findings. AJR Am J Roentgenol. 2008;190(6):1521–6.
36. Ponec RJ, Saunders MD, Kimmey MB. Neostigmine for the treatment of acute colonic pseudo-obstruction. N Engl J Med. 1999;341(3):137–41.
37. Jain A, Vargas HD. Advances and challenges in the management of acute colonic pseudo-obstruction (Ogilvie syndrome). Clin Colon Rectal Surg. 2012;25(1):37–45.
38. Rex DK. Colonoscopy and acute colonic pseudo-obstruction. Gastrointest Endosc Clin N Am. 1997;7(3):499–508.
39. Horton KM, Fishman EK. Multi-detector row CT of mesenteric ischemia: can it be done? Radiographics. 2001;21:1463–73.
40. Goldberg MA, Mueller PR, Saini S, et al. Importance of daily rounds by the radiologist after interventional procedures of the abdomen and chest. Radiology. 1991;180:767–70.
41. Scholz FJ. Ischemic bowel disease. Radiol Clin N Am. 1993;31:1197–218.
42. Wiesner W, Khurana B, Ji H, Ros PR. CT of acute bowel ischemia. Radiology. 2003;226(3):635–50.
43. Cannon WB. Bodily changes in pain, hunger fear, and rage: an account of recent researches into the function

of emotional excitement New York. NY: Appleton; 1920.
44. Reilly PM, Bulkley GB. Vasoactive mediators and splanchnic perfusion. Crit Care Med. 1993;21:55–68.
45. Matthews JG, Parks TG. Ischaemic colitis in the experimental animal. I. Comparison of the effects of acute and subacute vascular occlusion. Gut. 1976;17:671–6.
46. Matthews JG, Parks TG. Ischaemic colitis in the experimental animal. II. Role of hypovolaemia in the production of the disease. Gut. 1976;17:677–84.
47. Bibbo C, Petschenik AJ, Reddell MT, et al. Bacterial translocation after mesenteric ligation in dogs. J Investig Surg. 1996;9:293–303.
48. Weixiong H, Aneman A, Nilsson U, Lundgren O. Quantification of tissue damage in the feline small intestine during ischaemia-reperfusion: the importance of free radicals. Acta Physiol Scand. 1994;150:241–50.
49. Haglund U, Bergqvist D. Intestinal ischemia: the basics. Langenbeck's Arch Surg. 1999;384:233–8.
50. Whitehead R. The pathology of ischemia of the intestines. Pathol Annu. 1976;11:1–52.
51. Longo WE, Ballantyne GH, Gusberg RJ. Ischemic colitis: patterns and prognosis. Dis Colon Rectum. 1992;35:726–30.
52. Acosta S. Epidemiology of mesenteric vascular disease: clinical implications. Semin Vasc Surg. 2010; 23(1):4–8.
53. Ahmed R, Malas M. Mesenteric vascular insufficiency. In: Kasper DL, Fauci AS, Hauser SL, Longo DL, Jameson JL, Loscalzo J, editors. Harrison's principles of internal medicine. 19th ed. New York City, NY: McGraw-Hill Education; 2015.
54. Higgins PDR, Davis KJ, Laine L. Systematic review: the epidemiology of ischaemic colitis. Aliment Pharmacol Ther. 2004;19:729–38.
55. Longstreth GF, Yao JF. Epidemiology, clinical features, high-risk factors, and outcome of acute large bowel ischemia. Clin Gastroenterol Hepatol. 2009;7(10):1075–80.
56. Angelelli G, Scardapane A, Memeo M, Stabile Ianora AA, Rotondo A. Acute bowel ischemia: CT findings. Eur J Radiol. 2004;50:37–47.
57. Rha SE, Ha HK, Lee SH, et al. CT and MR imaging findings of bowel ischemia from various primary causes. Radiographics. 2000;20:29–42.
58. Wallace AB, Raptis CA, Mellnick VM. Imaging of bowel ischemia. Curr Radiol Rep. 2016;4(6):29.
59. Vicente DC, Kazmers A. Acute mesenteric ischemia. Curr Opin Cardiol. 1999;14:453–8.
60. Furukawa A, Yamasaki M, Furuichi K, et al. Helical CT in the diagnosis of small bowel obstruction. Radiographics. 2001;21:341–55.
61. Balthazar EJ, Birnbaum BA, Megibow AJ, Gordon RB, Whelan CA, Hulnick DH. Closed-loop and strangulating intestinal obstruction: CT signs. Radiology. 1992;185:769–75.
62. Moschetta M, Stabile Ianora AA, Pedote P, Scardapane A, Angelelli G. Prognostic value of multidetector computed tomography in bowel infarction. Radiol Med. 2009;114:780–91.
63. Oliva IB, Davarpanah AH, Rybicki FJ, et al. ACR Appropriateness Criteria® imaging of mesenteric ischemia. Abdom Imaging. 2013;38(4):714–9.
64. Kirkpatrick ID, Kroeker MA, Greenberg HM. Biphasic CT with mesenteric CT angiography in the evaluation of acute mesenteric ischemia: initial experience. Radiology. 2003;229(1):91–8.
65. Menke J. Diagnostic accuracy of multidetector CT in acute mesenteric ischemia: systematic review and meta-analysis. Radiology. 2010;256(1):93–101.
66. Gore RM, Yaghmai V, Thakrar KH, et al. Imaging in intestinal ischemic disorders. Radiol Clin N Am. 2008;46:845–75.
67. Furukawa A, Kanasaki S, Kono N, et al. CT diagnosis of acute mesenteric ischemia from various causes. AJR Am J Roentgenol. 2009;192(2):408–16.
68. Schieda N, Fasih N, Shabana W. Triphasic CT in the diagnosis of acute mesenteric ischaemia. Eur Radiol. 2013;23:1891–900.
69. Horton KM, Eng J, Fishman EK. Normal enhancement of the small bowel: evaluation with spiral CT. J Comput Assist Tomogr. 2000;24:67–71.
70. Wittenberg J, Harisinghani MG, Jhaveri K, Varghese J, Mueller PR. Algorithmic approach to CT diagnosis of the abnormal bowel wall. Radiographics. 2002;22(5):1093–107.
71. Horton KM, Fishman EK. Multidetector CT angiography in the diagnosis of mesenteric ischemia. Radiol Clin N Am. 2007;45:275–88.
72. Wiesner W, Mortelé KJ, Glickman JN, Ji H, Ros PR. Pneumatosis intestinalis and portomesenteric venous gas in intestinal ischemia: correlation of CT findings with severity of ischemia and clinical outcome. AJR. 2001;177:1319–23.
73. Liebman PR, Patten MT, Manny J, Benfield JR, Hechtman HB. Hepatic-portal venous gas in adults: etiology, pathophysiology and clinical significance. Ann Surg. 1978;187:281–7.
74. Faberman RS, Mayo-Smith WW. Outcome of 17 patients with portal venous gas detected by CT. AJR Am J Roentgenol. 1997;169:1535–8.
75. Chou CK. CT manifestations of bowel ischemia. AJR. 2002;178:87–91.
76. Bradbury MS, Kavanagh PV, Bechtold RE, et al. Mesenteric venous thrombosis: diagnosis and noninvasive imaging. Radiographics. 2002;22: 527–41.
77. Hounsfield GN. Computerized transverse axial scanning (tomography). I. Description of system. Br J Radiol. 1973;46(552):1016–22.
78. Alvarez RE, Macovski A. Energy-selective reconstructions in X-ray computerized tomography. Phys Med Biol. 1976;21(5):733–44.
79. Johnson TR. Dual-energy CT: general principles. Am J Roentgenol. 2012;199(5 Suppl):S3–8.
80. Otrakji A, Digumarthy SR, Gullo RL, Flores EJ, Shepard JO, Kalra MK. Dual-energy CT: spec-

trum of thoracic abnormalities. Radiographics. 2016;36(1):38–52.
81. Potretzke TA, Brace CL, Lubner MG, Sampson LA, Willey BJ, Lee FT Jr. Early small-bowel ischemia: dual-energy CT improves conspicuity compared with conventional CT in a swine model. Radiology. 2015;275(1):119–26.
82. Johnson TR, Krauss B, Sedlmair M, et al. Material differentiation by dual energy CT: initial experience. Eur Radiol. 2007;17(6):1510–7.
83. Graser A, Johnson TRC, Chandarana H, Macari M. Dual energy CT: preliminary observations and potential clinical applications in the abdomen. Eur Radiol. 2009;19(1):13–23.
84. Macari M, Spieler B, Kim D, et al. Dual-source dual-energy MDCT of pancreatic adenocarcinoma: initial observations with data generated at 80 kVp and at simulated weighted-average 120 kVp. AJR Am J Roentgenol. 2010;194(1):W27–32.
85. Robinson E, Babb J, Chandarana H, Macari M. Dual source dual energy MDCT: comparison of 80 kVp and weighted average 120 kVp data for conspicuity of hypo-vascular liver metastases. Investig Radiol. 2010;45(7):413–8.
86. Laissy JP, Trillaud H, Douek P. MR angiography: noninvasive vascular imaging of the abdomen. Abdom Imaging. 2002;27(5):488–506.
87. Carlos RC, Stanley JC, Stafford-Johnson D, Prince MR. Interobserver variability in the evaluation of chronic mesenteric ischemia with gadolinium-enhanced MR angiography. Acad Radiol. 2001;8(9):879–87.
88. Shetty AS, Mellnick VM, Raptis C, Loch R, Owen J, Bhalla S. Limited utility of MRA for acute bowel ischemia after portal venous phase CT. Abdom Imaging. 2015;40(8):3020–8.
89. Edelman RR, Sheehan JJ, Dunkle E, et al. Quiescent-interval single-shot unenhanced magnetic resonance angiography of peripheral vascular disease: technical considerations and clinical feasibility. Magn Reson Med. 2010;63(4):951–8.
90. Balthazar EJ, Yen BC, Gordon RB. Ischemic colitis: CT evaluation of 54 cases. Radiology. 1999;211(2):381–8.
91. Cruz C, Abujudeh HH, Nazarian RM, Thrall JH. Ischemic colitis: spectrum of CT findings, sites of involvement and severity. Emerg Radiol. 2015;22(4):357–65.
92. Rogers AI, David S. Intestinal blood flow and diseases of vascular impairment. In: Haubrich WS, Schaffner F, Berk JE, editors. Gastroenterology. 5th ed. Philadelphia, PA: Saunders; 1995. p. 1212–34.
93. Feuerstadt P, Brandt LJ. Colon ischemia: recent insights and advances. Curr Gastroenterol Rep. 2010;12(5):383–90.
94. Brandt LJ, Boley SJ. Colonic ischemia. Surg Clin North Am. 1992;72:203–29.
95. Romano S, Lassandro F, Scaglione M, Romano L, Rotondo A, Grassi R. Ischemia and infarction of the small bowel and colon: spectrum of imaging findings. Abdom Imaging. 2006;31:277–92.
96. Brandt LJ, Feuerstadt P, Blaszka MC. Anatomic patterns, patient characteristics, and clinical outcomes in ischemic colitis: a study of 313 cases supported by histology. Am J Gastroenterol. 2010;105(10):2245–52.
97. Hohenwalter EJ. Chronic mesenteric ischemia: diagnosis and treatment. Semin Interv Radiol. 2009;26(4):345–51.
98. Goodman GH. Angina abdominis. Am J Med Sci. 1918;155:524–8.
99. Ujiki M, Kibbe MR. Mesenteric ischemia. Perspect Vasc Surg Endovasc Ther. 2005;17:309–18.
100. Sreenarasimhaiah J. Chronic mesenteric ischemia. Best Pract Res Clin Gastroenterol. 2005; 19(2):283–95.
101. Cognet F, Ben Salem D, Dranssart M, et al. Chronic mesenteric ischemia: imaging and percutaneous treatment. Radiographics. 2002;22(4):863–79.
102. Kougias P, El Sayed HF, Zhou W, Lin PH. Management of chronic mesenteric ischemia. The role of endovascular therapy. J Endovasc Ther. 2007;14:395–405.
103. Cleveland TJ, Nawaz S, Gaines PA. Mesenteric arterial ischaemia: diagnosis and therapeutic options. Vasc Med. 2002;7:311–21.
104. Roobottom CA, Dubbins PA. Significant disease of the celiac and superior mesenteric arteries in asymptomatic patients: predictive value of Doppler sonography. AJR Am J Roentgenol. 1993;161:985–8.
105. Atkins MD, Kwolek CJ, LaMuraglia GM, et al. Surgical revascularization versus endovascular therapy for chronic mesenteric ischemia: a comparative experience. J Vasc Surg. 2007;45:1162–71.
106. Landis MS, Rajan DK, Simons ME, et al. Percutaneous management of chronic mesenteric ischemia: outcomes after intervention. J Vasc Interv Radiol. 2005;16:1319–25.

7 MR Imaging of Acute Appendicitis

Victoria Chernyak

Abstract

Magnetic resonance imaging (MRI) is highly accurate for the diagnosis of acute appendicitis. Lack of ionizing radiation and high contrast resolution makes MRI an attractive alternative to ultrasound and CT in pediatric and pregnant patients. This chapter discusses the literature supporting use of MRI in diagnosis of acute appendicitis, proper MRI technique essential for maximizing diagnostic accuracy, the MRI findings of acute appendicitis, and potential cases of false-positive and false-negative results.

Keywords

Acute appendicitis · Magnetic resonance imaging · Pediatric population · Appendicitis in pregnancy

7.1 Background

Acute appendicitis is a common clinical condition with a lifetime cumulative incidence rate estimated as high as 9% [1]. Imaging plays an important role in the diagnosis of acute appendicitis and its associated potential complications. Computed tomography (CT), the most commonly utilized examination for assessment of suspected appendicitis, while accurate and easily obtainable, has the drawback of ionizing radiation. Ultrasound offers a radiation-free alternative, but is heavily operator dependent and has limited performance in larger and pregnant patients. In the past decade, magnetic resonance imaging (MRI) emerged as an attractive option for pediatric and pregnant patients suspected to have acute appendicitis, due to absence of ionizing radiation and high diagnostic performance. For example, in the clinical setting of right lower quadrant pain, fever, and leukocytosis, the Appropriateness Criteria expert panel of the American College of Radiology assigned MRI a rating of 7 (usually appropriate) for pregnant women, and a rating of 5 (may be appropriate) for children and young adults [2].

High diagnostic performance of MRI has been demonstrated in various patient populations. Meta-analyses performed in the general population reported MRI to have a pooled sensitivity of 96–97% and a pooled specificity of 96% for the diagnosis of acute appendicitis [3, 4]. In patients younger than 30 years old, nonenhanced MRI has a sensitivity of 97% and a specificity of 99% for the diagnosis of acute appendicitis [5]. In the pediatric population, MRI has a sensitivity of 96–97%, a specificity of 96–97%, a positive predictive value of 92–93%, and a negative predictive value of 98–99% for the diagnosis of acute appendicitis [4, 6–8]. In pregnant patients, MRI has an accuracy of 88–99%, a sensitivity

V. Chernyak, M.D., M.S.
Department of Radiology, Montefiore Medical Center, Bronx, NY, USA

M. Patlas et al. (eds.), *MDCT and MR Imaging of Acute Abdomen*,
https://doi.org/10.1007/978-3-319-70778-5_7

of 60–100%, a specificity of 92–99%, a positive predictive value of 50–92%, and a negative predictive value of 94–100% for the diagnosis of acute appendicitis [4, 9–12].

Another advantage of MRI, particularly compared with ultrasound, is that it can offer an alternate diagnosis for a patient's symptoms up to 50% or more of the time [5]. MRI reveals an alternate diagnosis in 12–43% of pregnant patients, and in approximately 20% of pediatric patients [6, 8–10, 13, 14]. The proportion of noncontrast MRI examinations with identifiable alternative diagnoses is similar to that of CT [15]. In children with equivocal ultrasound, MRI is equally as effective as CT for diagnosis of acute appendicitis [15, 16]. Furthermore, the diagnostic performance of nonenhanced MRI is comparable to that of CT for the detection of appendiceal perforation, with a sensitivity of 57–90% and a specificity of 86% [15, 17].

An interpreting radiologist's proficiency in abdominal MRI is associated with a more accurate and reproducible interpretation of various abdominal and pelvic examinations [18–21]. In this respect, MRI for acute appendicitis is no different, and the diagnostic accuracy improves with the level of the radiologist's expertise. For example, inexperienced MR interpreters have sufficient sensitivity of 89% for MRI in suspected appendicitis, but the accuracy of MR-expert radiologists is higher, at 97% [22].

The use of MRI in suspected appendicitis has a positive effect on patient outcomes. Inclusion of MRI in the decision-making process decreases the rate of negative laparotomies without a significant change in the rate of perforation, and allows earlier planning for patients with an equivocal clinical picture [23, 24]. Pregnant patients who undergo MRI rather than ultrasound are 65% more likely to be discharged from the emergency department (ED) and have approximately 50% reduction in the length of stay in the ED [25].

7.2 MR Protocol

Anatomic coverage of the acquired MR sequences should include pelvis and upper abdomen, together with the gallbladder and kidneys, to ensure imaging of the appendix and areas which may provide an alternate cause for patient's signs and symptoms. Furthermore, in the second and third trimesters, the cecum and appendix are often displaced by the uterus, and therefore coverage of the upper abdomen can improve the rates of appendix detection. Multiple imaging planes are essential, because of numerous variations in the position and length of the appendix [26]. Depending on its orientation, orthogonal imaging planes are often complementary in displaying the appendix (Fig. 7.1).

The protocols of MRI for acute appendicitis vary among various institutions and practices, with the choice of included sequences being influenced by the available equipment and radiologist's preferences. The common goal, however, is to keep the examination as short as possible while maintaining sufficiently high image quality. Patients with suspected acute appendicitis may have reduced ability to comply with required breath holding and may not be able to lie motionless on the MR scanner table for prolonged periods of time. Therefore, acquisition times of the individual sequences should be kept to a minimum.

MRI protocol for evaluation of acute appendicitis typically includes T2-weighted sequences and T1-weighted sequences with and without IV gadolinium (Table 7.1) [27–30]. Post-gadolinium images are omitted in pregnant patients. T2-weighted sequences are fluid-sensitive and therefore are able to demonstrate a fluid-filled inflamed appendix, periappendiceal inflammation, and fluid collections. Single-shot fast spin echo (SSFSE) acquisitions are the central component of most protocols since it allows for very fast motion-resistant acquisition of T2-weighted images [6]. Motion resistance of SSFSE is so substantial that inability to breath-hold is not a contraindication for MRI to evaluate acute appendicitis [31]. An alternative acquisition of fluid-sensitive images is balanced steady-state free precession sequences (SSFP), which have mixed T1 and T2 properties that allows excellent visualization of bowel-wall morphology and are resistant to motion degradation [30, 32]. Fat saturation can be applied to both SSFSE and balanced SSFP sequences to improve fluid depiction.

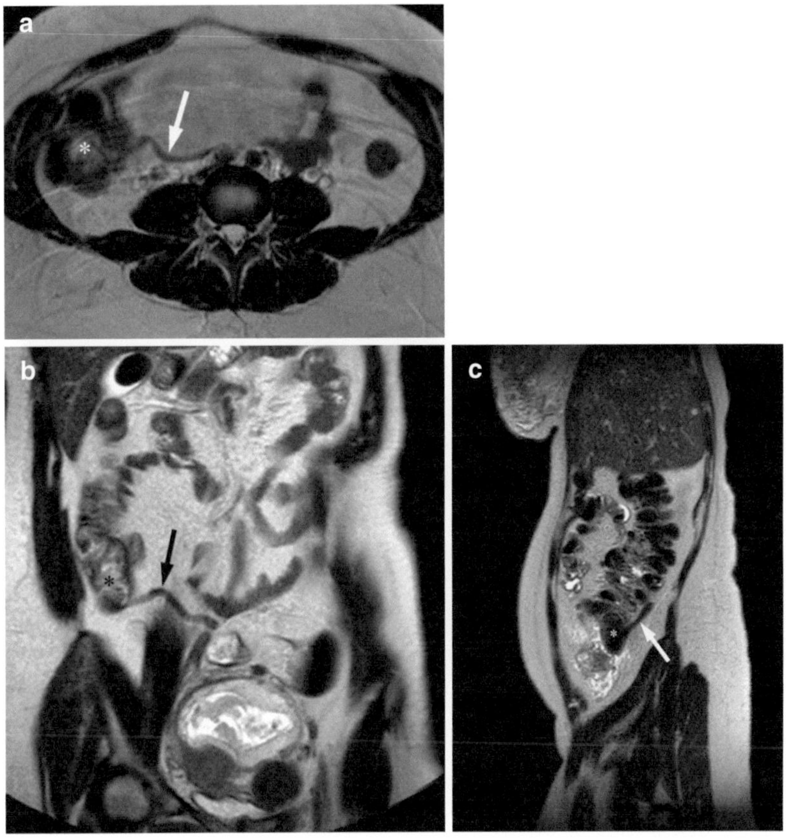

Fig. 7.1 Normal appendix on T2-weighted images. Axial (**a**), coronal (**b**), and sagittal (**c**) single-shot fast spin echo sequences in three different patients, all with a normal appendix. Normal appendix appears as a blind-ending hypointense structure with the diameter <7 mm (*arrows*) in continuity with the cecum (*). Note the plane of imaging on which the appendix is best seen varies among the patients and is dependent on the appendiceal location and course

Table 7.1 Sample MRI protocol for evaluation of acute appendicitis

Sequence	FOV (cm)	TR (ms)	TE (ms)	Matrix	Slice thickness/ gap (mm)	Flip angle
2D SSFSE						
Axial	25–30	312–648.3	80	128 × 128	4/0.4	90
Coronal[a]	30–34	368.5–815.7	80	128 × 128	4/0.4	90
Sagittal	34	364.8–678.6	80	128 × 128	4/0.4	90
Balanced SSFP axial	27–30	3.3–3.7	1.7–1.9	128 × 128	4/0.4	90
3D T1-weighted with fat saturation[b]						
Axial	25–28	2.1–3.1	Minimum	128 × 128–144 × 144	3.5–4/1.75–2	15
Coronal	30–34	2.3–3.6	Minimum	128 × 128–144 × 144	4/2	10–15

FOV field of view, *TR* time to repeat, *TE* time to echo, *SSFSE* single-shot fast spin echo, *SSFP* steady-state free precession

[a]Acquired with and without frequency-selective fast saturation

[b]Acquired as modified Dixon technique; postcontrast imaging is acquired in nonpregnant patients

Fat saturation results in a low signal arising from the intraperitoneal fat, which improves delineation of periappendiceal edema and/or abscess formation (Fig. 7.2).

3-D T1-weighted sequences typically are acquired with high spatial resolution. Precontrast T1-weighted fat-suppressed images help characterize tissues with intrinsic high signal on T1-weighted images (e.g., subacute blood or fluid with high protein content), which can be particularly helpful in identifying other causes of acute abdominal and pelvic pain. The addition

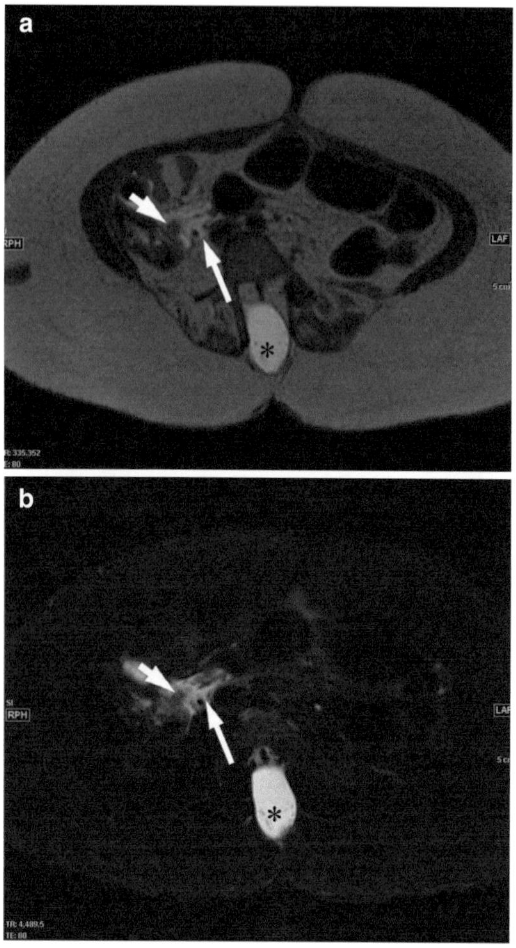

Fig. 7.2 Periappendiceal fluid assessment with and without fat saturation in a 31-year-old woman with acute appendicitis. Axial single-shot fast spin echo (SSFSE) images without fat saturation (**a**) and with fat saturation (**b**) demonstrate free fluid (*long arrow*) in the right lower quadrant, adjacent to a thickened appendix (*short arrow*). Note how suppression of the signal from fat allows easier depiction of the fluid. Note an incidental finding of posterior spinal defect with a meningocele (*)

of intravenous (IV) gadolinium, whenever possible, is helpful for identifying subtle mucosal enhancement of an inflamed appendix and for detecting complications of appendicitis, including mucosal discontinuity and periappendiceal abscesses [30, 32]. Multiple studies have demonstrated the utility of IV gadolinium in pediatric patients with suspected acute appendicitis. For instance, equivocal results were shown to be four times more common without the use of IV contrast [33]. However, the use of IV contrast is associated with increased cost and increased examination time. If "live" review of the acquired precontrast images is feasible, selective administration of IV contrast for patients where the diagnosis is inconclusive on precontrast images can reduce the number of unequivocal results, and has resulted in 80% reduction of contrast use in the literature [33].

It should be noted that IV gadolinium contrast is currently contraindicated in pregnancy, and therefore postcontrast images are not obtained in pregnant patients. However, as discussed earlier, noncontrast MRI in pregnant patients is both sensitive and accurate for the diagnosis of acute appendicitis. Furthermore, one retrospective study demonstrated that the accuracy of MR examinations which included both T2-weighted images and IV contrast-enhanced images was not significantly different than that for either the IV contrast-enhanced or the T2-weighted sequences alone, indicating that T2-weighted imaging alone may be adequate for assessment of acute appendicitis in the ED [27]. Interestingly, balanced steady-state free precession sequences were somewhat less accurate compared with postcontrast sequences, whereas the accuracy of T2-weighted sequences was equal to that of the postcontrast sequences [27].

Some studies have advocated the inclusion of diffusion-weighted images (DWI) in the MR protocol for assessment of acute appendicitis. DWI takes advantage of restricted diffusion of the water molecules that occurs in tissues with high cellularity (e.g., inflammation and malignancy). In addition, DWI is acquired using echoplanar techniques with fat suppression and relatively long time-to-echo (TE) [31]. Therefore, acute appendicitis will have high signal intensity on DWI because of the combination of restricted diffusion and edema that has high signal intensity with prolonged TE [31]. The addition of DWI may improve diagnostic performance of nonenhanced MRI for diagnosis of acute appendicitis [34, 35]. Furthermore, DWI, as a part of rapid noncontrast

MRI, can help to reveal drainable fluid collections in post-appendectomy patients [36]. If DWI is included in the protocol, at least two b values should be acquired: 0 s/mm^2 and ≥500 s/mm^2.

7.3 Findings

The normal appendix is seen on MRI in approximately 56–75% of pediatric patients [8, 15, 37]. In pregnant patients, the normal appendix is seen on MRI in approximately 69–80%, compared to only approximately 7% on ultrasound in some studies [10, 13]. Women in whom the appendix is not visualized on MRI are more likely to be beyond the first trimester [13]. This is thought to be at least in part secondary to the appendix and cecum being displaced from its usual location by the enlarging uterus. Even when the appendix is not directly visualized, appendicitis can be excluded with a high degree of accuracy if no secondary MR signs of appendicitis (e.g., more than physiologic free fluid, right lower quadrant inflammation, thickening of the terminal ileum, or abscess) are present [9, 38].

On MRI, a normal appendix has a mean diameter of 5–6 mm, no adjacent inflammatory changes, no contrast enhancement, and no related surrounding free fluid [37, 39]. On T2-weighted images, a normal appendix appears as a blind-ending hypointense structure arising from the base of the cecum (Fig. 7.1) [39]. Hyperintense signal may be seen on T1-weighted images in 51% of patients with normal appendices, and only in 4.5% of patients with acute appendicitis [40]. The presence of T1-hyperintense signal in the appendix has a positive predictive value of 98% for a normal appendix [40].

Table 7.2 summarizes the findings of acute appendicitis on MRI. Similar to other imaging modalities, the diagnosis of acute appendicitis on MRI rests on the identification of a dilated hyperemic appendix with adjacent inflammation, and possible abscess formation. Fluid within the appendiceal lumen and edema/fluid in the periappendiceal fat appear as high signal intensity on fluid-sensitive T2-weighted sequences. Appendicolith(s) may be present, which appears as rounded or ovoid structure(s) with low signal intensity on T2-weighted images (Fig. 7.3). Following administration of IV contrast, mucosal hyperemia will manifest as marked enhancement of the appendiceal wall (Fig. 7.4). On DWI with b value ≥500 s/mm^2, up to 99% of inflamed appendices appear hyperintense, and apparent diffusion coefficient (ADC) values are lower in acute appendicitis compared with in normal appendices [35, 41]. Appendiceal diameter >7 mm, periappendiceal fat infiltration, and restricted diffusion of the appendiceal wall are independent predictors of acute appendicitis [42]. If any one of these features is present on MRI, the probability of acute appendicitis is 88% [42]. The probability of acute appendicitis increases to 94% if any two MRI features are present, and to 96% if all three features are present [42]. Absence of all three features virtually excludes acute appendicitis, with a probability of only 2% [42].

Table 7.2 Key MRI features of acute appendicitis

	MRI Findings
Acute appendicitis	• Appendiceal dilatation >7 mm • Appendicolith • High signal intensity within the appendiceal lumen on fluid-sensitive sequences • Thickening of the appendiceal wall >2 mm • Enhancement of the appendiceal wall on postcontrast T1-weighted sequences • Restricted diffusion of the appendiceal wall • Increased signal intensity on fluid-sensitive sequences in the periappendiceal fat
Perforation	• Defect in appendiceal wall • Restricted diffusion within periappendiceal fluid • Extraluminal air (signal void, particularly on gradient echo sequences) • Periappendiceal abscess • Peritoneal enhancement

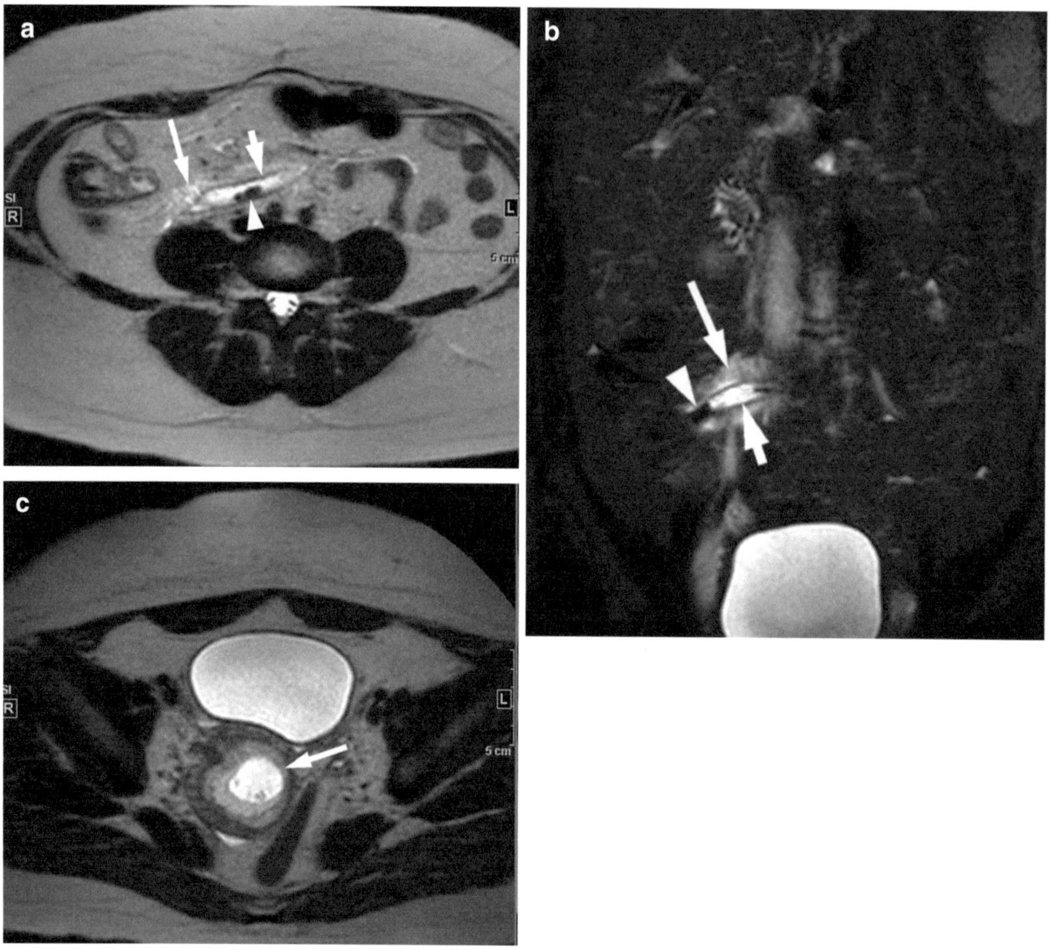

Fig. 7.3 Acute appendicitis in a 27-year-old pregnant woman. Axial single-shot fast spin echo (SSFSE) (**a**) and coronal SSFSE with fat saturation (**b**) images demonstrate a dilated fluid-filled appendix (*short arrow*) with multiple appendicoliths (*arrowheads*) and adjacent fluid (*long arrow*). A gestational sac (*arrow*) is seen in the uterus more inferiorly (**c**)

The patients with perforated appendicitis have larger appendiceal diameters compared with patients without perforation (mean diameters 12 vs. 8 mm, respectively) [41]. Other MRI signs which are associated with perforation are appendiceal restricted diffusion, wall defect, appendicolith, periappendiceal fluid, remote free fluid, restricted diffusion within periappendiceal fluid, abscess formation, peritoneal enhancement, ileocecal wall thickening, and ileus (Figs. 7.5 and 7.6) [41]. The presence of four or more of any of these findings has a sensitivity of 82% and a specificity of 85% for perforation [41]. ADC values in the perforated acute appendicitis tend to be lower than those of nonperforated appendicitis, although the exact ADC values are heavily dependent on the individual MR scanner [43].

7.4 Potential Pitfalls

Overall, MRI for acute appendicitis has very low false-negative rates [9]. False-negative results for acute appendicitis are usually a con-

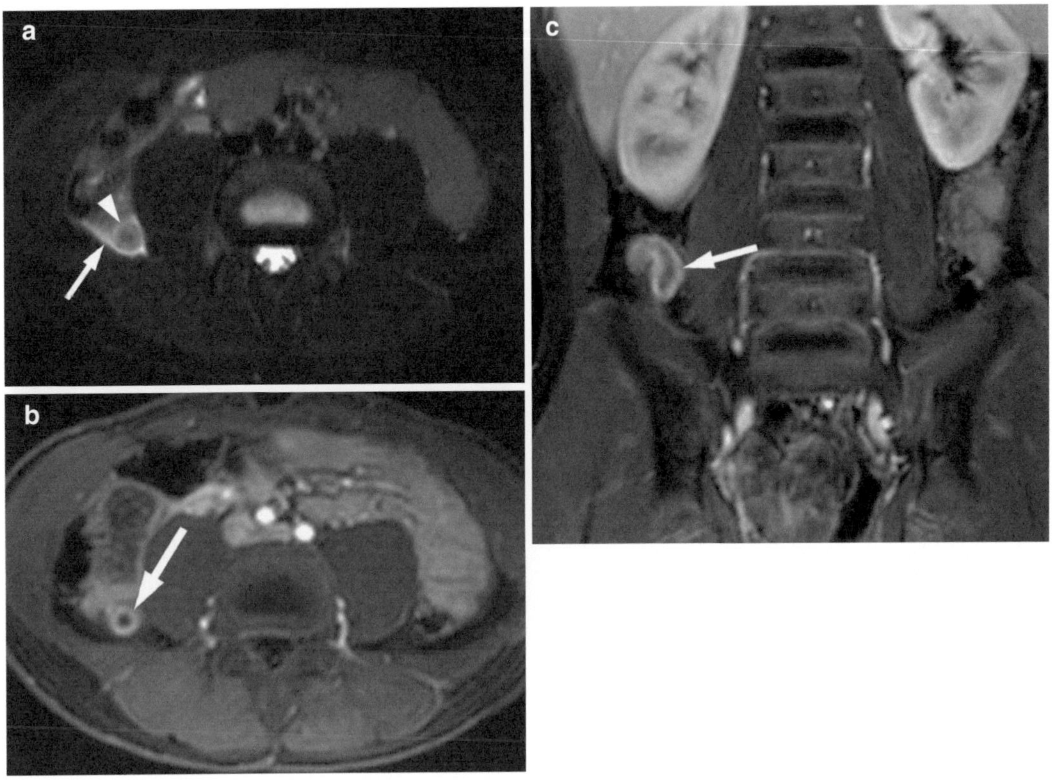

Fig. 7.4 Acute appendicitis in a 14-year-old boy. Axial single-shot fast spin echo with fat saturation image (**a**) demonstrates free fluid (*arrow*) adjacent to a thickened appendix (*arrowhead*). Axial (**b**) and coronal (**c**) postcontrast T1 with fat suppression images demonstrate avid enhancement of the appendiceal wall (*arrow*)

sequence of improper technique. For instance, incorrect anatomic coverage where only the pelvis is imaged may exclude the inflamed appendix in an unusually high location. Additionally, the absence of fat saturation increases the risk of false-negative results; periappendiceal fluid may not be easily detected on T2-weighted images without fat suppression, and incomplete fat saturation on T1-weighted images may result in observation of appendiceal wall enhancement to be obscured by the hyperintense mesenteric fat. Finally, excessive motion artifact may degrade the MR examination so that the images become nondiagnostic.

Interpretive errors also may lead to false-negative MR results for acute appendicitis. A distended fluid-filled appendix may be mistaken for the terminal ileum. Ascites from a comorbid condition can obscure periappendiceal inflammation. Periappendiceal inflammation may not be recognized due to the paucity of intraperitoneal fat. Finally, if the appendix is not traced to its tip, there is a potential to misdiagnose tip appendicitis.

False-positive MR results occur when regional inflammation from other causes is misinterpreted as acute appendicitis. Pericecal inflammation may be unrelated to acute appendicitis; for instance, it may be a result of active Crohn ileocolitis (Fig. 7.7). Cecal or small bowel diverticulitis may result in pericecal inflammation and abscess formation, and therefore be mistaken for acute appendicitis. Additionally, a fluid-filled terminal ileum may be mistaken for a dilated appendix. Finally, fluid in the right lower quadrant may originate from other causes (e.g., a

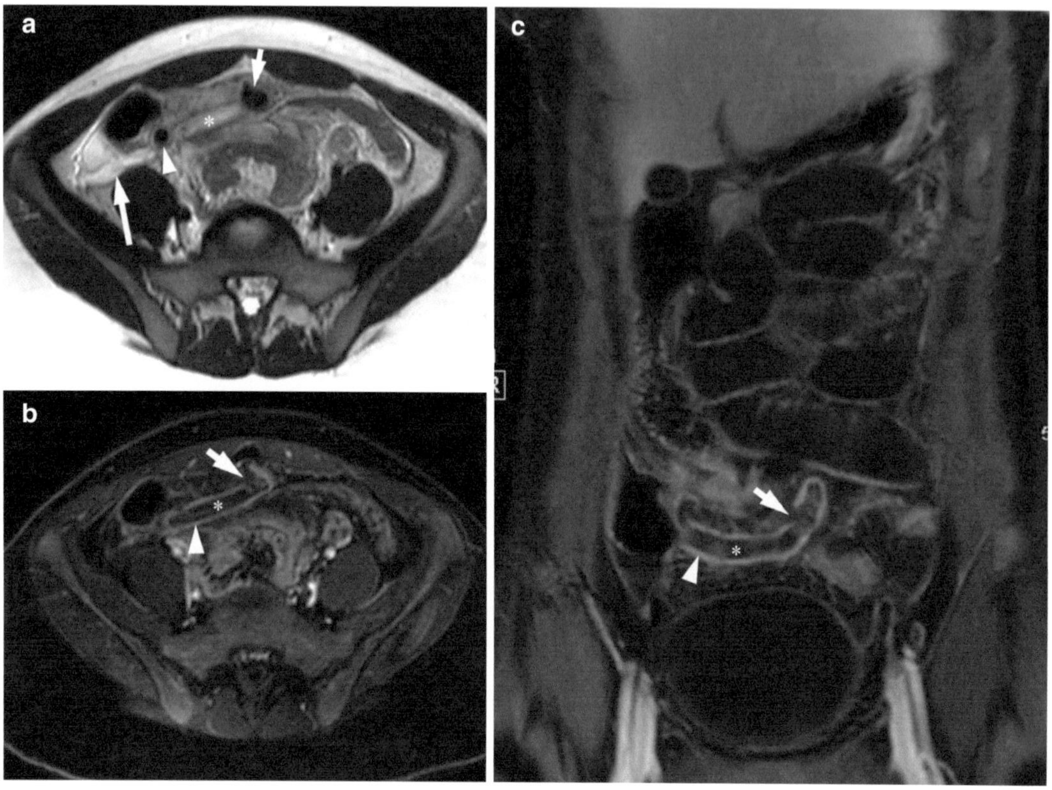

Fig. 7.5 Perforated acute appendicitis in a 15-year-old girl. Axial single-shot fast spin echo (SSFSE) image (**a**) demonstrates a dilated fluid-filled appendix (*) with an appendicolith at its base (*arrowhead*) and adjacent fluid (*long arrow*), representing acute appendicitis. Axial (**b**) and coronal (**c**) postcontrast T1 with fat suppression images demonstrate the dilated appendix (*) with hyperemia of its wall (*arrowhead*). Near the tip, there is discontinuity of the wall (*short arrow*, **b** and **c**), with the luminal contents extending beyond the confines of the wall (*short arrow*, **a**), representing perforation

ruptured right ovarian cyst, or generalized intra-abdominal ascites).

False-negative MR results for an alternate diagnosis may be a result of satisfaction of search, where identification of a normal appendix decreases the radiologist's attention to other potential causes of the patient's pain. Additionally, lack of familiarity with appearance of alternate diagnoses on MRI may contribute to misinterpretation of the examination (Fig. 7.8).

Finally, high cost of the MRI, limited availability, long acquisition times, and the need for greater patient cooperation compared with CT and ultrasound currently prevent its widespread use as the primary imaging modality for suspected acute appendicitis. For example, a prospective randomized pediatric cohort study comparing rapid MRI to ultrasound demonstrated ED length of stay on average to be 100 min longer in the MRI group compared with the ultrasound group [44]. Furthermore, MRI was associated with ED charges on average $4887 higher compared with ultrasound [44]. The authors concluded that in the diagnosis of

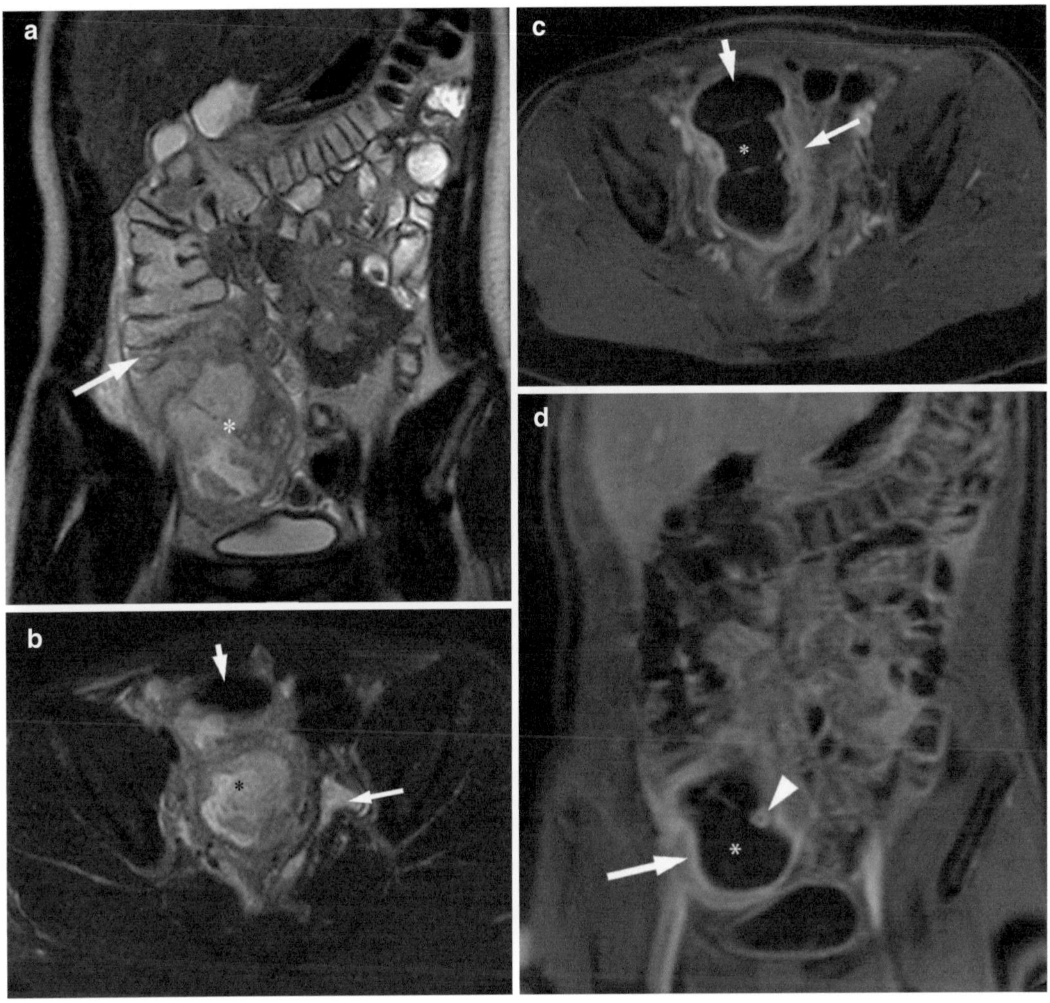

Fig. 7.6 Perforated acute appendicitis with a periappendiceal abscess in a 14-year-old girl. Coronal single-shot fast spin echo (SSFSE) image (**a**) demonstrates a large complex fluid collection (*) in close proximity with the cecum (*arrow*). Axial SSFSE with fat saturation image (**b**) demonstrates free fluid (*arrow*) adjacent to the collection (*), as well as nondependent signal void within the collection (*short arrow*), consistent with air. Axial (**c**) and coronal (**d**) postcontrast T1 with fat suppression images demonstrate avid enhancement of the wall (*long arrow*), and nondependent air (*short arrow*) in the collection (*). The collection wraps around a thickened hyperenhancing appendix (*arrowhead*)

appendicitis in young patients, ultrasound-first imaging is more time-efficient and less costly than rapid MRI despite inconclusive examinations with US [44]. The authors further speculated that ultrasound should be the first-line imaging modality for acute appendicitis unless the process of obtaining a rapid MRI becomes more efficient and less expensive [44].

7.5 Summary

In conclusion, MRI is a highly accurate imaging technique for the diagnosis of acute appendicitis. The advantage of lack of ionizing radiation and high contrast resolution makes MRI a promising imaging modality in pediatric and pregnant patients.

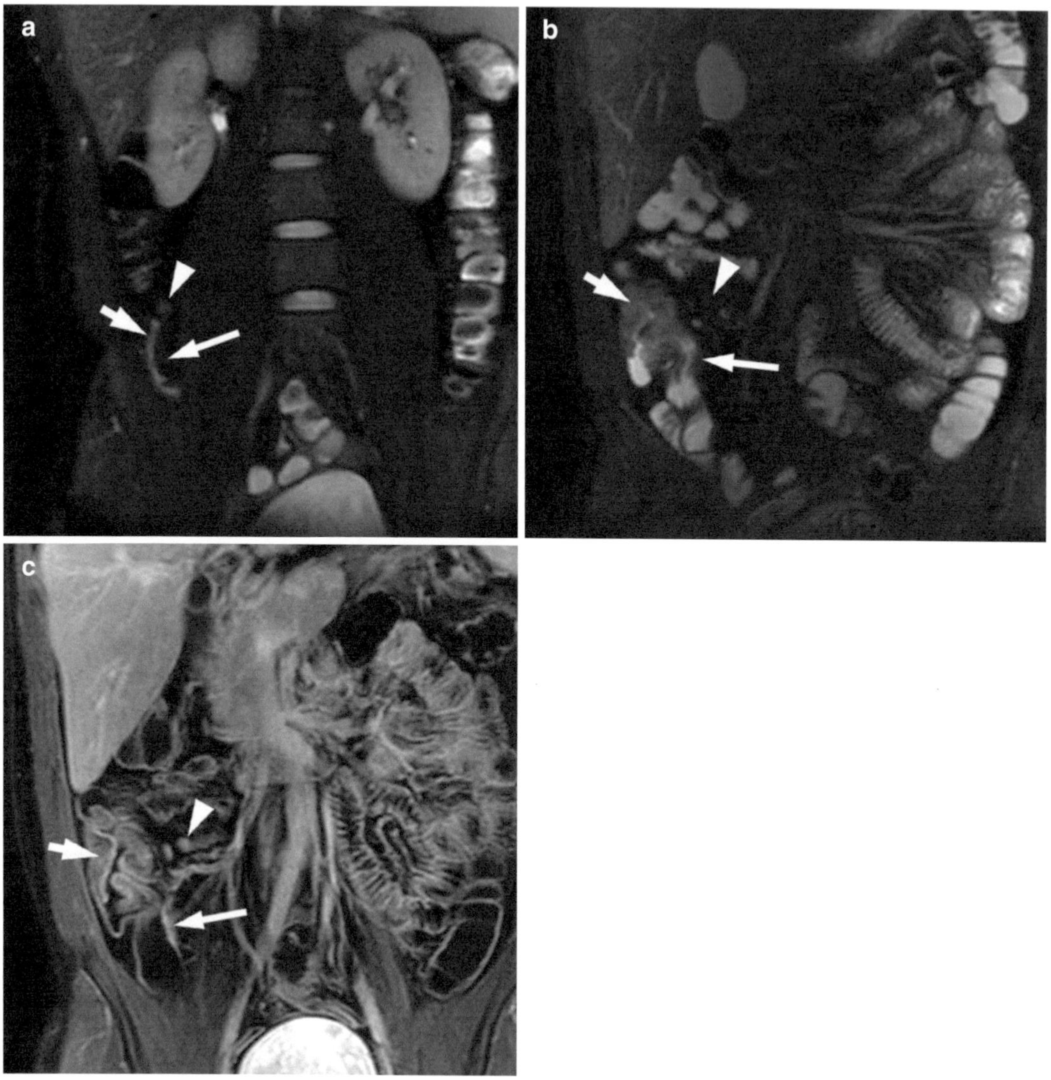

Fig. 7.7 Acute Crohn ileocolitis in a 24-year-old man. Coronal single-shot fast spin echo (SSFSE) with fat saturation image (**a**) demonstrates a fluid-filled appendix (*short arrow*) with adjacent mild inflammatory changes (*long arrow*), which could be mistaken for acute appendicitis. More anteriorly, coronal SSFSE with fat suppression (**b**) and postcontrast T1-weighted with fat suppression (**c**) images demonstrate thickening and avid mucosal enhancement of the terminal ileum (*long arrow*) and the cecum (*short arrow*), confirming the diagnosis of active Crohn ileocolitis. Note reactive right lower quadrant lymphadenopathy (*arrowhead* all images)

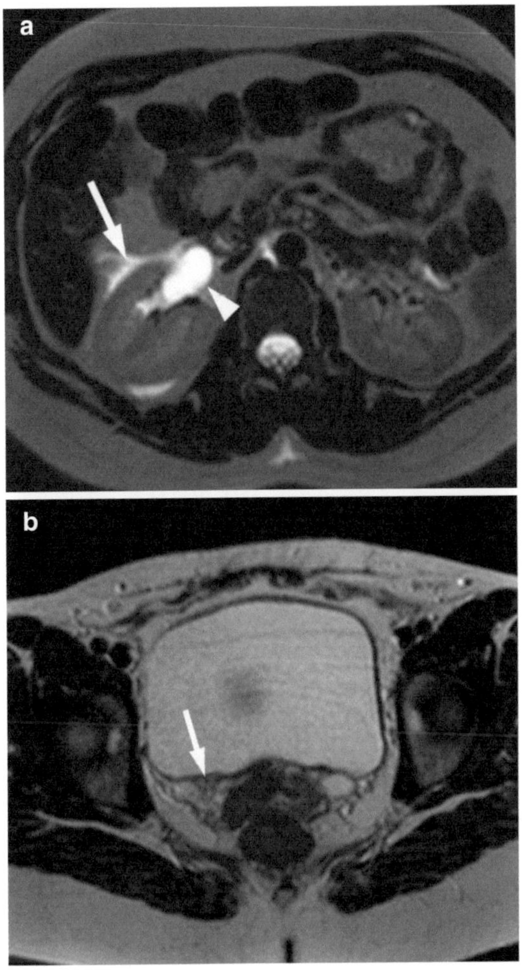

Fig. 7.8 Axial single-shot fast spin echo (SSFSE) image (**a**) demonstrates mild right hydronephrosis and perinephric fluid (*arrowhead*). More inferiorly, axial SSFSE image (**b**) demonstrates a small signal void (*arrow*) in the distal right ureter, representing an obstructing calculus. The appendix was normal (Fig. 7.1a)

References

1. Anderson JE, Bickler SW, Chang DC, Talamini MA. Examining a common disease with unknown etiology: trends in epidemiology and surgical management of appendicitis in California, 1995-2009. World J Surg. 2012;36(12):2787–94.
2. Smith MP, Katz DS, Lalani T, Carucci LR, Cash BD, Kim DH, et al. ACR appropriateness criteria(R) right lower quadrant pain--suspected appendicitis. Ultrasound Q. 2015;31(2):85–91.
3. Repplinger MD, Levy JF, Peethumnongsin E, Gussick ME, Svenson JE, Golden SK, et al. Systematic review and meta-analysis of the accuracy of MRI to diagnose appendicitis in the general population. J Magn Reson Imaging. 2016;43(6):1346–54.
4. Duke E, Kalb B, Arif-Tiwari H, Daye ZJ, Gilbertson-Dahdal D, Keim SM, et al. A systematic review and meta-analysis of diagnostic performance of MRI for evaluation of acute appendicitis. AJR. 2016;206(3):508–17.
5. Petkovska I, Martin DR, Covington MF, Urbina S, Duke E, Daye ZJ, et al. Accuracy of unenhanced MR imaging in the detection of acute appendicitis: single-institution clinical performance review. Radiology. 2016;279(2):451–60.
6. Moore MM, Kulaylat AN, Hollenbeak CS, Engbrecht BW, Dillman JR, Methratta ST. Magnetic resonance imaging in pediatric appendicitis: a systematic review. Pediatr Radiol. 2016;46(6):928–39.
7. Kulaylat AN, Moore MM, Engbrecht BW, Brian JM, Khaku A, Hollenbeak CS, et al. An implemented MRI program to eliminate radiation from the evaluation of pediatric appendicitis. J Pediatr Surg. 2015;50(8):1359–63.
8. Koning JL, Naheedy JH, Kruk PG. Diagnostic performance of contrast-enhanced MR for acute appendicitis and alternative causes of abdominal pain in children. Pediatr Radiol. 2014;44(8):948–55.
9. Burke LM, Bashir MR, Miller FH, Siegelman ES, Brown M, Alobaidy M, et al. Magnetic resonance imaging of acute appendicitis in pregnancy: a 5-year multiinstitutional study. Am J Obstet Gynecol. 2015;213(5):693 e1–6.
10. Konrad J, Grand D, Lourenco A. MRI: first-line imaging modality for pregnant patients with suspected appendicitis. Abdom Imaging. 2015;40(8):3359–64.
11. Patel D, Fingard J, Winters S, Low G. Clinical use of MRI for the evaluation of acute appendicitis during pregnancy. Abdom Radiol. 2017;42(7):1857–63.
12. Amitai MM, Katorza E, Guranda L, Apter S, Portnoy O, Inbar Y, et al. Role of emergency magnetic resonance imaging for the workup of suspected appendicitis in pregnant women. Isr Med Assoc J. 2016;18(10):600–4.
13. Theilen LH, Mellnick VM, Longman RE, Tuuli MG, Odibo AO, Macones GA, et al. Utility of magnetic resonance imaging for suspected appendicitis in pregnant women. Am J Obstet Gynecol. 2015;212(3):345 e1–6.
14. Moore MM, Kulaylat AN, Brian JM, Khaku A, Hulse MA, Engbrecht BW, et al. Alternative diagnoses at paediatric appendicitis MRI. Clin Radiol. 2015;70(8):881–9.
15. Dillman JR, Gadepalli S, Sroufe NS, Davenport MS, Smith EA, Chong ST, et al. Equivocal pediatric appendicitis: unenhanced MR imaging protocol for nonsedated children-A clinical effectiveness study. Radiology. 2016;279(1):216–25.

16. Leeuwenburgh MM, Wiarda BM, Wiezer MJ, Vrouenraets BC, Gratama JW, Spilt A, et al. Comparison of imaging strategies with conditional contrast-enhanced CT and unenhanced MR imaging in patients suspected of having appendicitis: a multicenter diagnostic performance study. Radiology. 2013;268(1):135–43.
17. Leeuwenburgh MM, Wiezer MJ, Wiarda BM, Bouma WH, Phoa SS, Stockmann HB, et al. Accuracy of MRI compared with ultrasound imaging and selective use of CT to discriminate simple from perforated appendicitis. Br J Surg. 2014;101(1):e147–55.
18. Rosenkrantz AB, Ginocchio LA, Cornfeld D, Froemming AT, Gupta RT, Turkbey B, et al. Interobserver reproducibility of the PI-RADS version 2 lexicon: a multicenter study of six experienced prostate radiologists. Radiology. 2016;280(3):793–804.
19. Davenport MS, Khalatbari S, Liu PS, Maturen KE, Kaza RK, Wasnik AP, et al. Repeatability of diagnostic features and scoring systems for hepatocellular carcinoma by using MR imaging. Radiology. 2014;272(1):132–42.
20. Puylaert CA, Tielbeek JA, Bipat S, Boellaard TN, Nio CY, Stoker J. Long-term performance of readers trained in grading Crohn disease activity using MRI. Acad Radiol. 2016;23(12):1539–44.
21. Purysko AS, Bittencourt LK, Bullen JA, Mostardeiro TR, Herts BR, Klein EA. Accuracy and interobserver agreement for prostate imaging reporting and data system, version 2, for the characterization of lesions identified on multiparametric MRI of the prostate. AJR. 2017;209(2):339–49.
22. Leeuwenburgh MM, Wiarda BM, Jensch S, van Es HW, Stockmann HB, Gratama JW, et al. Accuracy and interobserver agreement between MR-non-expert radiologists and MR-experts in reading MRI for suspected appendicitis. Eur J Radiol. 2014;83(1):103–10.
23. des Ziedses Plantes CM, van Veen MJ, van der Palen J, Klaase JM, Gielkens HA, Geelkerken RH. The effect of unenhanced MRI on the surgeons' decision-making process in females with suspected appendicitis. World J Surg. 2016;40(12):2881–7.
24. Rapp EJ, Naim F, Kadivar K, Davarpanah A, Cornfeld D. Integrating MR imaging into the clinical workup of pregnant patients suspected of having appendicitis is associated with a lower negative laparotomy rate: single-institution study. Radiology. 2013;267(1):137–44.
25. Fonseca AL, Schuster KM, Kaplan LJ, Maung AA, Lui FY, Davis KA. The use of magnetic resonance imaging in the diagnosis of suspected appendicitis in pregnancy: shortened length of stay without increase in hospital charges. JAMA Surg. 2014;149(7):687–93.
26. Lee SM, Ku YM, Choi BG, Byun JY. In vivo location of the vermiform appendix in multidetector CT. J Korean Soc Radiol. 2014;70(4):283–9.
27. Rosines LA, Chow DS, Lampl BS, Chen S, Gordon S, Mui LW, et al. Value of gadolinium-enhanced MRI in detection of acute appendicitis in children and adolescents. AJR. 2014;203(5):W543–8.
28. Singh A, Danrad R, Hahn PF, Blake MA, Mueller PR, Novelline RA. MR imaging of the acute abdomen and pelvis: acute appendicitis and beyond. Radiographics. 2007;27(5):1419–31.
29. Tkacz JN, Anderson SA, Soto J. MR imaging in gastrointestinal emergencies. Radiographics. 2009;29(6):1767–80.
30. Martin DR, Danrad R, Herrmann K, Semelka RC, Hussain SM. Magnetic resonance imaging of the gastrointestinal tract. Top Magn Reson Imaging. 2005;16(1):77–98.
31. Kinner S, Repplinger MD, Pickhardt PJ, Reeder SB. Contrast-enhanced abdominal MRI for suspected appendicitis: how we do it. AJR. 2016;207(1):49–57.
32. Heverhagen JT, Klose KJ. MR imaging for acute lower abdominal and pelvic pain. Radiographics. 2009;29(6):1781–96.
33. Lyons GR, Renjen P, Askin G, Giambrone AE, Beneck D, Kovanlikaya A. Diagnostic utility of intravenous contrast for MR imaging in pediatric appendicitis. Pediatr Radiol. 2017;47(4):398–403.
34. Bayraktutan U, Oral A, Kantarci M, Demir M, Ogul H, Yalcin A, et al. Diagnostic performance of diffusion-weighted MR imaging in detecting acute appendicitis in children: comparison with conventional MRI and surgical findings. J Magn Reson Imaging. 2014;39(6):1518–24.
35. Inci E, Kilickesmez O, Hocaoglu E, Aydin S, Bayramoglu S, Cimilli T. Utility of diffusion-weighted imaging in the diagnosis of acute appendicitis. Eur Radiol. 2011;21(4):768–75.
36. Lee MH, Eutsler EP, Sheybani EF, Khanna G. Rapid non-contrast magnetic resonance imaging for post appendectomy intra-abdominal abscess in children. Pediatr Radiol. 2017;47(8):935–41.
37. Swenson DW, Schooler GR, Stamoulis C, Lee EY. MRI of the normal appendix in children: data toward a new reference standard. Pediatr Radiol. 2016;46(7):1003–10.
38. Kearl YL, Claudius I, Behar S, Cooper J, Dollbaum R, Hardasmalani M, et al. Accuracy of magnetic resonance imaging and ultrasound for appendicitis in diagnostic and nondiagnostic studies. Acad Emerg Med. 2016;23(2):179–85.
39. Lam M, Singh A, Kaewlai R, Novelline RA. Magnetic resonance of acute appendicitis: pearls and pitfalls. Curr Probl Diagn Radiol. 2008;37(2):57–66.
40. Shin I, An C, Lim JS, Kim MJ, Chung YE. T1 bright appendix sign to exclude acute appendici-

tis in pregnant women. Eur Radiol. 2017;27(8):3310–6.
41. Rosenbaum DG, Askin G, Beneck DM, Kovanlikaya A. Differentiating perforated from non-perforated appendicitis on contrast-enhanced magnetic resonance imaging. Pediatr Radiol. 2017;47(11):1483–90.
42. Leeuwenburgh MM, Jensch S, Gratama JW, Spilt A, Wiarda BM, Van Es HW, et al. MRI features associated with acute appendicitis. Eur Radiol. 2014;24(1):214–22.
43. Avcu S, Cetin FA, Arslan H, Kemik O, Dulger AC. The value of diffusion-weighted imaging and apparent diffusion coefficient quantification in the diagnosis of perforated and nonperforated appendicitis. Diagn Interv Radiol. 2013;19(2):106–10.
44. Imler D, Keller C, Sivasankar S, Wang NE, Vasanawala S, Bruzoni M, et al. Magnetic resonance imaging versus ultrasound as the initial imaging modality for pediatric and young adult patients with suspected appendicitis. Acad Emerg Med. 2017;24(5):569–77.

8 Advances in MDCT and MRI of Renal Emergencies

Daniel Barkmeier and Suzanne Chong

Abstract

Acute renal conditions account for a notable volume of Emergency Department visits and often lead to imaging. Urolithiasis is the most commonly encountered etiology but a wide range of conditions including infection, inflammation, and hemorrhage can also cause acute pain. Ultrasound and computed tomography (CT) are the most commonly utilized imaging modalities for the kidneys while the role of dual-energy CT is expanding as a problem-solving tool. Management of acute renal conditions ranges from emergent intervention to medical management and may be determined by the imaging findings. Therefore, accurate and timely diagnoses are critical to expedite appropriate clinical management.

Keywords

Renal · Emergency · Urolithiasis · Infection Obstruction · Hemorrhage · Dual-energy CT

D. Barkmeier, M.D., Ph.D • S. Chong, M.D., M.S. (✉)
Department of Radiology, University of Michigan, Ann Arbor, MI, USA
e-mail: suzchong@med.umich.edu

8.1 Introduction

The kidneys are bilateral, paired retroperitoneal organs with important filtration, endocrine, and excretory functions. The kidneys maintain electrolyte and acid-base balance, secrete hormones including erythropoietin, calcitriol, and renin, and are a key excretory pathway for removing many waste products from the blood. Structurally, the kidneys are composed of the inner medullary pyramids and an outer cortex layer, surrounded by a capsule. Centrally, the renal sinus contains fat surrounding the collecting system and the renal hilum where arteries, veins, and nerves enter the kidney. Immediately surrounding the kidney is a layer of fat bounded by Gerota's fascia, which comprises the perirenal space (Fig. 8.1). Anterior to Gerota's fascia is the anterior pararenal space while posterior to the fascia is the posterior pararenal space.

Non-traumatic, non-vascular renal emergencies can be divided into three main categories: (1) acute obstruction (urolithiasis), (2) inflammatory/infectious processes, and (3) renal cysts and tumors which present urgently, usually due to hemorrhage, or which are detected incidentally in patients being imaged for other reasons in the emergency setting. Computed tomography (CT) and ultrasound (US) are the primary imaging modalities for renal abnormalities in the emergency setting due to a combination of their ubiquity, cost, and ability to demonstrate the majority

M. Patlas et al. (eds.), *MDCT and MR Imaging of Acute Abdomen*,
https://doi.org/10.1007/978-3-319-70778-5_8

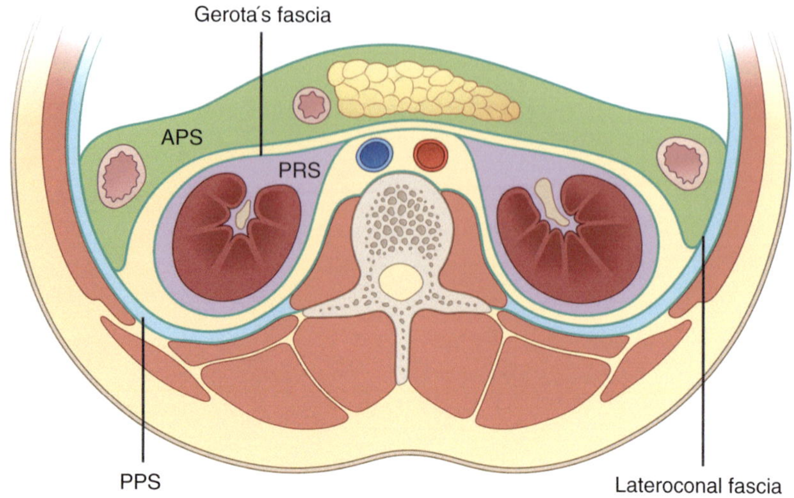

Fig. 8.1 *Retroperitoneal spaces*. The pararenal space (PRS) consists of a layer of fat immediately encircling both kidneys, bound by Gerota's fascia (GF). Anterior to Gerota's fascia is the anterior perirenal space (APS) while posterior to the fascia is the posterior pararenal space (PPS). The lateroconal fascia is created by fusion of the anterior and posterior pararenal spaces

of urgent renal etiologies. Magnetic resonance imaging (MRI) is generally not an appropriate modality for emergent renal imaging but is instead better suited for follow-up or problem-solving on a nonemergent basis in selected circumstances. Abdominal radiography has a largely historic role in the evaluation of urolithiasis. CT is more sensitive for urolithiasis and ongoing advances in dose reduction techniques have significantly reduced the radiation dose of CT compared to radiography.

8.2 Urolithiasis

Urolithiasis is a commonly encountered entity in the emergency department. The estimated costs of diagnosis and treatment approached $2.1 billion in the year 2000 which represented a greater than 50% increase from the prior decade [1]. Approximately 2–3% of the population will develop urinary tract calculi and up to 12% will experience an obstructing calculus in their lifetime. Recurrence rates in patients with renal and ureteral calculi approach 50%. The incidence appears to be increasing overall and there has also been an increase in the proportion of women with urinary calculus disease [1, 2]. Common risk factors for urolithiasis include male sex, increasing age, obesity, diabetes mellitus, and dehydration, in addition to numerous metabolic and digestive disorders [3–5].

Patients with urolithiasis classically present with acute, colicky flank pain which may radiate to the groin. Nausea and vomiting not associated with an acute abdomen may also be present. As the calculus descends toward the ureterovesical junction, the pain can radiate toward the urethra; symptoms may then include dysuria, urinary frequency, and urinary urgency, mimicking cystitis. Patients with obstructing calculi may have tenderness in the costovertebral angle or in the lower abdomen on physical examination. Although the majority of patients with acute renal and ureteral calculi have hematuria, it is frequently absent and therefore generally not used to determine whether a calculus is present.

Noncontrast CT is the imaging test of choice for the detection of urinary tract calculi, with reported sensitivities, specificities, and accuracies ranging from 97–100%, 94–98%, and 96–98%, respectively. This clearly outperforms conventional radiography, which depicts only 45–59% of calculi, and replaces intravenous urography, which was the preferred test in the past. Noncontrast CT is rapid, widely available, cost-effective, does not require contrast material, and can depict noncalculi causes of flank pain. The disadvantage is the use of ionizing radiation, but ongoing improvements in hardware and software have significantly reduced patient doses.

This is important since many patients with urolithiasis are young, and some will undergo multiple CT examinations in their lifetimes due to recurrent symptoms. Ultrasound may also be used to evaluate the kidneys and urolithiasis in the emergency setting, is widely available, does not confer ionizing radiation, and is relatively inexpensive. The disadvantages of sonography are its operator-dependent nature, insensitivity for ureteral calculi, and insensitivity for small calculi. While ultrasound can depict collecting system dilatation in the setting of obstruction and renal calculi larger than 5 mm, gray-scale ultrasound has reported sensitivities for ureteral calculi of only 11–24%. Use of the "twinkling" artifact on color Doppler imaging (a focus of alternating colors observed when insonating certain rough surfaces) increases sensitivity for detection of renal calculi to approximately 80% [6, 7] and can also be useful in identifying calculi in the distal ureter which are located near or at the ureterovesical junction [8, 9].

The most specific CT sign of urolithiasis is direct visualization of the calculus in the ureter. Thin-section CT images, typically less than 5 mm thickness and reconstructed at less than 5 mm intervals, allow the radiologist to track the ureter throughout its course and to detect renal and ureteral calculi as small as 2–3 mm. Obstructing ureteral calculi tend to lodge at the three points of anatomic ureteral narrowing: the ureterovesical junction (most commonly), the ureteropelvic junction, and the pelvic brim (Fig. 8.2). These regions should therefore be carefully evaluated. The vast majority of renal and ureteral calculi are hyperattenuating on CT and easily visible. Calcium-based calculi and struvite calculi (magnesium ammonium phosphate) are radiodense and are the most commonly encountered types, accounting for 70–80% and 15–20% of all calculi, respectively [10, 11]. Uric acid calculi account for 5–10% of all urinary calculi, and while radiolucent on radiograph, can be readily identified on CT. Relatively low attenuation (<500 HU) of a calculus on CT is suggestive of uric acid composition [12]. Cystine calculi are relatively rare, accounting for only 1–3% of all urinary calculi, and are primarily seen in patients with cystinuria. In rare instances, urease-producing bacteria can lead to the production of matrix calculi of soft-tissue attenuation which can be difficult or impossible to visualize on CT. Finally, some medications can crystallize in the urine and produce soft-tissue attenuation calculi which are not well visualized. This was classically described with the protease inhibitor indinavir but can also occur with other protease inhibitors

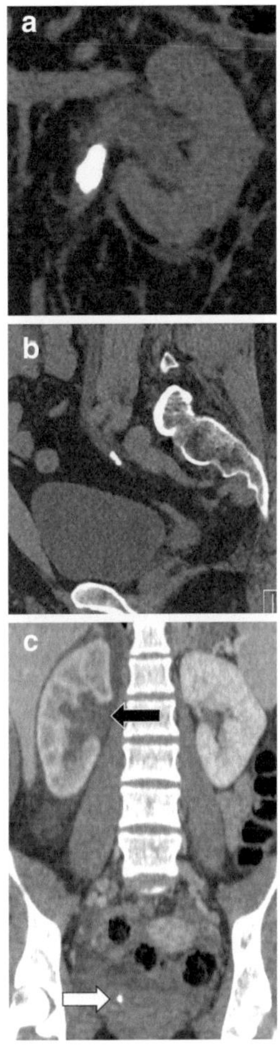

Fig. 8.2 *Most common sites of obstructing urolithiasis.* Coronal non-contrast CT image (**a**) shows a large obstructing calculus at the left ureteropelvic junction, causing collecting system dilation. Sagittal non-contrast CT image (**b**) in a different patient shows a calculus at the pelvic brim causing upstream left ureteral dilation. Coronal IV contrast-enhanced CT image (**c**) demonstrates a calculus at the right ureterovesical junction (white arrow) resulting in collecting system dilation and a delayed right nephrogram (black arrow)

which are in more widespread use today, such as atazanavir.

Secondary CT signs are often extremely helpful in making the diagnosis of obstructing urolithiasis and include renal collecting system and ureteral dilatation, perinephric and/or periureteral edema, and enlargement and decreased attenuation of the obstructed kidney. Urine within the dilated ureter or collecting system should be simple fluid attenuation. If urine measures higher than expected for fluid, blood or pus may be present and should be noted. Urothelial thickening is often present but is nonspecific and usually indicates co-existent inflammation or infection. One of the most commonly encountered challenges in interpreting urinary calculus CT examinations is differentiating ureteral calculi from phleboliths. Phleboliths are venous calcifications that can occur in any veins of the abdomen or pelvis but are most frequently encountered in the pelvis near the distal ureters. Multiplanar reformats, especially in the coronal plane, may be beneficial for differentiating ureteral calculi from phleboliths in some patients but are not always diagnostic. This is most problematic for patients in whom the distal ureters cannot be identified, such as those with a paucity of retroperitoneal fat or who do not have ureteral dilatation. In problematic patients, two other CT signs may be used: the rim sign and the comet tail sign. The rim sign refers to a circumferential ring of soft-tissue attenuation surrounding the ureteral calculus which represents the inflamed ureter at the site of calculus impaction. The comet tail sign is a triangular or tubular area of soft-tissue attenuation adjacent to a calcification which indicates the collapsed or thrombosed parent vein. Unfortunately, neither CT sign is very sensitive or specific, and there is significant interobserver variability [13]. A radiolucent center within a calcification also favors phlebolith over a ureteral calculus but this is more commonly seen on radiography and not usually appreciated on CT [14].

Another problem in interpreting urinary calculus CT examinations is when secondary signs are present but no obstructing calculus is visualized. In these patients, several diagnoses must be considered: a recently passed calculus, an alternative cause of urinary tract obstruction (such as a urothelial cancer), infection, renal vein thrombosis, acute renal emboli, renal infarction, and, most rarely, a low-attenuation calculus. Follow-up intravenous (IV) contrast-enhanced CT may be helpful in these instances to better depict the renal parenchyma and vascular structures. A diagnostic pitfall to consider is when CT images are obtained following intravenous contrast administration and contrast is excreted into the collecting system, high attenuation calculi can be obscured.

Management options for urolithiasis depend on calculus size, location, composition, and complications. In general, the smaller the calculus and the more distally the calculus is located, the sooner and more likely it will pass spontaneously. Approximately two-thirds of renal calculi measuring less than 5 mm on CT will pass spontaneously within 4 weeks. Many impacted ureteral calculi can be extracted ureteroscopically while some may require shock wave lithotripsy. Struvite calculi are amenable to fragmentation by lithotripsy, while cysteine and calcium oxalate monohydrate calculi are more resistant to fragmentation [15–17]. Uric acid calculi can be managed with oral medications. Complications of obstructing stone disease including pyonephrosis or collecting system rupture require more urgent intervention such as stent placement.

Given the differing management options based on calculus composition, dual-energy CT (DECT) is becoming increasingly utilized as a problem-solving tool (Fig. 8.3). DECT is a newer technology which works by passing X-rays beams at two different spectra (higher and lower kVp) through a material and evaluating the energy-dependent changes in attenuation values. This method has been shown to reliably differentiate uric acid from non-uric acid calculi, and more recent work suggests that dual-energy CT may be able to further subcharacterize non-uric acid calculi [18–26]. Radiation dose is currently comparable to standard CT, so this technique should be considered in patients with a strong pretest probability of an obstructing calculus.

Noncalculus causes of flank pain are present in 12–45% of nonenhanced CT examinations

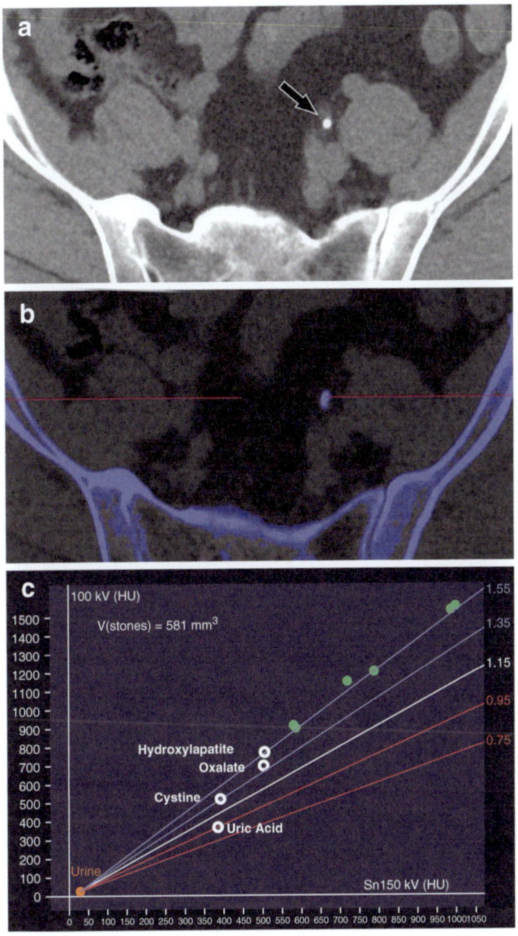

Fig. 8.3 *Dual-energy CT for calculus composition.* A 53-year-old man presented with acute left flank pain. An obstructing calculus in the distal left ureter (**a**) is detected and colored blue by the analysis software (**b**). A plot of attenuation values at two different energies of this calculus as well as additional nonobstructing renal calculi (green circles) indicate that these calculi are comprised of hydroxyapatite (**c**)

performed for flank pain due to suspected urolithiasis. The shared innervation of the genitourinary and gastrointestinal systems can result in overlap of clinical symptoms, with symptoms from one system referred to the other. Acute pelvic or abdominal conditions may present with symptoms of colicky, flank pain, mimicking a ureteral calculus (Fig. 8.4). Renal capsular distention from hydronephrosis may result in nausea and vomiting. The most common alternative diagnoses encountered on CT examinations performed for suspected urolithiasis include adnexal

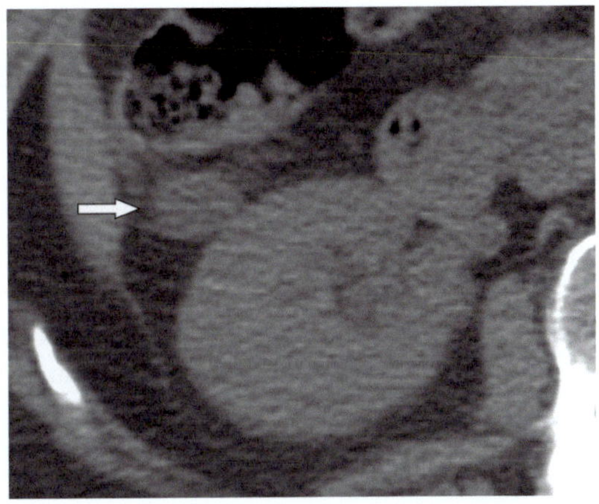

Fig. 8.4 *Appendicitis mimicking an acute renal condition.* A 58-year-old woman presented with right flank and groin pain. A noncontrast CT was obtained to evaluate for obstructive urolithiasis. Both kidneys are normal, but an inflamed appendix (arrow) lied anterior to the right kidney and was the cause of the right flank pain

masses, appendicitis, and diverticulitis. Occasionally, patients with suspected urinary tract calculi may instead have abdominal aortic aneurysms or aortic dissections which may necessitate further evaluation with IV contrast-enhanced CT (CECT).

8.3 Inflammatory and Infectious Disorders

8.3.1 Acute Pyelonephritis

Acute pyelonephritis is the infection of renal parenchyma, typically due to ascending bacterial infection from the urinary bladder. Females are affected five times more commonly than males, with an overall incidence of 15–17 cases per 10,000 females and 3–4 cases per 10,000 males [27]. At least 250,000 patients with pyelonephritis are diagnosed annually in the United States. The vast majority of infections are due to *Escherichia coli* and less commonly, by coagulase-negative staphylococci, *Proteus mirabilis*, klebsiella species, enterococci, among others [28]. Acute pyelonephritis is usually diagnosed based on clinical presentation (flank pain and fevers) and laboratory test results (pyuria and leukocytosis). Imaging is generally reserved for patients with acute pyelonephritis who do not respond well to appropriate antibiotic therapy, such as persistent fevers after 72 h or rapid recurrence of symptoms. Complications including urinary tract obstruction or abscess formation should be suspected in these patients. Factors that predispose patients to developing complications include advanced age, diabetes, and immunosuppression. These complications are readily identified on any cross-sectional imaging modality which may also help guide subsequent percutaneous intervention.

At some institutions and practices, IV contrast-enhanced CT is generally preferred due to its higher sensitivity for the depiction of complicated pyelonephritis. Acute pyelonephritis is usually unilateral but within the kidney can be diffuse or focal, resulting in different imaging manifestations. On CECT, there may be a classic "striated nephrogram" in which linear bands of low attenuation representing the poorly enhancing tubules alternate with more normally enhancing renal parenchyma (Fig. 8.5a). Diffuse, acute pyelonephritis may also manifest as only an enlarged, edematous kidney on any imaging modality. Comparison to prior imaging and with the contralateral kidney is beneficial, as is evaluation for any secondary signs of inflammation that may be present. Common ancillary findings in both focal and diffuse pyelonephritis include perinephric infiltration and urothelial thickening or enhancement (Fig. 8.5b). Focal, acute pyelonephritis appears as a wedge-shaped or rounded area of poor or streaky enhancement that is best identified on the nephrographic phase of contrast enhancement. These regions can appear mass-like and mimic a solid renal neoplasm (Fig. 8.6). On noncontrast CT, often ordered to evaluate for calculi in the setting of flank pain, uncomplicated pyelonephritis can easily be overlooked. Images should be carefully inspected for renal enlargement, perinephric stranding, and fascial or urothelial thickening. Occasionally, wedge-shaped or linear areas of high attenuation may be observed, which likely represent foci of hemorrhage.

Ultrasound in the setting of acute pyelonephritis can be normal in up to 75% of patients

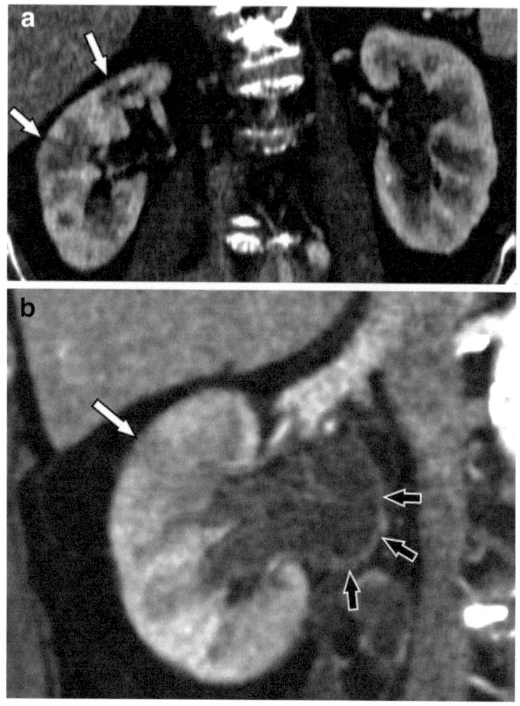

Fig. 8.5 *Acute pyelonephritis on IV contrast-enhanced CT.* An 83-year-old man presented with acute onset abdominal pain. The right kidney shows a striated nephrogram (**a**), with multiple linear low-attenuation areas in the cortex (white arrows). Contrast-enhanced CT in a 75-year-old patient with a history of bladder cancer following cystectomy with ileal conduit formation, undergoing routine surveillance (**b**), also has a low-attenuation region in the cortex (white arrow), as well as urothelial thickening and enhancement (black arrows). The findings were compatible with pyelonephritis and pyelitis

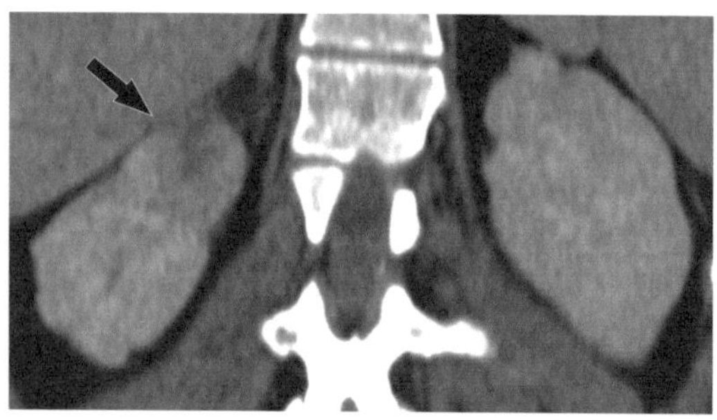

Fig. 8.6 *Focal, mass-like pyelonephritis.* A 24-year-old woman with history of HIV presented with right upper quadrant pain and dysuria, and an IV contrast-enhanced CT was performed. A focal, mass-like hypoattenuating area in the superior pole of the right kidney could not be distinguished from a renal mass on CT. The patient's young age and presenting symptoms of flank pain and dysuria favored pyelonephritis and a course of antibiotics was instituted. This finding resolved on follow-up CT three weeks later (not shown)

[29, 30]. When findings are present, focal pyelonephritis may cause wedge-shaped or rounded regions of either decreased (edema) or increased (hemorrhage) echogenicity. Perfusion is typically decreased on both color and power Doppler imaging due to edema and increased pressure within an encapsulated organ. Urothelial thickening, decreased corticomedullary differentiation, or debris within the collecting system may be seen in focal or diffuse pyelonephritis.

MRI findings are similar to those on CECT including striated areas of hypoenhancement, renal enlargement, urothelial thickening or enhancement, and perinephric/periureteral stranding. Additionally, the local edema caused by parenchymal inflammation may cause increased T2-weighted signal and restricted diffusion in the foci of infection. Subtraction images can make regions of decreased enhancement more apparent.

Acute pyelonephritis is mainly a clinical diagnosis but imaging plays an important role in identifying complications, which impact management. A complicating renal abscess appears as a focal hypoechoic area without color Doppler flow on US, and as a rim-enhancing, low-attenuation mass on CECT. On MR, abscesses are typically hypointense on T1-weighted images and hyperintense on T2-weighted images, with rim enhancement, restricted diffusion, and adjacent edema. In rare instances, gas may be present within the abscess. Another potential complication is calyceal or collecting system rupture which can allow the infection to spread into the pararenal and retroperitoneal spaces.

One of the challenges in establishing the diagnosis of pyelonephritis is that the CT findings are nonspecific. Other entities including glomerulonephritis and interstitial nephritis due to noninfectious causes including sarcoidosis, medications, or immune or metabolic-related conditions may have similar appearances, with areas of low attenuation in the renal parenchyma. Lymphoma can cause renal enlargement. Perinephric infiltration may be seen with recent trauma, prior infection, or vascular diseases, including vasculitides and renal vein thrombosis. Correlation of the CT findings with the clinical presentation and laboratory values is therefore critical to narrow the differential diagnosis.

8.3.2 Acute Pyelitis, Ureteritis, and Pyonephrosis

Pyelitis and ureteritis refer to infections of the renal collecting system and ureter, respectively. These processes typically produce urothelial thickening on all imaging modalities, often with post-contrast enhancement of the urothelium on CT and MR. Pyonephrosis refers to the accumulation of purulent material in the renal collecting system and/or ureter. Pyonephrosis usually requires IV antibiotics and immediate drainage to prevent permanent renal parenchymal destruction and life-threatening sepsis. The most common underlying cause of pyonephrosis is obstructing renal calculi but tumors, iatrogenic strictures, and retroperitoneal fibrosis should be considered as well. Imaging findings of pyonephrosis include collecting system dilatation, urothelial thickening and/or enhancement, and sometimes fluid-debris levels within the collecting system (Fig. 8.7). Debris within the dilated collecting system is often seen as low-level echoes on US and can increase the attenuation value to higher than simple fluid on CT. Early investigative efforts into the use of diffusion-weighted MR to distinguish pyonephrosis from hydronephrosis suggest that pyonephrosis tends to have more restricted diffusion and lower ADC values than simple hydronephrosis [31, 32]. The renal parenchyma may or may not be involved, i.e., concomitant pyelonephritis.

8.3.3 Emphysematous Pyelonephritis

Emphysematous pyelonephritis refers to infection of the renal parenchyma by a gas-producing organism, usually *E. coli* (70%), *Klebsiella pneumoniae*, or *Proteus mirabilis*. This should be distinguished from emphysematous pyelitis, which is a gas-forming infection restricted to the collecting system. In contrast to emphysematous

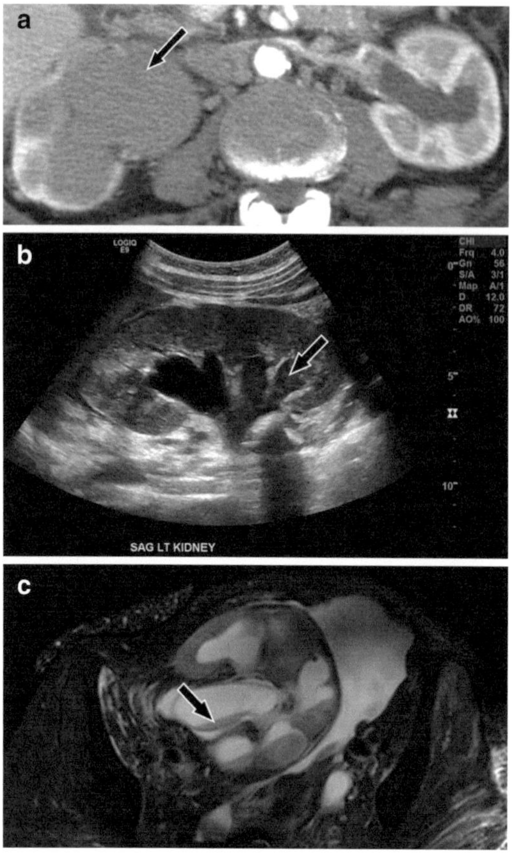

Fig. 8.7 *Pyonephrosis*. (**a**) IV contrast-enhanced CT in an 86-year-old woman with peritoneal carcinomatosis and abdominal pain shows that the collecting system of the right kidney is asymmetrically dilated and is higher in attenuation (arrow) than the left. (**b**) A 27-year-old woman with no past medical history presented to the Emergency Department with left-sided back pain. Ultrasound shows a dilated collecting system with layering, echogenic debris in the pelvis and lower pole calyces (arrow). (**c**) A 42-year-old woman with history of recurrent urinary tract infections and lupus nephritis following renal transplant presented with acute kidney injury. T2-weighted, fat-saturated MR image of a right lower quadrant transplanted kidney shows an enlarged kidney with a dilated collecting system, urothelial thickening, and layering debris (arrow)

pyelonephritis, emphysematous pyelitis is a much less severe infection which usually responds well to antibiotics. Emphysematous pyelonephritis, on the other hand, carries significant mortality risk, with rates as high as 11–42% [33–35]. Emphysematous pyelonephritis is usually unilateral, is more common in women, and occurs almost exclusively (80–100%) in patients with uncontrolled diabetes. Nondiabetic patients are typically either immunocompromised or have associated urinary tract obstruction. Physical examination reveals a palpable flank mass representing the involved kidney in 50% of patients. Crepitus over the flank or thigh may also be present.

Several classification systems have been proposed to correlate imaging findings with subsequent prognosis and management. The initial system proposed by Wan categorizes this entity into two types: Type 1 is characterized primarily by renal parenchymal destruction, with streaky or mottled areas of gas within the parenchyma but no intra- or extrarenal fluid collections. Type 2 emphysematous pyelonephritis is characterized by renal or perirenal fluid collections which are directly associated with bubbly or loculated gas, or by gas within the urinary collecting system [36]. Type 1 has a much more severe clinical course, classically requiring more aggressive intervention, i.e., nephrectomy. Type 2 emphysematous pyelonephritis is more amenable to urgent percutaneous drainage and antibiotics. The other proposed classification system by Huang and Tseng [34] described four classes of severity ranging from the least severe, emphysematous pyelitis (class 1), to bilateral emphysematous pyelonephritis or a solitary kidney with emphysematous pyelonephritis (class 4). Overall, while emergent nephrectomy was the mainstay of treatment for emphysematous pyelonephritis, an initial trial of percutaneous drainage with antibiotic therapy and aggressive fluid resuscitation is becoming much more common, and mortality rates appear to be improving [37–39].

The key imaging finding on all modalities is gas within the renal parenchyma (Fig. 8.8). On ultrasound, there will be nondependent echogenic foci in the renal parenchyma with reverberation artifact and low-level echoes ("dirty" shadowing). CT is the modality of choice for identifying and categorizing emphysematous pyelonephritis, and will show mottled or bubbly foci of low attenuation in the kidney. The

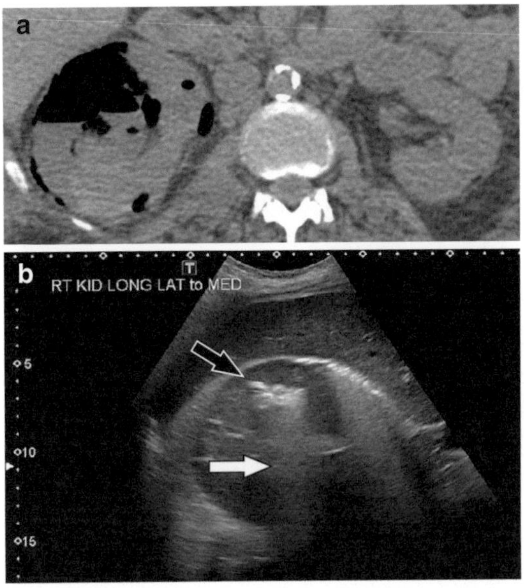

Fig. 8.8 *Emphysematous pyelonephritis*. A 60-year-old woman with history of diabetes mellitus presented with fever, fatigue, and vomiting, and was found to be in septic shock. Axial CT image (**a**) shows gas both within the right renal collecting system and the renal parenchyma. Ultrasound in the same patient (**b**) demonstrates echogenic foci in the renal parenchyma (black arrow) with posterior "dirty" shadowing (white arrow), representing gas

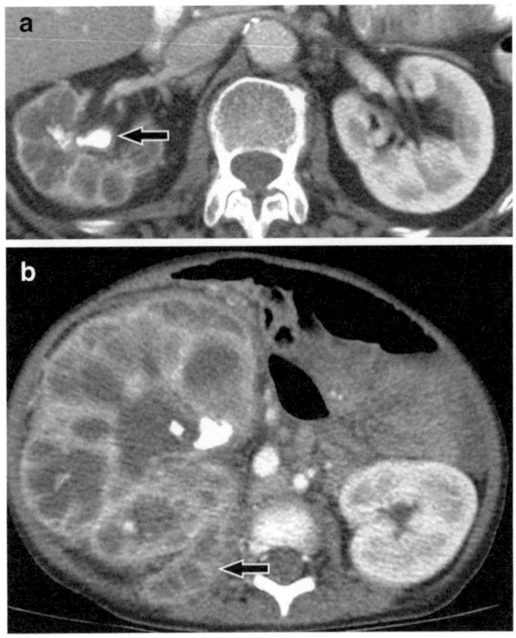

Fig. 8.9 *Xanthogranulomatous pyelonephritis on IV contrast-enhanced CT*. (**a**) An 80-year-old woman with metastatic colon cancer underwent surveillance CT. The right kidney contains a large, central calculus (arrow) with numerous low-attenuation foci in the surrounding renal parenchyma, delay of the nephrogram indicating reduced renal function, and perinephric stranding. Renal enlargement is a typical finding, but was not present in this patient. (**b**) A 2-year-old girl was referred by her primary care physician for fever, elevated white blood cell count, and a palpable abdominal mass. IV contrast-enhanced CT shows typical findings of XGP, with renal enlargement, a central calculus, delayed nephrogram, and low-attenuation foci in a radial pattern. Extension to the right psoas muscle with abscess formation (arrow) is also present. In this example, the young age of the patient is very unusual for this entity

presence of collections of fluid or fluid and gas within or adjacent to the kidney is vital to report in order to classify, prognosticate, and treat.

8.3.4 Xanthogranulomatous Pyelonephritis

Xanthogranulomatous pyelonephritis (XGP) is a relatively rare, chronic infection of the kidney characterized by destruction of renal parenchymal and replacement by lipid-laden macrophages. XGP results from long-standing obstruction of the collecting system, usually from a staghorn calculus and superimposed chronic bacterial infection, which provokes an atypical immune response with accumulation of lipid-laden macrophages (xanthoma cells). The most commonly implicated bacteria are *E. coli* and *P. mirabilis*. There is a female predilection (F:M = 2:1) and diabetes is a predisposing factor. XGP occurs most commonly in middle aged patients but any age may be affected. Symptoms are often nonspecific, including low-grade fevers and malaise, but flank pain and hematuria may direct imaging evaluation to the urinary tract.

XGP often has a characteristic appearance on imaging (Fig. 8.9). Obstructing calculi are usually identified in the affected renal collecting system, often of the staghorn type. The renal pelvis and calyces are dilated, sometimes massively, from a combination of urinary tract obstruction and accumulation of pus and debris in the renal collecting system. The affected kidney is diffusely enlarged while its reniform contour is preserved, and there is often perinephric inflammatory change. CT is the mainstay of diagnostic imaging for XGP because many patients demonstrate specific findings and because surgical planning requires accurate assessment of the presence and extent of extrarenal disease. Infected, loculated fluid collections are frequently found in the adjacent tissues including in the perirenal space, the anterior and posterior pararenal spaces, and the psoas muscles (Fig. 8.9b). In some patients, fistulae to the skin or gastrointestinal tract may develop. By the time of diagnosis, renal function on the affected side is significantly impaired so contrast excretion is delayed or absent. XGP is usually diffuse but can also have focal involvement in about 10%, resulting in localized renal swelling that can be mistaken for a solid renal mass [40].

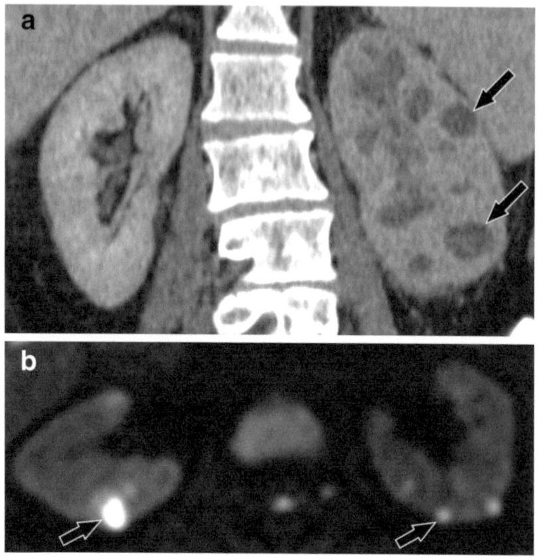

Fig. 8.10 *Renal microabscesses.* A 60-year-old man with history of CLL was recently treated for pyelonephritis, but returned for persistent flank pain and intermittent hematuria despite antibiotic therapy. Coronal contrast-enhanced CT image (**a**) shows multiple rounded, low-attenuation foci centered in the renal cortex which are not continuous with the collecting system more centrally. (**b**) A 55-year-old man with history of autoimmune hepatitis on immunosuppressive medications presented with a diffuse, painful, erythematous rash. Multimodality evaluation eventually resulted in an MRI to further characterize renal lesions seen on ultrasound. Axial diffusion-weighted MRI in another patient shows numerous foci of restricted diffusion in the periphery of both kidneys (arrows) compatible with microabscesses

8.3.5 Opportunistic and Human Immunodeficiency Virus–Related Renal Conditions

HIV can affect every organ system in the body, either via the virus directly, from the opportunistic infections and malignancies for which HIV patients are at increased risk, or from side effects of HIV therapy. HIV-associated nephropathy is a glomerulopathy caused directly by HIV. In the ED setting, this can result in renal failure, which prevents the use of intravenous contrast material in many of these patients. Kidneys affected by HIV nephropathy appear enlarged at imaging, with markedly echogenic renal cortex on US, a striated pattern of enhancement at CECT, and loss of corticomedullary differentiation on MR. Imaging findings are nonspecific and the definitive diagnosis can only be made histologically.

Patients with AIDS or other forms of significant immunosuppression are susceptible to opportunistic infections from organisms including *Pneumocystis jirovecii* and candida, aspergillus, and mycobacterial species. *P. jirovecii* is the most common opportunistic infection in patients with HIV and is typically seen when CD4 counts are lower than 200. Renal involvement is uncommon and is almost always associated with *Pneumocystis* pneumonia. Renal infection may show multiple hyperechoic foci in the cortex and medulla on US, eventually leading to punctate cortical calcifications in the later phase, although the appearance is not specific [41]. Disseminated fungal infections can occur in immunosuppressed patients of any cause and can result in microabscesses in the kidneys (Fig. 8.10). These manifest as hypoechoic foci on US, low-attenuation, hypoenhancing foci on CT, and are often associated with collecting system dilatation. MR findings are similar to CECT, showing multiple foci of poor enhancement, collecting system dilatation, and heterogeneous signal on T2-weighted images. Fungus balls (mycetomas) can develop in the renal collecting systems and ureters, causing obstruction, and manifesting as filling defects on all modalities. In mycobacterial infection, the renal tract is the second most commonly affected site, usually due to disseminated pulmonary tuberculosis. Disseminated tuberculosis has a similar appearance in the acute phase to disseminated fungal infections, resulting in hypoechoic, hypoattenuating, hypoenhancing multifocal abscesses that may have thick walls. In the chronic phase, the kidneys may become scarred, shrunken, and calcified. Stricturing of any portion of the collecting system or ureter may occur.

Multifocal infections need to be differentiated from renal and perirenal neoplasms, which are also common in patients infected with HIV, especially high-grade non-Hodgkin's lymphoma. Patients undergoing therapy with highly activate antiretroviral medications have an increased incidence of urolithiasis and can present with acute urinary tract obstruction and flank pain. As previously mentioned, these calculi are composed of drug crystals and may not be hyperattenuating.

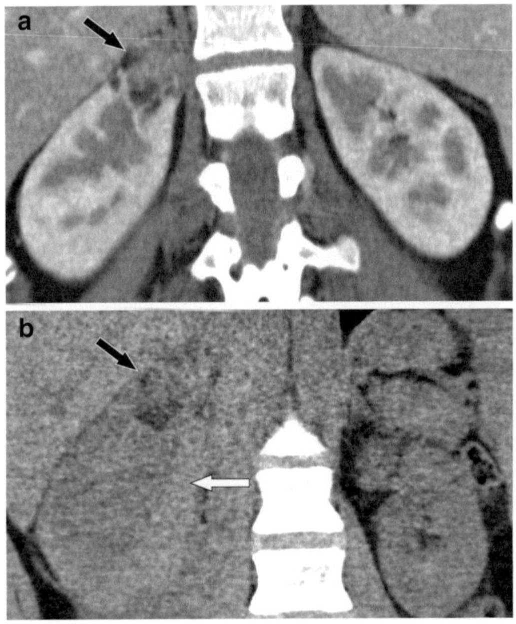

Fig. 8.11 *Hemorrhage into an underlying renal mass.* Prior to acute presentation, this patient had a known angiomyolipoma in the right upper pole (**a**, arrow). The patient presented with acute right flank pain, and noncontrast CT (**b**) revealed that the angiomyolipoma (black arrow) had bled. Blood product fill much of the right pararenal space (white arrow)

8.4 Renal Masses Presenting Urgently

Renal masses are often incidentally discovered when imaging the abdomen for other reasons or can present acutely with complications such as hemorrhage. Spontaneous (nontraumatic) renal hemorrhage may occur due to a number of causes but is usually the result of a ruptured tumor, most commonly a renal cell carcinoma, a simple renal cyst, or an angiomyolipoma (Fig. 8.11). A renal hematoma occurring after minimal trauma should raise suspicion of a pre-existing renal cyst. Spontaneous hemorrhage occurs more commonly in angiomyolipomas, benign fat-containing renal tumors. Large angiomyolipomas (>4 cm) are at much higher risk for spontaneous rupture and may lead to exsanguination, and it is recommended that these patients undergo prophylactic transarterial embolization [42, 43].

Incidentally discovered renal masses should be described and appropriate recommendations for follow-up made. Cystic masses should be graded and followed according to the Bosniak designation. A solid mass containing macroscopic fat without calcification is diagnostic of a benign angiomyolipoma and does not need active follow-up although the size should be included in the report due to the risk of hemorrhage in larger masses. Solid, enhancing masses in an adult must be regarded as renal cell carcinoma until proven otherwise. One problem in the emergency setting is that examinations are typically obtained in a single post-contrast phase, which makes it impossible to determine whether a mass is truly enhancing or simply hyperdense. The growing availability of DECT provides a solution to this problem. DECT can be used to create virtual noncontrast images, which allows the radiologist to

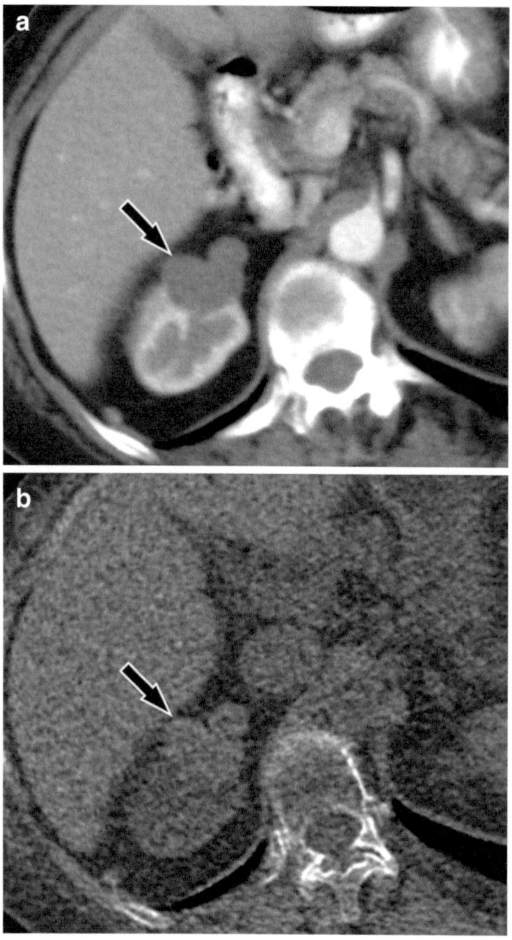

Fig. 8.12 *Dual-energy CT for mass characterization.* Corticomedullary phase axial CT image (**a**) shows a lobulated right renal mass (arrow), which measures greater than simple fluid attenuation, 55 HU. The examination was performed as a dual energy examination, allowing creation of an iodine-subtracted, virtual noncontrast image (**b**) which now shows an attenuation of 45 HU in this mass. The lesion is therefore nonenhancing, compatible with a hemorrhagic or proteinaceous cyst, and does not require follow-up. *Case courtesy of Dr. Ravi Kaza*

determine whether a renal mass is a benign hyperdense cyst or a solid, enhancing mass (Fig. 8.12) [44, 45].

Conclusion

A wide range of renal conditions can prompt emergency imaging, including obstructive, infectious, and inflammatory causes. Clinical management varies from emergent intervention to medical treatment or observation, depending on the cause. Familiarity with the clinical presentation and imaging manifestations of these conditions is vital to expedite appropriate patient management. CT and US are the primary imaging modalities for renal emergencies, with dual-energy CT increasingly used as a problem-solving tool.

References

1. Pearle MS, Calhoun EA, Curhan GC. Urologic diseases in America project: urolithiasis. J Urol. 2005; 173(3):848–57.
2. Scales CD Jr, Curtis LH, Norris RD, et al. Changing gender prevalence of stone disease. J Urol. 2007;177(3):979–82.
3. Bartoletti R, Cai T, Mondaini N, et al. Epidemiology and risk factors in urolithiasis. Urol Int. 2007;79 (Suppl 1):3–7.
4. Bihl G, Meyers A. Recurrent renal stone disease-advances in pathogenesis and clinical management. Lancet. 2001;358(9282):651–6.
5. Coe FL, Parks JH, Asplin JR. The pathogenesis and treatment of kidney stones. N Engl J Med. 1992;327(16):1141–52.
6. Kielar AZ, Shabana W, Vakili M, et al. Prospective evaluation of Doppler sonography to detect the twinkling artifact versus unenhanced computed tomography for identifying urinary tract calculi. J Ultrasound Med. 2012;31(10):1619–25.
7. Masch WR, Cohan RH, Ellis JH, et al. Clinical effectiveness of prospectively reported sonographic twinkling artifact for the diagnosis of renal calculus in patients without known urolithiasis. AJR Am J Roentgenol. 2016;206(2):326–31.
8. Moesbergen TC, de Ryke RJ, Dunbar S, et al. Distal ureteral calculi: US follow-up. Radiology. 2011;260(2):575–80.
9. Ripolles T, Martinez-Perez MJ, Vizuete J, et al. Sonographic diagnosis of symptomatic ureteral calculi: usefulness of the twinkling artifact. Abdom Imaging. 2013;38(4):863–9.
10. Cheng PM, Moin P, Dunn MD, et al. What the radiologist needs to know about urolithiasis: part 1—pathogenesis, types, assessment, and variant anatomy. AJR Am J Roentgenol. 2012;198(6):W540–7.
11. Van Arsdalen KN. Pathogenesis of renal calculi. Urol Radiol. 1984;6(2):65–73.
12. Garcia Marchinena P, Billordo Peres N, Liyo J, et al. CT scan as a predictor of composition and fragility of urinary lithiasis treated with extracorporeal shock wave lithotripsy in vitro. Arch Esp Urol. 2009;62(3):215–22. discussion 22
13. Guest AR, Cohan RH, Korobkin M, et al. Assessment of the clinical utility of the rim and comet-tail signs in differentiating ureteral stones from phleboliths. AJR Am J Roentgenol. 2001;177(6):1285–91.

14. Traubici J, Neitlich JD, Smith RC. Distinguishing pelvic phleboliths from distal ureteral stones on routine unenhanced helical CT: is there a radiolucent center? AJR Am J Roentgenol. 1999;172(1):13–7.
15. Marcovich R, Smith AD. Renal pelvic stones: choosing shock wave lithotripsy or percutaneous nephrolithotomy. Int Braz J Urol. 2003;29(3):195–207.
16. Massoud AM, Abdelbary AM, Al-Dessoukey AA, et al. The success of extracorporeal shock-wave lithotripsy based on the stone-attenuation value from non-contrast computed tomography. Arab J Urol. 2014;12(2):155–61.
17. Williams JC Jr, Saw KC, Paterson RF, et al. Variability of renal stone fragility in shock wave lithotripsy. Urology. 2003;61(6):1092–6. discussion 7
18. Acharya S, Goyal A, Bhalla AS, et al. vivo characterization of urinary calculi on dual-energy CT: going a step ahead with sub-differentiation of calcium stones. Acta Radiol. 2015;56(7):881–9.
19. Duan X, Li Z, Yu L, et al. Characterization of urinary stone composition by use of third-generation dual-source dual-energy CT with increased spectral separation. AJR Am J Roentgenol. 2015;205(6):1203–7.
20. Fung GS, Kawamoto S, Matlaga BR, et al. Differentiation of kidney stones using dual-energy CT with and without a tin filter. AJR Am J Roentgenol. 2012;198(6):1380–6.
21. Hidas G, Eliahou R, Duvdevani M, et al. Determination of renal stone composition with dual-energy CT: in vivo analysis and comparison with X-ray diffraction. Radiology. 2010;257(2):394–401.
22. Li XH, Zhao R, Liu B, et al. Determination of urinary stone composition using dual-energy spectral CT: initial in vitro analysis. Clin Radiol. 2013;68(7):e370–7.
23. Spek A, Strittmatter F, Graser A, et al. Dual energy can accurately differentiate uric acid-containing urinary calculi from calcium stones. World J Urol. 2016;34(9):1297–302.
24. Stolzmann P, Kozomara M, Chuck N, et al. vivo identification of uric acid stones with dual-energy CT: diagnostic performance evaluation in patients. Abdom Imaging. 2010;35(5):629–35.
25. Thomas C, Patschan O, Ketelsen D, et al. Dual-energy CT for the characterization of urinary calculi: in vitro and in vivo evaluation of a low-dose scanning protocol. Eur Radiol. 2009;19(6):1553–9.
26. Zhang GM, Sun H, Xue HD, et al. Prospective prediction of the major component of urinary stone composition with dual-source dual-energy CT in vivo. Clin Radiol. 2016;71(11):1178–83.
27. Czaja CA, Scholes D, Hooton TM, et al. Population-based epidemiologic analysis of acute pyelonephritis. Clin Infect Dis. 2007;45(3):273–80.
28. Hooton TM. The current management strategies for community-acquired urinary tract infection. Infect Dis Clin North Am. 2003;17(2):303–32.
29. June CH, Browning MD, Smith LP, et al. Ultrasonography and computed tomography in severe urinary tract infection. Arch Intern Med. 1985;145(5):841–5.
30. Vourganti S, Agarwal PK, Bodner DR, et al. Ultrasonographic evaluation of renal infections. Radiol Clin North Am. 2006;44(6):763–75.
31. Chan JH, Tsui EY, Luk SH, et al. MR diffusion-weighted imaging of kidney: differentiation between hydronephrosis and pyonephrosis. Clin Imaging. 2001;25(2):110–3.
32. Cova M, Squillaci E, Stacul F, et al. Diffusion-weighted MRI in the evaluation of renal lesions: preliminary results. Br J Radiol. 2004;77(922):851–7.
33. Falagas ME, Alexiou VG, Giannopoulou KP, et al. Risk factors for mortality in patients with emphysematous pyelonephritis: a meta-analysis. J Urol. 2007;178(3 Pt 1):880–5. quiz 1129
34. Huang JJ, Tseng CC. Emphysematous pyelonephritis: clinicoradiological classification, management, prognosis, and pathogenesis. Arch Intern Med. 2000;160(6):797–805.
35. Wan YL, Lo SK, Bullard MJ, et al. Predictors of outcome in emphysematous pyelonephritis. J Urol. 1998;159(2):369–73.
36. Wan YL, Lee TY, Bullard MJ, et al. Acute gas-producing bacterial renal infection: correlation between imaging findings and clinical outcome. Radiology. 1996;198(2):433–8.
37. Chen MT, Huang CN, Chou YH, et al. Percutaneous drainage in the treatment of emphysematous pyelonephritis: 10-year experience. J Urol. 1997;157(5):1569–73.
38. Kangjam SM, Irom KS, Khumallambam IS, et al. Role of conservative management in emphysematous pyelonephritis—a retrospective study. J Clin Diagn Res. 2015;9(11):PC09–11.
39. Tsu JH, Chan CK, Chu RW, et al. Emphysematous pyelonephritis: an 8-year retrospective review across four acute hospitals. Asian J Surg. 2013;36(3):121–5.
40. Craig WD, Wagner BJ, Travis MD. Pyelonephritis: radiologic-pathologic review. Radiographics. 2008;28(1):255–77. quiz 327-8
41. Symeonidou C, Standish R, Sahdev A, et al. Imaging and histopathologic features of HIV-related renal disease. Radiographics. 2008;28(5):1339–54.
42. Oesterling JE, Fishman EK, Goldman SM, et al. The management of renal angiomyolipoma. J Urol. 1986;135(6):1121–4.
43. Sooriakumaran P, Gibbs P, Coughlin G, et al. Angiomyolipomata: challenges, solutions, and future prospects based on over 100 cases treated. BJU Int. 2010;105(1):101–6.
44. Chandarana H, Megibow AJ, Cohen BA, et al. Iodine quantification with dual-energy CT: phantom study and preliminary experience with renal masses. AJR Am J Roentgenol. 2011;196(6):W693–700.
45. Kaza RK, Platt JF. Renal applications of dual-energy CT. Abdom Radiol (NY). 2016;41(6):1122–32.

9 Vascular Emergencies of the Retroperitoneum: Recent Advances in MDCT and Interventional Radiology

Anna Maria Ierardi, Francesca Iacobellis, Gianpaolo Carrafiello, Filippo Pesapane, Refky Nicola, and Mariano Scaglione

Abstract

Vascular emergencies of the retroperitoneum can arise from traumatic or nontraumatic arterial or venous injuries. Advances in interventional radiology technique have permitted less invasive alternative treatments to surgery for the management of aortic and inferior vena cava acute injuries. In this chapter, the MDCT findings of large-vessel vascular emergencies within the retroperitoneum are discussed, with correlative interventional findings and treatment.

Keywords

Vascular trauma · Vascular emergencies Retroperitoneal bleeding · Intramural hematoma · Pseudoaneurysm · Aortic aneurysm Artero-venous fistula · Aorto-caval fistula Aorto-enteric fistula · Inferior vena cava thrombosis

9.1 Introduction

Vascular emergencies of the retroperitoneum can arise from either traumatic or nontraumatic arterial or venous injuries. In patients with high-energy blunt polytrauma, vascular injuries are the second most common cause of death [1–3], so their identification is crucial for patient survival [4]. Vascular emergencies can occur spontaneously, particularly ruptured abdominal aortic aneurysm (AAA). The ruptured abdominal aortic aneurysm is one of the most serious emergencies, with a high morbidity and mortality rate.

The management of retroperitoneal vascular emergencies is challenging and requires a multidisciplinary approach. Advances in interventional radiology techniques allow a less invasive treatment as an alternative to surgery for the management of aortic, inferior vena cava, other retroperitoneal central vascular acute injuries, and other related conditions.

A. M. Ierardi • G. Carrafiello • F. Pesapane
Diagnostic and Interventional Radiology Department, University of Milan, San Paolo Hospital, Milan, Italy

F. Iacobellis
Department of Diagnostic Imaging, "Pineta Grande" Hospital, Castel Volturno, Caserta, Italy

Department of Radiology, University of Campania "L. Vanvitelli", Naples, Italy

R. Nicola
Department of Radiology, University of Massachusetts, Memorial Medical Center, Worcester, MA, USA

M. Scaglione (✉)
Department of Diagnostic Imaging, "Pineta Grande" Hospital, Castel Volturno, Caserta, Italy

Department of Radiology, City Hospitals Sunderland, NHS Foundation Trust, Sunderland, UK

M. Patlas et al. (eds.), *MDCT and MR Imaging of Acute Abdomen*,
https://doi.org/10.1007/978-3-319-70778-5_9

In this chapter, the MDCT findings of large-vessel emergencies of the retroperitoneum are discussed, with correlative interventional radiology findings and treatment.

9.2 Multidetector CT (MDCT) Diagnosis

MDCT with intravenous contrast is the primary imaging modality for the assessment of suspected vascular injuries and other related acute conditions, to assess whether medical, interventional, or surgical management is necessary [4].

9.2.1 MDCT Protocol

The MDCT protocol includes two acquisitions. The arterial phase is acquired after the injection of 100–120 mL of iodinated intravenous (iv) contrast medium (cm) injected at 4–5 mL/s. In our practice, this is followed by 40 mL of saline chaser at the same flow rate. Automated bolus tracking is used, with a region of interest placed in the aortic arch at an attenuation threshold of 100 HU. To evaluate the aorto-iliac axis and the central venous vessels in their entire length, the venous phase is acquired at a 60–70 s delay from the end of the injection.

The examination is supervised by a consultant radiologist, who reviews the images before the patient leaves the CT scanner.

Three-dimensional multiplanar reformation (MPR) and maximum intensity projection (MIP) images are also obtained to display the anatomy, including anatomic variants.

9.3 Traumatic Vascular Emergencies

9.3.1 Trauma Mechanisms

Arterial injuries are caused by either blunt or penetrating trauma.

Blunt traumatic aortic injuries arise from sudden stretching mechanism of the vessels on a fixed axis [4]. Blunt traumatic abdominal aortic injury is an uncommon occurrence and is typically associated with other abdominal injuries [5, 6]. The severity of injury varies from a simple subtle intimal flap to a complete transection [7] and may arise from direct trauma to the abdominal aorta (e.g., a seat belt injury) or from indirect forces transmitted to the aorta through contiguous organs [6, 7]. Also, visceral branches may be involved, including the renal, mesenteric, and iliac arteries [8], the latter of which are associated with pelvic fractures [6] (Fig. 9.1).

Penetrating trauma involving the great vessels of the retroperitoneum is caused by a stab wound to the back, flank, or more commonly due to a gunshot wound [9]. The mechanism of injury, the velocity of the object, and the trajectory can all be used to predict the severity of injury [9]. MDCT is useful for assessing the course of the penetrating injury. It also offers valuable information on the location and extent of the injured vessel, as well as on associated parenchymal and other injuries [10]. Large arterial vascular injuries due to penetrating trauma are associated with pseudoaneurysms and/or active contrast extravasation [6, 11] (Fig. 9.1). According to Azizzadeh et al. [12], traumatic aortic injuries are classified into four degrees of severity: grade I (intimal tear), grade II (intramural hematoma), grade III (pseudoaneurysm), and grade IV (rupture).

9.3.2 Management

The management of retroperitoneal vascular trauma, especially in the emergency setting, is challenging and requires a multidisciplinary approach [13].

Within the past decade, endovascular techniques performed by interventional radiologists have become an alternative to surgery at many level-1 trauma centers [14].

Regardless of the etiology of the retroperitoneal bleeding (RB), all patients should initially be managed in an intensive care unit, with careful monitoring, fluid resuscitation, blood transfusion, and normalization of coagulation factors [15]. There are no specific guidelines to suggest when

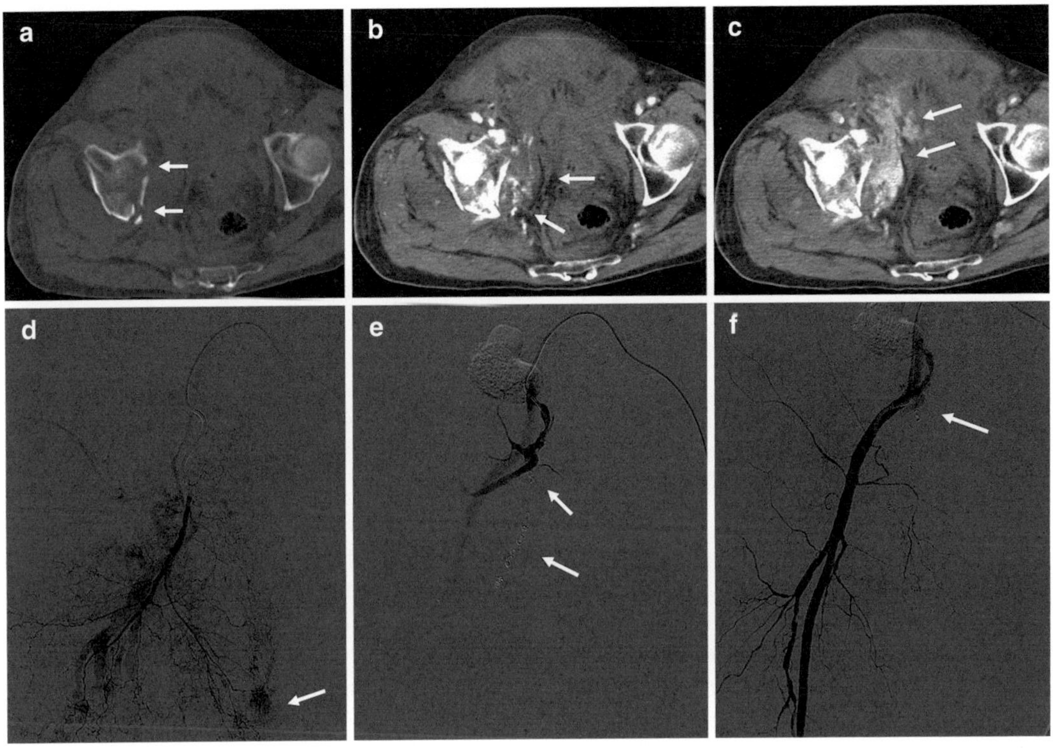

Fig. 9.1 Active arterial bleeding in the obturator region related to pelvic trauma treated with endovascular embolization, in an 81-year-old man. (**a**) Axial nonenhanced CT image showing acetabular fracture (arrows); (**b**) axial IV contrast-enhanced CT image in the arterial phase showing a hematoma adjacent to the acetabular fracture, with active bleeding (arrows); (**c**) axial IV contrast-enhanced CT image in the venous phase showing an increase of the hemorrhage due to obturator artery injury (arrows); (**d**) selective angiogram of the right internal iliac artery showing active extravasation of contrast from the distal branches of right obturator artery (arrow); (**e**) superselective embolization of the bleeding vessel with multiple steel coils (3-mm diamond-shaped), followed by gelfoam suspension embolization (arrow); (**f**) postprocedural selective angiogram of the right internal iliac artery, showing complete exclusion of bleeding (arrow). *Fig. 1 is reprinted with permission from Carrafiello G, Mangini M, Ierardi AM, Recaldini C, Cotta E, Piacentino F, Fugazzola C. Vascular Emergencies of the Retroperitoneum. Book chapter in: M. Scaglione* et al., *Emergency Radiology of the Abdomen, Medical Radiology. Diagnostic Imaging Editor: Springer-Verlag Berlin Heidelberg 2012; pp. 189–205*

an endovascular versus surgical intervention is recommended, to our knowledge. However, if the patient is hemodynamically stable without evidence of obvious hemorrhage, nonsurgical management or careful observation should be considered [7].

Currently there is a growing trend in the use of interventional radiology (IR) techniques as an alternative to open surgery in the management of retroperitoneal hemorrhage in trauma patients. The advancement in endovascular techniques over the last few decades has enabled hemostasis to be achieved safely and rapidly, by using several methods including embolization, balloon occlusion, and stent-grafting [15, 16].

Intra-arterial transcatheter embolization (TAE) is being used with increasing frequency in patients whose angiograms show active bleeding sites [17]. Coils are probably the safest agents (Fig. 9.1), but Isokangas and Perala [17] have commented that proximal coiling of the bleeding artery is not sufficient with retroperitoneal hemorrhage, where there is a rich network of collateral arteries, and new arterial pathways may develop after obliteration of the lumbar arteries. It is critical to place embolic agents both proximally and distally relative to the bleeding site, to prevent re-occurrence of hemorrhage. The indications for embolization are based on the hemodynamic stability of the patient and the extent of hemorrhage [7].

These advancements have become a useful adjunct in the treatment of persistent or recurrent bleeding and have also been used as a primary therapeutic approach in selected patients [18].

9.3.3 Arterial Injuries

9.3.3.1 Intimal Tear

Intimal disruption is one of the most common types of blunt aortic injuries detected in patients with blunt trauma [6]. It is due to an injury of the intima, while the media and adventitia remain intact, so a focal detachment of the internal aortic layer occurs [4]. The intimal flap, dissected by the blood flow, may lead to thrombosis [6] due to the exposure of thrombotic subintimal factors, or can progress into a complete vessel dissection [4].

On MDCT, an intimal tear is identified as a linear endoluminal defect connected with the inner layer of the aortic wall [4, 7]. If the intimal flap measures less than 10 mm, conservative management is usually performed, and short-term follow-up imaging is indicated [4, 5]. If the flap evolves into a dissection, endovascular intervention is recommended.

9.3.3.2 IR Management

Appropriate management of traumatic aortic dissection isolated to the abdomen is not well defined to our knowledge [15]. The failure of a nonoperative approach to this condition suggests that disease progression may be inevitable [15]. Some authors suggest that all traumatic abdominal aortic injuries should be treated either by endovascular stenting, if feasible, or by conventional prosthetic graft replacement in selected patients [19]. In comparison with spontaneous abdominal aortic dissection, which will be described later in the chapter, the surgical mortality is higher in trauma because of associated retroperitoneal venous injury and sepsis [20, 21]. Emergency surgery is recommended when medically uncontrolled hemodynamic shock, lower limb acute ischemia, proven ischemic medullar paraplegia, or tortuous iliac arteries are present [19].

Excluding these conditions, IR techniques provide a less invasive alternative [16]. Several studies [22–26] provide encouraging results with regard to IR treatment of acute traumatic dissection of the retroperitoneal aorta, especially in the inferior inframesenteric segment. Nevertheless, the potential complexity of the entry-re-entry scenario, and the risk of aortic wall injury, may require immediate laparotomy [27].

Deployment of an endoluminal stent-graft in a dissected abdominal aorta is challenging and has a high morbidity. Most of the problems occur from the anatomical variability, where the dissection flap can propagate distally [28]. As a result, the true and false lumens may appear in complex configurations, and the branch vessel origins may be distributed in unpredictable patterns, occasionally in association with life-threatening ischemia of the viscera and extremities. It is imperative to locate the primary entry tear, as aortic rupture is most frequent cause of death in patients with abdominal aortic dissection [29, 30].

In 1995, Peterson et al. [8] and Nishimura et al. [24] successfully treated an aortic dissection by percutaneous balloon fenestration followed by stent placement. In both patients, lower limb ischemia was relieved, and a 2-year follow-up did not reveal any abnormality. Later, Berthet et al. [19] published their results of small series of patients with traumatic abdominal aortic dissection who were treated using endovascular techniques by percutaneous stent placement. No deaths were related to the aortic dissection or its treatment, and no patient underwent endovascular fenestration. The authors proposed that isolated fenestration only treats the ischemic consequences of the dissection without treating the cause; however, this is useful when the dissection extends above the renal arteries.

The placement of an aortic stent within the dissection is an alternative to fenestration, and experimental studies [31, 32] have demonstrated that stenting is more efficient if stents are inserted at the site of the intimal tear and cover the entire dissected lumen.

IR treatment could be the first therapeutic option for the following reasons:

- endovascular approach may be performed immediately after closure of a laparotomy for septic injuries [19]
- a less invasive technique avoids aortic cross-clamping and retroperitoneal dissection [19]
- the limited length of dissection is a characteristic feature of aortic injuries, making it easier to cover the whole dissection by stenting [23]
- the use of short stent-grafts and deployment far from the T8 to L2 vertebrae further minimize the risk of paraplegia, as compared with the risk of surgical aortic replacement and graft interposition [29, 30]

Endoluminal stent placement is a faster method than conventional surgery because it avoids the need for circulatory arrest and cross-clamping of the aorta, and the associated ischemia and reperfusion injury [28].

9.3.3.3 Intramural Hematoma

Intramural hematoma of the abdominal aorta may be due to blunt trauma, and arises from a minimal intimal tear causing bleeding in the media tunic of the vessel wall [4, 34]. The sensitivity of MDCT for the depiction of intramural hematoma is high, as it appears as hyperdense mural vessel thickening (Fig. 9.2). On such scans a manual adjustment of the window settings is recommended. Intramural hematoma is needed to treat because it can progress to frank aortic dissection [4, 33, 34].

9.3.3.4 IR Management

Intramural hematoma (IMH) of the aorta is a variant of dissection with no entry or false lumen flow and typically occurs in hypertensive patients with severe atherosclerotic disease [35]. Traumatic IMH of the aorta is a relatively rare, but potentially life-threatening disease. Blunt trauma patients with upper or lower back pain should be considered as possibly having IMH of the descending aorta (IMH—type B) in the emergency department until it is diagnosed or excluded with imaging [36]. Fewer than 10% will resolve spontaneously [37], whereas 16–47% will progress to frank dissection [29]. Mortality may be reduced by early diagnosis and adequate treatment [7].

Indications for endovascular treatment of traumatic IMH depend on symptomatic presentation, diameter increase, pseudoaneurysm formation,

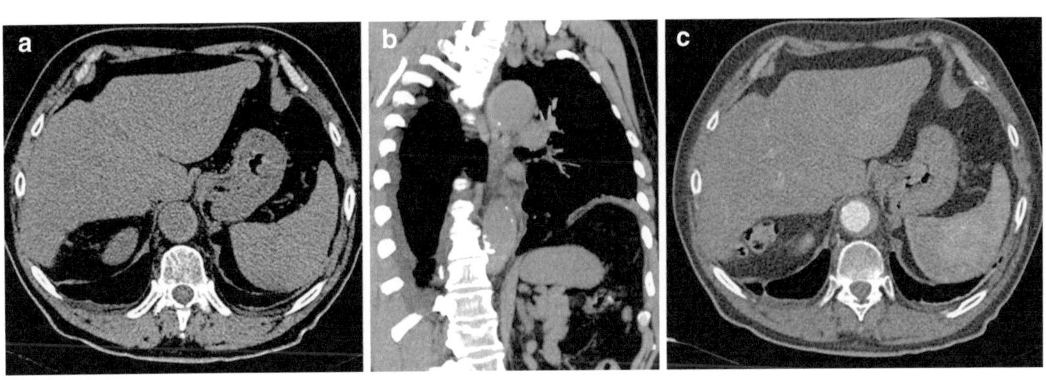

Fig. 9.2 Intramural hematoma following blunt trauma, in a 57-year-old man. Nonenhanced CT images in axial (**a**) and in coronal planes (**b**) show hyperdense mural thickening due to the recent bleeding, extending from the aortic arch to the abdominal aorta; (**c**) axial IV contrast-enhanced CT image shows that the hematoma does not enhance after contrast administration, and no intimal flap is seen. *Figure 2 is reprinted with permission from Carrafiello G, Mangini M, Ierardi AM, Recaldini C, Cotta E, Piacentino F, Fugazzola C. Vascular Emergencies of the Retroperitoneum. Book chapter in: M. Scaglione* et al., *Emergency Radiology of the Abdomen, Medical Radiology. Diagnostic Imaging Editor: Springer-Verlag Berlin Heidelberg 2012; pp. 189–205*

or progression into acute aortic dissection during follow-up imaging. MDCT can depict the entrance tear, and endovascular aortic repair aims to close the entrance tear, with complete stent-graft coverage of the IMH having the best therapeutic outcome [33, 36].

Most studies describing IMH have looked at small patient populations due to its relative rarity [38, 39]. Thus, the optimal therapy for this condition is still largely unknown to our knowledge [38, 40]. Trauma patients with IMH present with subacute or acute pain, which can progress to aortic dissection and can eventually rupture. Dilatation of 60 mm and above should undergo surgical treatment [41]. Uncomplicated IMH is treated conservatively with blood pressure regulation and serial MDCT scans [42, 43]. Uncomplicated stable patients with retroperitoneal IMH can be treated using endovascular techniques [44, 45]. In a study [46] which compared early medical therapy with medical plus IR treatment in IMH complicated by intimal tear, at a mean follow-up of 17.6 months, 10 of 11 medically treated patients demonstrated regression, and 5 of these patients (45%) had complete resolution of their IMH. All those treated with endovascular management had resolution. Song et al. compared medical therapy with endovascular therapy in 56 patients with IMH with a thickness more than 10 mm, or with sustained chest or back pain despite maximal medical therapy. The technical success was 100%, with no progression or mortality [47].

9.3.3.5 Pseudoaneurysms

A pseudoaneurysm is false aneurysm due to the disruption of the arterial wall layer, in which the blood flow is only contained by the connective tissue surrounding the vessel [34].

On MDCT, a pseudoaneurysm is an outpouching of the arterial wall, which is well defined, with endoluminal enhancement synchronous with those of the other arterial vessels. They may occur at the aorta or may involve other splanchnic arterial vessels due to blunt or penetrating trauma. They can also occur as a sequela of prior injury [48]. The majority of blunt trauma pseudoaneurysms occur in the thoracic aorta. Post-traumatic aortic pseudoaneurysm in the abdomen is very uncommon. Post-traumatic abdominal aortic pseudoaneurysm occurs due to penetrating injury of the upper abdomen, such as from a gunshot or knife wound [11]. Multiphasic CT is helpful for correct identification, and to distinguish them from active bleeding, as a pseudoaneurysm does not change its shape and decreases in attenuation value on delayed scans, and is isodense to the arterial structures [4, 49]. Pseudoaneurysms need to be treated because several complications can occur, including rupture, fistula, mass effect upon the surrounding structures, infection, or thromboembolic events. The most severe and most common complication is rupture due to increase of the endoluminal pressure [31, 51].

9.3.3.6 IR Management

Traumatic aortic pseudoaneurysm is a potentially lethal condition [52–54]. Advances in endovascular techniques have provided options to treat traumatic pseudoaneurysms of the abdominal aorta and have led to a marked decrease in the morbidity and mortality rates [52]. A complete work-up to determine the location of the pseudoaneurysm and to evaluate surrounding structures and relevant vascular anatomy is essential for treatment, which should be tailored to the site, rupture risk, and clinical setting of the pseudoaneurysm, as well as to patient comorbidities [55]. IR management serves to exclude a pseudoaneurysm from the circulation and has the advantage of accessibility to most locations of the arterial system, without the potential morbidity of open surgical repair. Baltacioglu et al. [56] reported 100% technical success in the treatment of 17 retroperitoneal pseudoaneurysms with covered stents.

Selecting the optimal method depends on the size of the pseudoaneurysm neck and the expendability of the donor artery [57]. There are several visceral arteries which have a well-established collateral supply, including the gastroduodenal, hepatic, and splenic arteries, and other upper gastrointestinal arteries [55]. When embolizing arteries with numerous collateral vessels, one must embolize both proximal and distal to the pseudoaneurysm, to completely exclude it from the circulation, by preventing backflow from the collateral circulation [57]. A pseudoaneurysm arising from an inexpendable donor artery must be excluded from the circulation, while preserving the donor artery [55]. The width of the pseudoaneurysm neck relative to the diameter of the donor artery is the determining factor in the method used. A vital donor artery may be embolized in certain emergent situations (e.g., rupture with active bleeding) [55]. If the neck is narrow, the pseudoaneurysm may be embolized with catheter-directed delivery of coils (the preferred embolization material) into the sac itself [55].

In IR, coils fall into two main categories: nondetachable and detachable [55]. The nondetachable coils reassume their shape immediately after deployment from the catheter. These coils are available in a wide array of diameters and lengths. They are made of either stainless steel or, more recently, of platinum, which allows them to be softer and have a more complex (helical) shape. Consequently, such coils conform to the shape of and fill the pseudoaneurysm sac, so fewer coils are needed for the embolization [55]. However, because platinum coils are softer, initial placement of stainless steel coils may be required to act as a scaffolding. Detachable coils are held to the pusher guide wire by either a mechanical or an electrochemically dissolvable connection, which is released to deploy the coil [55]. This facilitates more accurate deployment and the possibility of readjusting the position of the coil before its final deployment [55]. A disadvantage of using coils as an embolization material is the potential for recanalization of the embolized sac, if the coils are not tightly packed [55]. However, this drawback has been largely overcome with the use of soft helical coils, which may be tightly packed in the pseudoaneurysm sac [58]. Agents such as thrombin or N-butyl 2-cyanoacrylate (glue) may also be used, either alone or in addition to coils [57, 59]. Moreover, if the neck is wide, the pseudoaneurysm can still be embolized with catheter-directed delivery of embolization materials, but remodeling is required to prevent outflow of these materials into and distal embolization of the donor artery, and to ensure adequate embolization of the pseudoaneurysm sac [55]. This remodeling may be performed with the use of a stent cage, or by trapping the coils by means of temporary balloon occlusion of the donor artery between coil deployments [60]. If distal arterial embolization is a concern, detachable balloons may be used as the embolic agent [61]. Another option, if the pseudoaneurysm neck is wide, is stent-graft placement across the neck to exclude the pseudoaneurysm [60], although this procedure requires a higher profile and a stiffer delivery system than does catheter-directed coil embolization. As a result, the arterial anatomy and the caliber of the arteries leading to and at the pseudoaneurysm site should be favorable (i.e., reduced arterial tortuosity and large-diameter arteries). An additional reason for placing stent-grafts only in larger arteries is that in small arteries they pose a higher risk of thrombosis [55]. Visceral pseudoaneurysms, which are usually smaller and located off small and tortuous donor arteries, pose a particular challenge for stent-graft placement.

Endovascular techniques have a lower complication rate for the treatment of visceral pseudoaneurysms than surgical management [59, 61]. The main complication of IR techniques is intraprocedural rupture of the pseudoaneurysm [62]. Rare cases of recanalization of the embolized vessel and reconstitution of arterial flow to the pseudoaneurysm have also been reported [62].

9.3.3.7 Artero-venous Fistula

Penetrating trauma may cause abnormal communications between arteries and veins. In the retroperitoneum, aorto-caval fistulas may be detected following trauma or interventional procedures [63].

At MDCT, these may be seen only if an arterial phase is performed; they appear as early venous opacification in the arterial phase. Furthermore, obliteration of the fat planes between the aorta and the vena cava may be detected and, less commonly, visualization of the abnormal communication may be identified [64]. Small fistulas may be asymptomatic but may enlarge over time, increasing the venous return and causing severe hemodynamic alterations with congestive heart failure [64–66].

9.3.3.8 IR Management

Penetrating injury remains the most common cause of abdominal and pelvic arterio-venous fistulae [67]. Although ACF due to penetrating wounds frequently have a severe acute presentation, iatrogenic fistulae produce less acute symptoms than traumatic and spontaneous aortic or iliac fistulae [7].

Surgical treatment includes repair of the fistula, usually with direct suture and reconstruction of the aortoiliac aneurysm with a dacron graft [68]. Venous bleeding from the sac of the aneurysm can be excessive, and careful and expeditious control of the bleeding using digital compression, sponge sticks, or balloon catheters is imperative. Blood salvage and rapid return of the autologous blood in these patients can be lifesaving [7]. As in other complications of AAA, open surgical repair is associated with high morbidity and mortality, which will be affected by the acute presentation and the preoperative recognition of the ACF. There are considerable difficulties with the open repair of central abdominal fistulae, which are related to the arterialization of venous structures and perivascular inflammation, resulting in an increased risk of substantial blood loss and pulmonary embolization [69].

The significance of this condition in the modern era, where endovascular aortic reconstruction (EVAR) is often performed, is when an ACF is an unexpected finding during open repair of ruptured abdominal aortic aneurysms (rAAA), this is a situation where exsanguinating hemorrhage may occur [69].

Endovascular stent-grafting offers an attractive therapeutic alternative to the open repair of ACF because it does not involve a laparotomy, there is less blood loss, it does not require general anesthesia, and therefore postoperative complication rates and costs are reduced [69]. Boudghene et al. [70] reported successful treatment of ACF with percutaneous stent-grafts in an experimental study in which the ACF was created percutaneously in eight sheep. According to the literature review reported by Antoniou et al. [71] the technical success rate is 96%; however, the mean follow-up was only 9 months, with only one study reporting a follow-up of 24 months. The most common procedure-related complication was a type II endoleak, which was found in 22% of the patients examined, but no standardized imaging modality was used at follow-up. This event was either self-limiting or required minimal percutaneous intervention to correct [71]. Lau et al. [72] summarized that endovascular repair reduces blood loss and may reduce the significant morbidity and mortality rates often associated with open surgery. In cases of rAAA with associated ACF, the technique may offer its greatest benefits. From the reported literature, it seems that endovascular repair has a higher success rate with regard to morbidity and mortality, but there is no consistency in patient selection or analysis as to whether these patients were operated on in an emergency setting or electively. In 2009, a new hybrid technique was performed to treat a patient presenting with hemodynamic instability in the context of an acute ACF complicating a large AAA which was unsuitable for standard endovascular repair. Siepe et al. treated this fistula by placing a large covered aortic stent into the inferior vena cava (IVC) [73]. This was successful in reducing central pressures, stabilizing arterial blood pressure, and allowing inotropic support to be weaned. With the patient thus stabilized, standard open surgery on the AAA was performed, without the risk of massive blood loss from the large defect that was noted in the IVC covered by the stent-graft, once the aneurysm sac was opened [73].

9.3.3.9 Bleeding

Active retroperitoneal bleeding (RB) may be seen after blunt or penetrating trauma; it represents an urgent condition that needs to be promptly treated. In blunt trauma, severe injuries to the abdominal aorta are uncommon due to the protected position of the abdominal aorta; the anatomic location of abdominal aortic injury is usually infrarenal. The most frequent sites of injury are at the level of the inferior mesenteric artery (33%), near the renal arteries (24%), and between the inferior mesenteric artery and the bifurcation (19%) [74]. In the arterial phase on CT, a focal disruption with active bleeding of the arterial wall can be detected, with hematoma in the retroperitoneal space. The extraluminal contrast medium extravasation increases, and changes its morphology in the portal venous and late acquisitions. Only occasionally, a transection or disruption of the aorta with exsanguinating hemorrhage may be seen, as these injuries quickly lead to death [6, 11].

9.3.3.10 IR Management

Traumatic RB is a life-threatening condition that requires prompt and accurate diagnosis and treatment [75]. The high morbidity (40–50%) and mortality (5–30%) rates are due to the inability to surgical control of such hemorrhage [7], which can be of arterial, venous, or osseous origin (the latter usually due to a pelvic fracture). Arterial injuries are the most common and the most severe [7].

Surgical exploration and controlling the bleeding vessels are particularly arduous for the retroperitoneum region [17]. Thus, once a bleeding artery is kept under control, collateral supply to the same territory may lead to new hemorrhage [75]. That is why most surgeons avoid exploration of the retroperitoneum in patients with RB [76]. Furthermore, surgery often carries the risk of lethal hemorrhage, by dissection of the retroperitoneal space and loss of passive tamponade of a hematoma [77].

When compared with surgical management, IR procedures are not only safe, fast, and less invasive, but also provide prompt treatment through trans-arterial embolization (TAE) of the bleeding vessel [78] (Fig. 9.3). Currently, therapeutic TAE is becoming increasingly used in the management of traumatic RB, either as definite method or as a surgical adjunct [79]. The efficacy of TAE in the management of RP due to arterial hemorrhage in trauma patients has been demonstrated by Papakostidis et al. [80], who reported a success rate, expressed in terms of hemorrhage control, and reduction in transfusion requirements, ranging from 85% to 100%. Recently, Velmahos et al. reviewed the medical records of 102 consecutive trauma patients who underwent TAE to stop RB, with angiographic and clinical bleeding control in 93 (91%). The

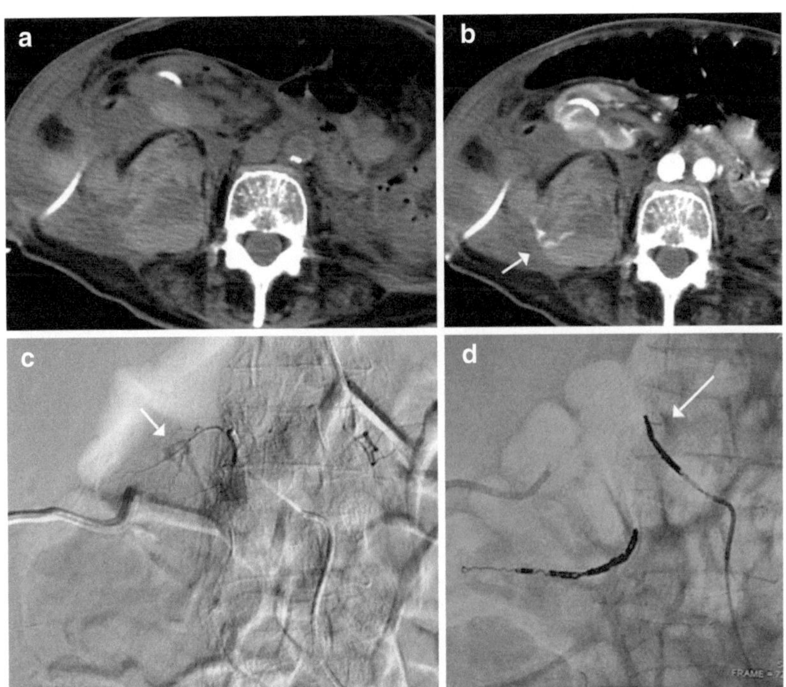

Fig. 9.3 Nonenhanced axial CT image shows retroperitoneal hematoma, in a 45-year-old man (**a**); arterial phase demonstrates active bleeding from a lumbar arterial vessel (**b**, arrow); selective lumbar arteriogram confirms blush (**c**, arrow); postprocedural angiography shows the embolization of the lumbar artery (**d**, arrow)

rate of successful hemostasis by TAE was identical in blunt and penetrating trauma patients. There was no major morbidity after TAE. No factors predicted patients with a high likelihood to have a positive angiogram. Patients who had AE before or after a period of attempted hemodynamic stabilization in the intensive care unit were no different with respect to hemodynamic parameters immediately before TAE or effectiveness of TAE for bleeding control [18]. Selective catheterization and TAE of the bleeding arterial branch should be carried out as quickly as possible, to avoid dangerous delays and complications related to multiple blood transfusions, prolonged hemodynamic compromise, and extensive blood loss [18, 77]. Therefore, timing is of particular importance for TAE, but there is no consensus to our knowledge regarding the best time for embolization [18, 75]. Early TAE may be used in selected patients as a front-line therapeutic intervention that offers expeditious hemostasis and prevents delays in definitive bleeding control [16]. Active RB due to an injury of small distal vessels can be treated by embolization using particles including polyvinylalcohol (150–300 μm), embospheres (300–500 μm), or gelfoam in small segments. Microcoils have to be customized to the vessel diameter [7].

There are a few heterogeneous case series or reports on stent-grafts in the management of RB. Watarida et al. [81] reported the successful use of a fenestrated stent-graft to manage a RB. Traumatic aortic rupture with retroperitoneal hematoma can also be treated with a combined operative and endovascular approach [82]. In conclusion, percutaneous control of RB is a valuable therapeutic option in trauma patient, especially with TAE, which is a rapid, effective, and minimally invasive technique.

9.4 Venous Injuries

Blunt injuries to the central retroperitoneal veins are very unusual and are usually associated with other abdominal injuries. Only a few cases have been reported in the literature of blunt inferior vena cava injuries, to our knowledge [83]. The mortality rate is high, ranging from 34% to 70% [84]. The CT findings depend on the location of the injury. Blunt IVC injuries can be difficult to diagnose, since the contrast material extravasation as direct evidence of vascular injury may be absent, and other extensive parenchymal injury may be associated. Retrohepatic IVC injury is usually associated with extensive liver lacerations into the porta hepatis and retrohepatic IVC region, or an irregular contour of the retrohepatic IVC [85, 86]. Injuries may vary from thrombosis to venous pseudoaneurysm formation, to active bleeding.

9.4.1 Thrombosis

Only a few cases of post-traumatic IVC thrombosis have been reported in the literature, to our knowledge [87]. There are several mechanisms that may be responsible, including endothelial injury of the caval wall with exposure of prothrombotic factors and secondary thrombus formation, caval stasis due to compression by a pericaval/retroperitoneal hematoma, hepatic vein thrombosis extending into the IVC, or a hypercoagulable state after major trauma [87]. The major risk of this condition is pulmonary embolism. Multiphasic MDCT examination represents the technique of choice for diagnostic purpose.

9.4.2 Traumatic Pseudoaneurysm

Similarly to arterial injuries, but much less commonly, veins may develop pseudoaneurysms after blunt or penetrating trauma due to an incomplete wall injury. Symptoms may include abdominal pain, IVC syndrome, tachycardia, upper gastrointestinal bleeding secondary to venobiliary fistulas, hemorrhagic shock secondary to rupture, and pulmonary embolus or other thromboembolic phenomenon secondary to IVC thrombosis [86]. These injuries need to be treated promptly, as they have high risk of a rupture with severe hemorrhage [88].

9.4.3 Bleeding

In IVC injury, active bleeding represents the most severe complication needing prompt treatment. At MDCT, this is evident as active extravasation of intravenous contrast media, vessel contour abnormality, and associated retroperitoneal hematoma [84].

9.5 Nontraumatic Vascular Emergencies

9.5.1 Arterial

Nontraumatic acute aortic syndromes are a spectrum of life-threatening aortic pathologies with significant implications for diagnosis, therapy, and management. There is a common etiology, leading to a breakdown of the aortic intima and media.

The subtypes of aortic syndromes are acute aortic dissection, penetrating atherosclerotic ulcer, and aortic aneurysm, with potential associated complications.

9.5.2 Management

Management of nontraumatic retroperitoneal vascular emergency is both difficult and challenging and requires a multidisciplinary approach. The control of RB can be accomplished by either surgical or endovascular approaches and, in specific circumstances (e.g., spontaneous bleeding), by conservative management. The results of surgical exploration and primary repair in hemodynamically unstable patients are well known [7]. This strategy is associated with a high mortality rate, ranging from 30% to 80%, regardless of the location [7]. The high mortality rate is linked to the opening of the retroperitoneum space, which leads to suppression of the tamponade effect, disruption of the hematoma, and destabilization of patient [16]. Embolization is becoming more common as an alternative to open surgery in the treatment of RB following iatrogenic injuries, procedures including percutaneous lumbar sympathectomy, renal biopsy, and percutaneous nephrostomy, or following iatrogenic iliofemoral vessel injuries [7]. Open surgery is indicated if the patient remains unstable despite adequate fluid and blood product resuscitation, or if IR is either not successful or is unavailable [7].

9.5.2.1 Acute Aortic Dissection

Acute aortic dissection is the most common acute aortic emergency condition. It arises from a separation of the layers of the aortic wall. Due to an intimal tear, the blood flow enters the media; this results in two lumina, a true and a false lumen. Then, pressure may increase in the false lumen, impairing the blood flow in the true lumen and its branches [6, 34, 89] (Fig. 9.4).

MDCT findings of acute aortic dissection are eccentric aortic wall calcification on nonenhanced MDCT, a double aortic lumen, and direct visualization of the media-intima entrance as an intimomedial flap defect on arterial-phase images. In the early angiographic phase, the true lumen appears smaller and more intensely opacified than the false lumen due to higher pressure and faster mixing with blood [6, 89] (Fig. 9.4). The venous phase may help in differentiating between the true lumen and partially thrombosed false lumen. Rarely, a re-entry tear may be identifiable as a small defect in the dissected intimal layer [6, 89].

IR Management

The optimal treatment strategy for patients with aortic dissection confined to the abdominal aorta remains controversial to our knowledge [90]. Despite remarkably improved operative techniques, surgical repair of the abdominal aorta is still associated with high morbidity and mortality [91]. Contemporary operative mortality rates of elective surgery range between 0% and 27%, but may exceed 50% in complicated dissection under emergency conditions [91, 92].

Currently, there is consensus that patients with otherwise uncomplicated abdominal aortic dissection should primarily be treated medically with tight blood pressure control, while reserving operative treatment for evolving complications [93]. Thus, the indications for operative treatment (open or endovascular repair of the abdominal aorta) of acute aortic dissection are basically the

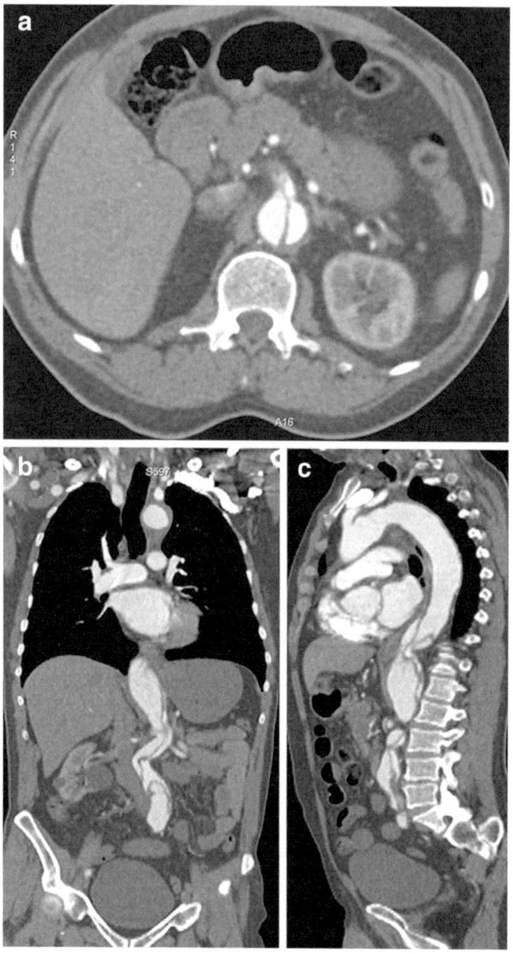

Fig. 9.4 Extensive dissection of the abdominal aorta in a 64-year-old man with abdominal pain. (**a**) IV contrast-enhanced axial CT image in the arterial phase shows the intimal flap of the abdominal aorta at the level of the superior mesenteric artery, with intraluminal thrombosis at the origin; (**b**) coronal and (**c**) sagittal MPR reformations permit better appreciation of the extension of the dissection. *Figure 4 is reprinted with permission from Carrafiello G, Mangini M, Ierardi AM, Recaldini C, Cotta E, Piacentino F, Fugazzola C. Vascular Emergencies of the Retroperitoneum. Book chapter in: M. Scaglione* et al., *Emergency Radiology of the Abdomen, Medical Radiology. Diagnostic Imaging Editor: Springer-Verlag Berlin Heidelberg 2012; pp. 189–205*

same as for IMH [34, 37], and included active rupture, lower extremity ischemia, unremitting pain, associated aortic aneurysm, and prevention of future aneurysm formation.

In 1999, endovascular stent-graft closure of the proximal entry tear was introduced as a new treatment option for patients with type B acute aortic dissection [29, 30]. Aortic remodeling is accomplished by sealing the proximal entry tear, at the same time avoiding the risks associated with open surgery [94]. This rationale was originally based on the clinical observation that patients with spontaneous thrombosis of the false lumen have a better long-term prognosis than those patients without thrombosis [90].

As dissection may extend to the iliac arteries, aorto-bi-femoral grafting is the procedure of choice [95]. Currently, endovascular treatment of isolated dissection has been associated with a high rate of technical and clinical success, with reduced morbidity and mortality rates at experienced institutions [19, 30]. A recent meta-analysis reported 30-day or in-hospital mortality for type B acute aortic dissection of 0–27% (median, 7%) for medical treatment, 13–17% (median, 16%) for open surgical procedures, and 0–18% (median, 6%) for endovascular aortic repair (EVAR) [39]. One study published in 2013 [96] compared 853 patients with medical management for type B dissection to 276 receiving EVAR in a propensity-matched analysis. Although EVAR patients presented with more complications (pulse deficit, malperfusion syndrome, shock, stroke, spinal cord ischemia, visceral ischemia, or renal failure), in-hospital mortality was not different, and 5-year cumulative probability of mortality was lower for EVAR than for medical management (15.5% vs. 29.0%, respectively). In 2005, Eggebrecht et al. [93] published a meta-analysis encompassing 609 type B dissection patients, demonstrating that endovascular stent-graft treatment of acute aortic dissection is feasible and can be performed with technical success rates of 95%. Furthermore, the acute and mid-term survival of about 90% at 2 years following stent-graft placement compares favorably with medically and surgically treated type B acute dissection patients.

Neurologic complications and paraplegia remain the most potential complications of stent-graft placement, as for surgical repair of type B dissection. Eggebrecht et al. showed that the overall risk of neurologic complications with stent-grafting ranged between 2.9% and 3.4%

[93]. The 1% risk of paraplegia appears to be very low, considering that contemporary studies have suggested the risk of paraplegia after surgical repair of the descending thoracic aorta to be between 7% and 36% [91].

Patients undergoing stent-graft placement for acute dissections were found to be at higher risk of death and major complications than those with chronic aortic dissection, regardless of their age [93]. However, it should be recognized that in patients with acute aortic dissection implantation of stent-grafts is often prompted by complications of the dissection, making this patients more prone for higher complications and lower survival when compared with stable patients with chronic disease undergoing elective stent-graft placement [93].

Recent data suggest a strong influence of the interventional radiologists' experience on the results of stent-graft placement [93]. Institutes that reported an overall endovascular experience of more than 20 patients treated with stent-grafts had higher success rates and fewer complications than less experienced centers [93].

Eggebrecht's meta-analysis highlights some technical limitations of endovascular stent-graft placement in abdominal aortic dissection [93]. Stent-grafting fails to abolish the false lumen in about a quarter of patients, suggesting that it perhaps may not be a definitive treatment for type B dissection. Even in the presence of a false lumen's thrombosis, the aorta may enlarge during follow-up. Thus, there is a continued risk of aortic rupture (about 2% during follow-up) after stent-graft placement, and the need for adjunctive stent-graft placement or conversion to open surgery in about 12% of patients over time [93]. Nevertheless, the incidence of aortic rupture and the need of repeat endovascular or surgical interventions may also be related to progression of the disease itself, and may not necessarily reflect treatment failure. This is supported by the fact that 11–20% and 10–44% of the patients with abdominal aortic dissection need repeat surgery when treated medically or surgically, respectively [91].

9.5.2.2 Penetrating Atherosclerotic Ulcer

Penetrating atherosclerotic ulcer (PAU) is an ulceration in an atherosclerotic plaque penetrating the elastic lamina leading to hematoma formation within the media tunic of the aortic wall [7, 33, 89] (Fig. 9.5). Nonenhanced MDCT shows high-density hematoma surrounding the ulceration. At enhanced MDCT, a PAU is seen as a focal contrast filled outpouching of the aortic wall in the setting of an atheroma [34] (Fig. 9.5).

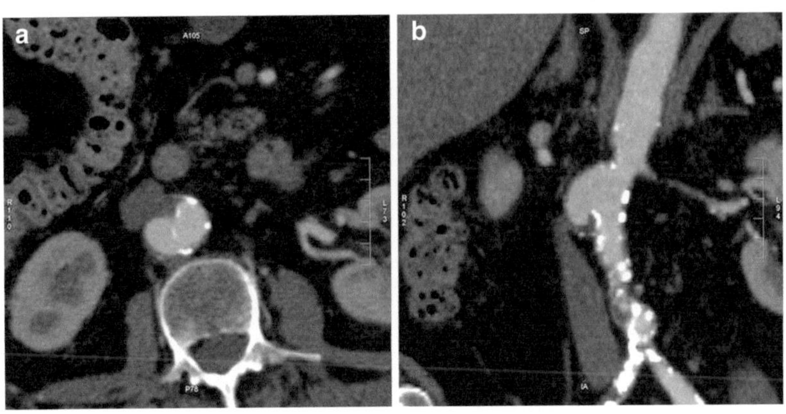

Fig. 9.5 Penetrating atherosclerotic ulcer of the abdominal aorta in a 76-year-old man. IV contrast-enhanced CT scans in the arterial phase in axial (**a**) and coronal planes (**b**) show endoluminal outpouching along the aortic borders, and focal thickening of the aortic wall due to intramural hematoma. *Figure 5 is reprinted with permission from Carrafiello G, Mangini M, Ierardi AM, Recaldini C, Cotta E, Piacentino F, Fugazzola C. Vascular Emergencies of the Retroperitoneum. Book chapter in: M. Scaglione et al., Emergency Radiology of the Abdomen, Medical Radiology. Diagnostic Imaging Editor: Springer-Verlag Berlin Heidelberg 2012; pp. 189–205*

IR Management

Penetrating atherosclerotic ulcers (PAUs) are most often found in patients with severe atherosclerosis, usually elderly patients with several comorbidities [33].

The indications and the techniques of PAUs treatment are still controversial to our knowledge. There is currently no clear cut-off for a PAU diameter (depth) or neck diameter which warrants treatment (in one publication a depth of >20 mm or a neck >10 mm was associated with higher complication rates) [97]. Although some authors believe immediate treatment is not always required [98], as most PAUs have a benign clinical courses, early intervention has been recommended when PAU is complicated by aneurysm expansion, regardless of size, rupture, embolic symptoms, or uncontrolled pain [99]. Open surgical repair with graft interposition has been used traditionally [66], but patients with PAU are generally not ideal candidates for open surgery because of patient age and poor general status [99].

Aortic stent-grafts have changed the management strategy for PAU. This less invasive procedure is suitable for these high-risk patients, and can be useful in cases of rupture [100]. PAUs are ideal for endovascular repair, since there is usually a focal abnormality [100]. If IMH is present, the hematoma may be relatively limited, possibly due to concomitant atherosclerotic lesions causing medial fibrosis of the surrounding aorta and preventing expansion [99]. Stent-grafting of the PAU seals the diseased segment of the aorta, which reduces the wall stress and may decrease the chance of a PAU evolving into a dissection, IMH, or aneurysm [99]. Therefore, endovascular stent-grafting has been developed, and several reports about this technique applied to the treatment of PAU have been published [100, 101]. Open surgical repair of the descending aorta requires clamping of the aorta, a large thoracotomy incision, possible cardiopulmonary bypass, and prolonged mechanical ventilation. Because endovascular surgery generally requires only a femoral or iliac arterial cut down for exposure, short operative times, and no clamping of the aorta, this less invasive procedure has the potential to substantially reduce the morbidity and mortality of definitive surgical correction of PAUs [98]. Between 2003 and 2005, 21 patients with aortic PAUs were treated with Gore TAG endoluminal stent-grafts as part of a single-center investigational device exemption protocol reported by Brinster et al. [98]. Despite the high number of comorbidities and advanced age in this patient population, there was no operative mortality. Postoperative morbidities included one re-operation for an occluded limb of an iliac–femoral bypass graft, but no perioperative myocardial infarctions, strokes, or paraplegias occurred. The use of just one device in 20 (95%) of 21 patients indicates that the focal nature of PAUs is optimal for treatment by endoluminal grafts. Additionally, because there has been a correlation between the length of the descending thoracic aorta covered by stent-grafts and paraplegia rate, the single application of a single graft may have reduced the risk of postoperative neurologic dysfunction. Freedom from end-point treatment failure was 100% [98].

These mid-term results of low morbidity and mortality compare favorably with previously published studies which have examined the use of stent-grafts in the treatment of PAU [100, 102], and indicate the success of EVAR for aorta PAU. The combined success rate approaches 100%, with very low morbidity and mortality compared to the traditional open techniques. PAUs may be uniquely suited for treatment with endovascular grafts in this patient population, by allowing a minimally invasive means to treat a focal anatomic disease.

9.5.2.3 Aortic Aneurysm Rupture

Abdominal aortic aneurysm occurs in 2–9% of the population >65 years. About 80% occur between the renal arteries and the bifurcation [7]; iliac aortic aneurysm is seen in 2–10% of patients with abdominal aortic aneurysm [7, 33, 89]. Most abdominal aortic aneurysms are true aneurysms, with aortic dilation caused by weakening of all the three layers. A true aneurysm involves all three layers (intima, media, and adventitia) of the arterial wall. Ninety percent of all aortic aneurysms are caused by atherosclerotic damage to the aortic wall. Other etiologies include mycotic and inflammatory [7, 34, 89]. In the abdominal aorta, aneurysms are defined by a diameter >30 mm, regardless of the age of the patient [34]. Rupture risk increases with the diameter, with upward of 30–33% risk of rupture for aneurysms larger than 70 mm [34].

Findings at MDCT of impending rupture include:

- size increase more than >10 mm/year
- focal new wall discontinuity of the intimal calcifications
- eccentric shape of the aortic lumen
- penetrating ulcer with intramural hematoma
- periaortic stranding [89] (Fig. 9.6)

The rupture may present as a contained rupture or free rupture. Differentiation between these two conditions is crucial in selecting proper treatment. Most commonly the rupture involves the posterolateral aorta with hemorrhage into the retroperitoneum; if the anterior or anterolateral wall is involved, an intraperitoneal rupture may occur [103]. A retroperitoneal hematoma adjacent to the aortic aneurysm is the most common CT finding of abdominal aortic aneurysm rupture [104]. Another important finding that may be seen in contained rupture is the "draped aorta" sign, where the aorta is draped over and inseparable from adjacent vertebrae [7, 104]. The "crescent sign," a peripheral crescent of increased

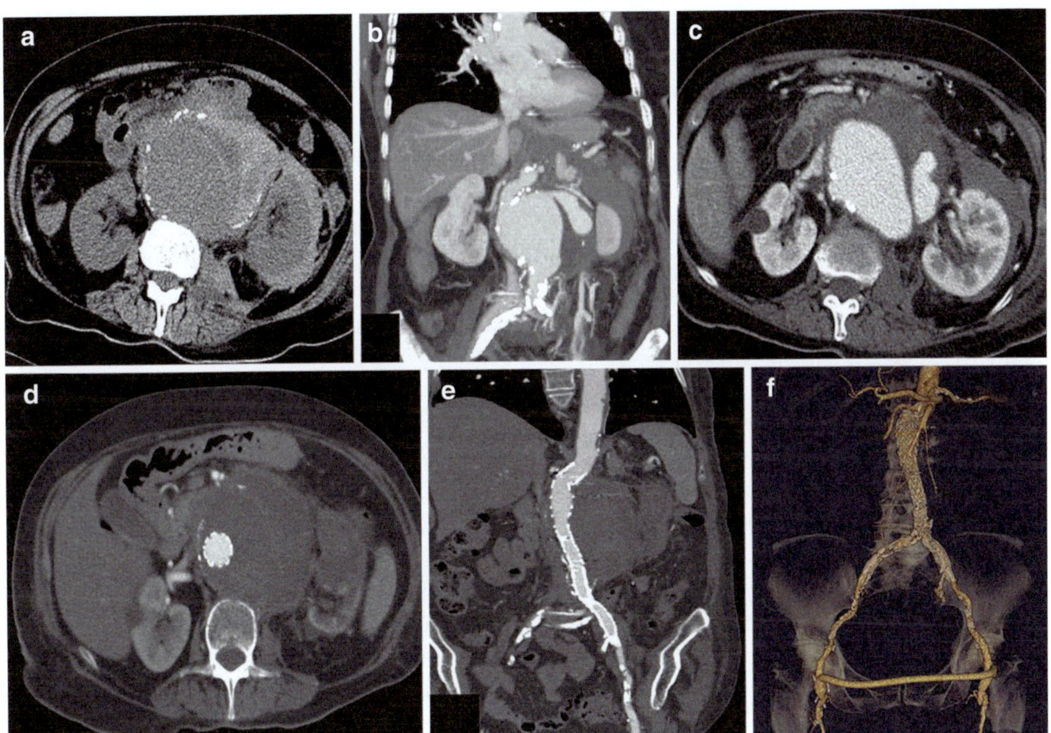

Fig. 9.6 Rupture of an abdominal aorta aneurysm in an 80-year-old woman with abdominal pain and hypotension. (**a**) Note on the nonenhanced axial CT image the "crescent sign" due to acute hematoma in the left aneurysm wall; (**b**) IV contrast-enhanced CT image in coronal plane showing active extravasation from the ruptured aneurysm, and associated retroperitoneal hemorrhage; (**c**) IV contrast-enhanced CT image in the coronal plane showing also the left perirenal hematoma; IV contrast-enhanced CT image in the axial plane (**d**), coronal plane (**e**), and 3D-volume rendering (**f**), showing the complete exclusion of the aneurysm after endoprosthesis positioning. *Figure 6 is reprinted with permission from Carrafiello G, Mangini M, Ierardi AM, Recaldini C, Cotta E, Piacentino F, Fugazzola C. Vascular Emergencies of the Retroperitoneum. Book chapter in: M. Scaglione* et al., *Emergency Radiology of the Abdomen, Medical Radiology. Diagnostic Imaging Editor: Springer-Verlag Berlin Heidelberg 2012; pp. 189–205*

attenuation within the thrombus of an aortic aneurysm, is a CT sign of acute or impending rupture, but it is not highly sensitive or specific as an isolated CT finding [7, 104] (Fig. 9.6). Signs of uncontained rupture are seen with active bleeding in the retroperitoneal or peritoneal spaces seen on arterial-phase images, which increases on the following phases.

IR Management

There is no universal agreement to our knowledge about the role of EVAR for the treatment of aortic aneurysm rupture [34], but it is established that open repair has been associated with significant morbidity and mortality, prolonged recovery, and some late complications [105, 106]. Because of these limitations, many patients and their physicians choose EVAR, which has become an effective alternative, and currently there are several studies which compared endovascular repair with surgical open repair [107–114]. Approximately 50% of all patients with rAAA are suitable for EVAR [34, 54, 115], which is less invasive and has lower overall treatment costs [116, 117], reduced morbidity and mortality, and has short- and long-time survival advantages over open surgery [105, 118]. The 30-day mortality after elective surgical repair in major randomized trials ranges from 2.7% to 5.8%, and is influenced by the volume of procedures performed at the institution and the expertise of the surgeon [116]. Logistics plays a central role in the management of traumatic patient with rAAA: EVAR may not be possible if CT angiography cannot be done immediately after the triage in emergency department and if an operating room is not available [119]. A large randomized trial of EVAR and open surgery for rAAA [119] underlined the importance of CT to confirm the suitability of endovascular repair of rAAA, without delaying treatment. Nevertheless, it is essential to have an early multidisciplinary approach [120], including a vascular surgeon, an interventional radiologist, emergency department physicians, anesthesiologists, operating room staff, and radiologic technologists [7]. Endovascular rAAA repair needs other validation in multicenter prospective studies, but is an evolving technique which offers the potential for improved outcomes in patients who otherwise have a high morbidity and mortality [15].

9.5.2.4 Aorto-enteric and Aorto-caval Fistulas

Aorto-enteric and aorto-duodenal fistulae are rare but frequently fatal complications which may follow open abdominal aneurism repair [121] or aneurysm infection. The perivascular inflammation may spread and involve the adjacent tissue leading to the formation of a fistula tract. Most of aorto-enteric fistulas involve the duodenum, most commonly its third and fourth portions. CT features of aorto-enteric fistulas include an abdominal aortic aneurysm, often with signs of rupture, and endoluminal and periaortic extraluminal gas, and contrast-enhanced CT may show contrast material extravasation from the aorta into the involved portion of the bowel [104, 121].

It has been reported that the overall prevalence of aorto-caval fistula is quite low, about 2–6%; such fistulas are caused by chronic perivascular inflammation, leading to erosion of the wall of the IVC. Aorto-caval fistula causes hemodynamic alteration with pulmonary congestion [122].

IR Management

Aorto-enteric fistulae (AEF) are rare but often fatal late complications of open repair with graft implantation or aneurysm infection [123]. The optimum management of AEF is currently not well defined to our knowledge, with a wide range of possible treatments. Several studies showed that replacement of the aneurysm with a prosthetic graft is preferable compared to other surgical treatment [124–126]. However, the mortality rates of in situ grafting remain 30–40% in the past decades. Axillobifemoral bypass is reserved for patients with extensive local sepsis, but this approach is associated with high mortality rates [127]. The advent of endovascular techniques has revolutionized the management of AEFs, especially for patients unsuitable for open surgery [128, 129]. Percutaneous aortic endografts are now widely used, and new endovascular approaches and other materials have been investigated [127]. A very recent systematic review by Kakkos et al. [130] showed that in a pooled analysis of 823 patients, EVAR was associated with a significantly reduced in-hospital mortality (7.1%) compared with open surgery (33.9%). Nevertheless, this difference mostly disappeared during the first 18–24 months after the procedure (2-year patient survival: 51% and 40%, respectively), concomitant with a high sepsis rate (2-year rates 42% vs. 19% for open surgery). A drawback of IR treatment is the increased risk of infection. Therefore, prophylactic broad-spectrum antibiotics should be instituted as soon as the diagnosis is suspected [127]. Moreover, patients who have undergone AAA repair may need periodic imaging to monitor treatment efficacy [128]. Endovascular closure of AEFs has proven to be less durable than other open surgery techniques, with a higher recurrence rate (100% at 2 years), which was also observed for in situ repair with homograft and impregnated prosthetic grafts (32% and 29%, respectively, at 2 years), both associated also with a poor overall survival rate (40% and 23%, respectively, at 2 years) [130]. As long-term use of multiple antibiotics cannot guarantee an uneventful outcome in patients undergoing endovascular repair [131], the correct management appears to consist of an urgent individualized interdisciplinary approach, potentially combining EVAR for bridging and open surgery (which has better results when performed in patients not actively bleeding) as the definitive treatment [34, 132]. The exact timing and also type of such a definite repair may be difficult to choose, but based on the results of the Kakkos' review [130], in situ repair with vein grafts or prosthetic grafts covered with omentum may be the best option, and can be performed within the first few weeks.

Primary aorto-caval fistulas (ACF) are a rare complication of AAA and involve fewer than 1% of all AAAs [69]. Penetrating traumatic injury is the most common cause of IVC fistulas. Their IR management has already been discussed.

9.5.2.5 Acute Thrombosis (Acute Leriche Syndrome)

Acute thrombosis of the aorta is a rare and severe disease, which is mostly seen in patients with severe atherosclerosis of the distal abdominal aorta and the iliac arteries. At MDCT, it is seen as an opacification defect in the arterial phase due to extensive endoluminal thrombosis (Fig. 9.7). It is important to evaluate the location of aortic stenosis, the extension of the occlusion, the involvement of visceral arteries, and the extent of collateralization [7].

IR Management

Acute thrombosis of the aorta is rare [133], and although it may cause major thromboembolic complications, there is no standardized treatment to our knowledge [134].

Thrombolysis and anticoagulation have been used with variable success, but they carry the risk of distal embolism caused by partial lysis and dislodgment of the thrombus [135]. Simple thrombectomy according to Fogarty has declined in importance because of the high recurrence rate [136]. Surgical removal is now recommended as the treatment of choice by some authors [135, 137]. However, the poor general condition of patients, especially those with associated cancer, may be less suited for standard surgery, and IR treatment will prove to be a preferred mode of management. Recently, several manuscripts have described the efficiency of stent-graft exclusion of the thrombus [138–142].

The advantages of IR techniques are not only to exclude the thrombus but also to cover the underlying atherosclerotic aortic wall to prevent recurrence [135]. Another benefit of IR is the possibility of combining the procedure with a peripheral embolectomy through the same surgical access. Shames et al. [138] performed endovascular stent-graft thrombus exclusion in eight patients at different locations with promising results. They observed no apparent embolic events during the stent implantation, and there was no evidence of recurrent emboli within a 12-month follow-up period, demonstrating the safety and efficacy and the safety of the procedure.

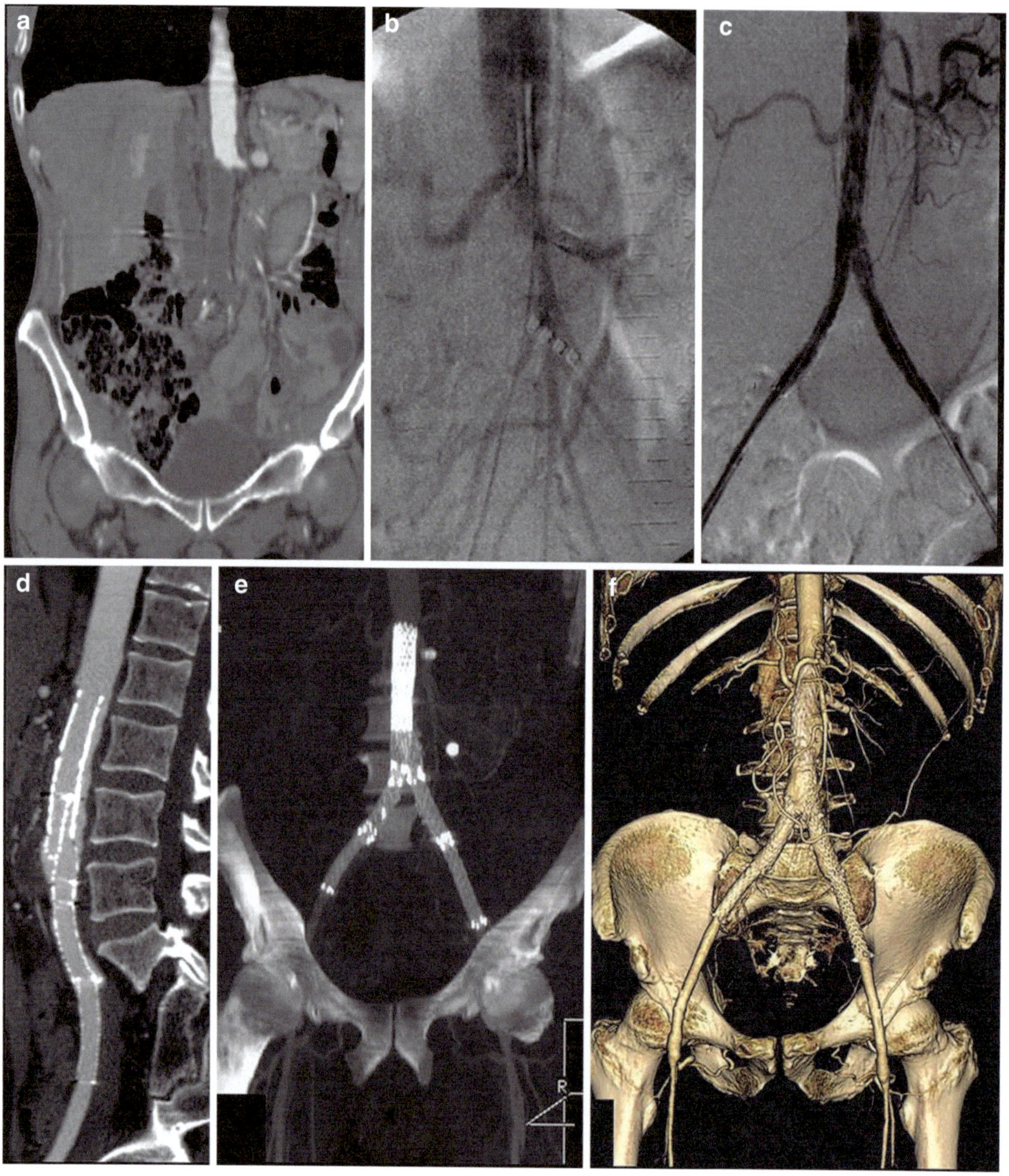

Fig. 9.7 Complete aorto-bi-iliac thrombosis in a 63-year-old man. (**a**) IV contrast-enhanced CT image in the coronal plane in the arterial phase shows complete aorto-bi-iliac thrombosis; (**b**) pretreatment intraoperative digital subtraction angiography (DSA) showing the complete occlusion of the distal abdominal aorta and of the iliac branches; (**c**) post-treatment DSA shows the recanalization of the treated vessels after stent-graft deployment; IV contrast-enhanced CT images in the arterial phase in the sagittal (**d**) and coronal (**e**) planes and with a 3D-volume rendering (**f**), showing the successful procedure. *Figure 7 is reprinted with permission from Carrafiello G, Mangini M, Ierardi AM, Recaldini C, Cotta E, Piacentino F, Fugazzola C. Vascular Emergencies of the Retroperitoneum. Book chapter in: M. Scaglione* et al., *Emergency Radiology of the Abdomen, Medical Radiology. Diagnostic Imaging Editor: Springer-Verlag Berlin Heidelberg 2012; pp. 189–205*

The disadvantages are the inability to perform a pathological examination (necessary to differentiate bland thrombus for aortic tumor), and the possible distal embolism and migration of the device caused by lodged thrombus between the stent-graft and the aortic wall [143]. Filter systems (e.g., temporary caval filters) are not appropriate for the aorta. Therefore, it is recommended that visceral and peripheral angiography should be routinely used at the end of the procedure, to identify potential embolic events caused by the intervention, so they can be treated simultaneously [140].

Because stent-graft placement for the acute aortic thrombosis has been rarely reported to our knowledge, there are no guidelines for the postoperative management regarding anticoagulation. Anticoagulation therapy should therefore be guided on an individual patient basis [143].

Concerning thrombosis of the superior mesenteric artery (SMA), the main nonsurgical treatments are endovascular stent placement, catheter-directed vasodilation, or thrombolytic therapy [144]. Limited studies, however, are available in the literature to our knowledge, and these procedures continue to be controversial [144]. Undoubtedly, as the average life expectancy increases and subsequently the number of elderly in our hospitals continues to grow, the need for endovascular thrombolytic therapy, angioplasty, and stent placement in either acute or chronic mesenteric ischemia will increase, especially when surgical therapy in some elderly is neither indicated nor safe [7, 144].

9.5.2.6 Spontaneous Bleeding

Spontaneous RB is a relatively uncommon but potentially lethal entity with a nonspecific presentation that can frequently lead to misdiagnosis and delayed treatment [145, 146]. If the patient is hemodynamically stable, the mainstay of management is a conservative approach, with withdrawal of anticoagulation therapy, correction of coagulopathy, volume resuscitation, and supportive measures [7, 146]. In some patients, IR procedures are necessary (Fig. 9.8). Surgery is rarely indicated and is reserved for patients with failed angiographic procedures, concurrent surgical

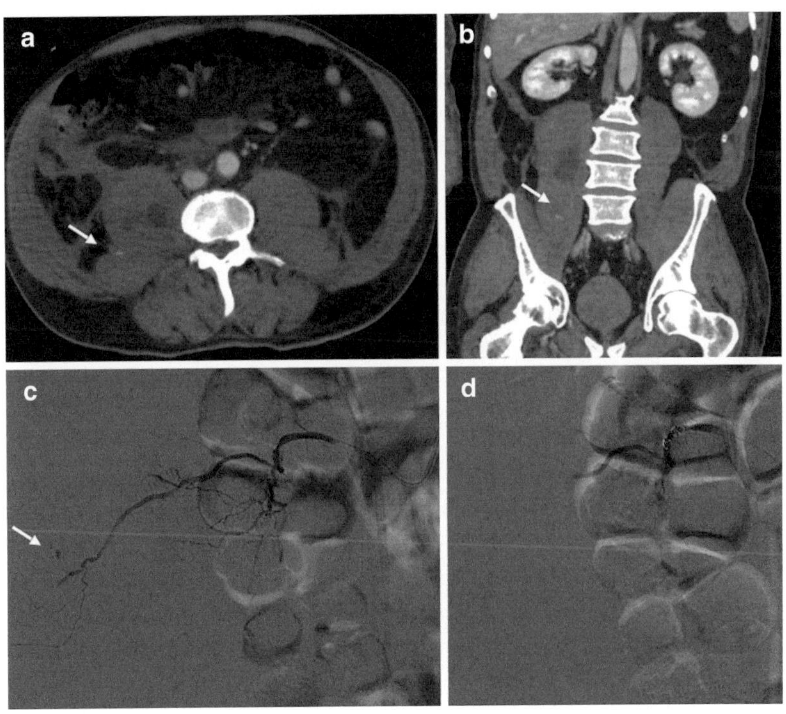

Fig. 9.8 Spontaneous active bleeding in a retroperitoneal hematoma in a 56-year-old man. IV contrast-enhanced CT images in the axial (**a**) and coronal (**b**) planes in the arterial phase show a right retroperitoneal hematoma, with active arterial bleeding; (**c**) selective angiogram of the feeding lumbar artery confirms a vascular "blush"; (**d**) angiogram performed at the end of the embolization with microcoils and sponge revealing complete embolization

conditions, or with significant compressive symptoms on nervous system structures from hematoma formation [146, 147].

There is a growing trend in the use of IR techniques as an alternative to open surgery in the management of RB, whatever the etiology [148]. The main options are selective intra-arterial embolization or stent-grafts to stop the bleeding. Intra-arterial embolization is being used with increasing frequency in patients where the angiogram shows active bleeding sites [17]. In a series reported by Isokangas et al., four patients were operated on prior to embolization, but surgery failed to control the bleeding. Embolization using a combination of agents, including coils, gelatin, and/or polyvinyl alcohol, has been used. Coils are probably the safest, but Isokangas et al. commented that proximal coiling of the bleeding artery may not be sufficient in the retroperitoneum, where there is a rich network of collateral arteries, and new arterial pathways may develop after obliteration of the lumbar arteries [6, 149], so the embolic agents should be placed both proximal and distal to the bleeding site to prevent re-bleeding.

Panetta et al. [150] stated that hemodynamic instability despite 4 or more units of blood transfusion within 24 h, or 6 or more units of blood transfusion within 48 h, is an indication for urgent investigation and IR treatment. Embolization should be performed whenever arterial extravasation is seen. Sharafuddin et al. [151] showed that selective arterial embolization was successful in a series of five patients, although re-bleeding occurred in one patient. Subsequent small case series have shown similar results [152].

9.6 Venous

9.6.1 Inferior Vena Cava Thrombosis

IVC thrombosis is a rare but severe disease which is associated with a high rate of mortality [153] (Fig. 9.9). IVC thrombosis may arise from an isolated thrombus, or may be due to propagation from the iliac veins. Isolated IVC thrombosis is commonly associated with outflow obstruction of the IVC, such as in Budd-Chiari syndrome, IVC anomalies from tumoral invasion, or from external compression by a mass or hematoma. IVC thrombosis can initially be asymptomatic and may be revealed after sudden pulmonary embolism [7, 153].

9.6.1.1 IR Management

IVC thrombosis is a rare but severe disease which is associated with a high rate of mortality. The management of IVCT has no universal agreement and continues to be the target of continued research [153]. Although anticoagulation therapy remains fundamental in treating IVCT, its inherent limitations have led to the use of minimally invasive, endovascular treatment options, including transcatheter thrombolysis, mechanical thrombectomy, or a combination of these techniques.

The primary goals of treatment for IVCT include prevention of pulmonary embolism, restoration of unobstructed venous return, prevention of recurrent deep venous thrombosis (DVT), and preservation of venous valve function [154].

To achieve these goals, the guidelines from the Society for Vascular Surgery and the American Venous Forum advocate early thrombus removal strategies for acute DVT [155], but these recommendations are mostly applicable for the treatment of primary IVCT.

The strategy of early deep venous thrombus removal is suggested if the selected patients meet the following criteria [155]:

- first episode of acute iliofemoral DVT
- fewer than 14 days of symptoms
- low risk of bleeding
- good functional capacity and acceptable life expectancy

The evidence for treatment of primary IVCT with IR procedures is predominantly extrapolated from lower extremity DVT treatment data [153]. Unless contraindicated by a significantly increased risk of RB, urgent endovascular treatment is recommended for those patients with severe acute DVT associated with

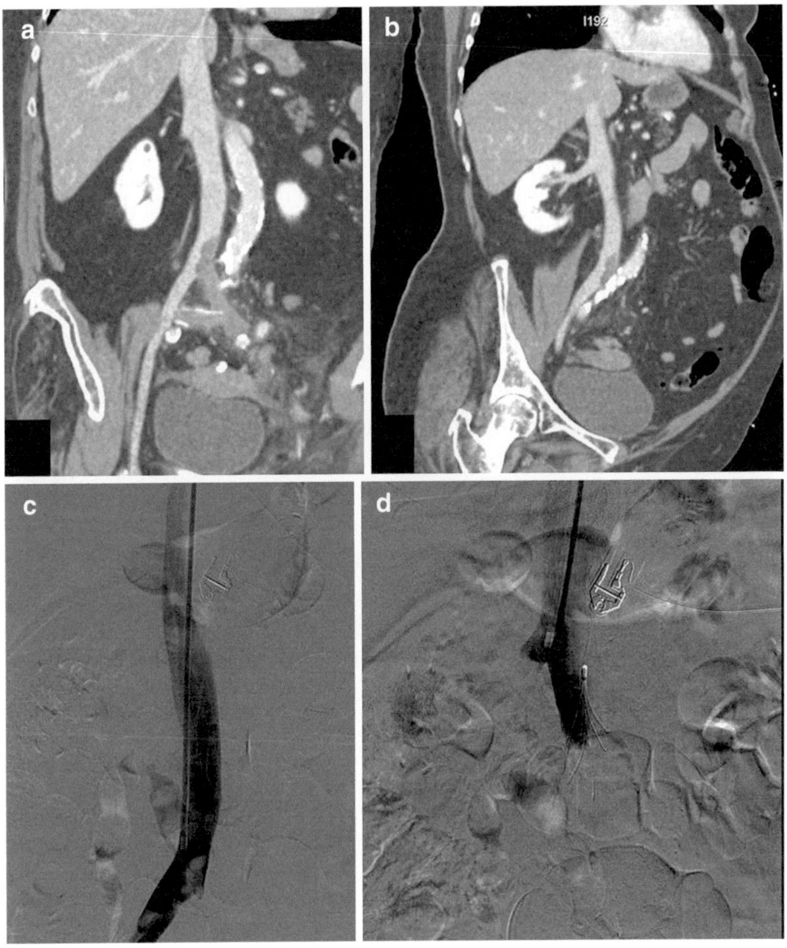

Fig. 9.9 Acute left iliac vein and IVC thrombosis in a 67-year-old woman. IV contrast-enhanced CT image in the coronal plane (**a**) and in a coronal MIP (**b**), showing thrombosis of the left iliac vein and IVC; (**c**) transjugular vein access DSA confirms the thrombosis; (**d**) postprocedural DSA after caval filter placement. *Figure 9 is reprinted with permission from Carrafiello G, Mangini M, Ierardi AM, Recaldini C, Cotta E, Piacentino F, Fugazzola C. Vascular Emergencies of the Retroperitoneum. Book chapter in: M. Scaglione* et al., *Emergency Radiology of the Abdomen, Medical Radiology. Diagnostic Imaging Editor: Springer-Verlag Berlin Heidelberg 2012; pp. 189–205*

limb-threatening compromise, or worsening IVCT despite anticoagulation therapy [156].

Alkhouli et al. [157] reported a total of 2674 patients with IVCT; among them 718 patients were treated with catheter-directed therapy, and the others were managed with anticoagulation alone. This study, along with the reports from the Catheter-Directed Venous Thrombolysis (CaVenT) trial [158], suggests the main benefit from IR treatment for IVCT patients is the reduced risk of developing post-thrombotic syndrome.

Limitations of the catheter-directed therapy include lengthy thrombolytic infusions in an intensive monitored setting with the inherent risks related to hemorrhage [153]. Among the 473 patients included in the national multicenter registry [156], bleeding complications were reported in 54 (11%), neurologic complications in 2 (0.4%), and death in 2 (0.4%) for the treatment of DVT.

Moreover, a current limitation is patient access to care, as not all healthcare facilities may have the availability to the endovascular interventionalists skilled in these advanced techniques to provide optimum management for IVCT [7, 153].

In conclusion, although there is a scarcity of data in the literature regarding the management of IVCT, and although there is no consensus regarding the most successful approach, accumulated evidence advocates endovascular strategies as a safe option for the treatment of IVCT [153].

Conclusion

Vascular emergencies of the retroperitoneum can be traumatic or nontraumatic, arterial, or venous in origin. Their management is challenging and requires multidisciplinary approach. MDCT with intravenous contrast is the primary imaging modality for the diagnosis of retroperitoneal vascular injuries, and to assess whether medical, interventional, or surgical management—or a combination of these—is necessary. Currently, there is a growing trend in the use of interventional radiology techniques as an alternative to open surgery. Advances in interventional radiology technique permit less invasive treatments for the management of retroperitoneal vascular emergencies, using several methods including embolization, balloon occlusion, and stent-grafting. Open surgery is still indicated if the patient remains hemodynamically unstable, or if IR techniques are either not successful or unavailable.

References

1. Pfeifer R, Tarkin IS, Rocos B, Pape HC. Patterns of mortality and causes of death in polytrauma patients—has anything changed? Injury. 2009;40:907–11.
2. Muckart DJ, Pillay B, Hardcastle TC, Skinner DL. Vascular injuries following blunt polytrauma. Eur J Trauma Emerg Surg. 2014;40:315–22.
3. Sobrino J, Shafi S. Timing and causes of death after injuries. Proc (Bayl Univ Med Cent). 2013;26:120–3.
4. Iacobellis F, Ierardi AM, Mazzei MA, Magenta Biasina A, Carrafiello G, Nicola R, Scaglione M. Dual-phase CT for the assessment of acute vascular injuries in high-energy blunt trauma: the imaging findings and management implications. Br J Radiol. 2016;89(1061):20150952.
5. Charlton-Ouw KM, DuBose JJ, Leake SS, et al. Observation may be safe in selected cases of blunt traumatic abdominal aortic injury. Ann Vasc Surg. 2016;30:34–9.
6. Genovese EA, Fonio P, Floridi C, et al. Abdominal vascular emergencies: US and CT assessment. Crit Ultrasound J. 2013;5(Suppl 1):S10.
7. Carrafiello G, Mangini M, Ierardi AM, et al. Vascular emergencies of the retroperitoneum. In: Scaglione M, et al., editors. Emergency radiology of the abdomen, medical radiology. Diagnostic imaging. Berlin Heidelberg: Springer-Verlag; 2012. p. 189–205.
8. Scaglione M, Romano L, Bocchini G, et al. Multidetector computed tomography of pancreatic, small bowel, and mesenteric traumas. Semin Roentgenol. 2012;47(4):362–70.
9. Romano F, Iacobellis F, Guida F, et al. Traumatic injuries: mechanisms of lesions. In: Miele V, Trinci M, editors. Diagnostic imaging in polytrauma patients. Berlin Heidelberg: Springer-Verlag; 2018. p. 35–55.
10. Bernstein MP, Mirvis SE. Penetrating trauma to the abdominal aorta: CT demonstration of active bleeding. Emerg Radiol. 2001;8:43–7.
11. Borioni R, Garofalo M, Seddio F, Colagrande L, Marino B, Albano P. Posttraumatic infrarenal abdominal aortic pseudoaneurysm. Tex Heart Inst J. 1999;26(4):312–4.
12. Azizzadeh A, Keyhani K, Miller CC 3rd, Coogan SM, Safi HJ, Estrera AL. Blunt traumatic aortic injury: initial experience with endovascular repair. J Vasc Surg. 2009;49(6):1403–8.
13. Ertel W, Keel M, Eid K, Platz A, Trentz O. Control of severe hemorrhage using C-clamp and pelvic packing in multiply injured patients with pelvic ring disruption. J Orthop Trauma. 2001;15(7):468–74.
14. Boufi M, Bordon S, Dona B, et al. Unstable patients with retroperitoneal vascular trauma: an endovascular approach. Ann Vasc Surg. 2011;25(3):352–8.
15. Nicholson AA. Vascular radiology in trauma. Cardiovasc Intervent Radiol. 2004;27(2):105–20.
16. Velmahos GC, Toutouzas KG, Vassiliu P, et al. A prospective study on the safety and efficacy of angiographic embolization for pelvic and visceral injuries. J Trauma. 2002;53(2):303–8. discussion 308
17. Isokangas JM, Perala JM. Endovascular embolization of spontaneous retroperitoneal hemorrhage secondary to anticoagulant treatment. Cardiovasc Intervent Radiol. 2004;27(6):607–11.
18. Velmahos GC, Chahwan S, Falabella A, Hanks SE, Demetriades D. Angiographic embolization for intraperitoneal and retroperitoneal injuries. World J Surg. 2000;24(5):539–45.
19. Berthet JP, Marty-Ane CH, Veerapen R, Picard E, Mary H, Alric P. Dissection of the abdominal aorta in blunt trauma: endovascular or conventional surgical management? J Vasc Surg. 2003;38(5):997–1003. discussion 1004
20. Sniderman KW, Sos TA, Gay WA Jr, Subramanian VA. Aortic dissection beginning in the abdomen. AJR. 1978;130(6):1115–8.
21. Arendrup H, Frimodt-Moller PC, Christensen JE. Acute dissection confined to the abdominal aorta. Scand J Thorac Cardiovasc Surg. 1983;17(2):121–3.
22. Picard E, Marty-Ane CH, Vernhet H, et al. Endovascular management of traumatic infrarenal abdominal aortic dissection. Ann Vasc Surg. 1998;12(6):515–21.
23. Vernhet H, Marty-Ane CH, Lesnik A, et al. Dissection of the abdominal aorta in blunt trauma: management by percutaneous stent placement. Cardiovasc Intervent Radiol. 1997;20(6):473–6.

24. Nishimura K, Kanaoka Y, Ikebuchi M, et al. Percutaneous balloon fenestration in a case of traumatic abdominal aortic dissection with lower extremity ischemia. J Vasc Surg. 2000;32(3):616–8.
25. Michaels AJ, Gerndt SJ, Taheri PA, et al. Blunt force injury of the abdominal aorta. J Trauma. 1996;41(1):105–9.
26. Maleux G, Soula P, Otal P, Colombier D, Cérène A, Joffre F, Rousseau H. Traumatic aortobiiliac dissection treated by kissing-stent placement. J Trauma. 1997;43(4):706–8.
27. Hahmann M, Richter GM, Schuhmacher H, Allenberg JR, Kauffmann GW. Post-traumatic dissection of the abdominal aorta. Radiologe. 2001;41(7):590–4.
28. Bortone AS, Schena S, Mannatrizio G, et al. Endovascular stent-graft treatment for diseases of the descending thoracic aorta. Eur J Cardiothorac Surg. 2001;20(3):514–9.
29. Nienaber CA, Sievers HH. Intramural hematoma in acute aortic syndrome: more than one variant of dissection? Circulation. 2002;106(3):284–5.
30. Dake MD, Kato N, Mitchell RS, et al. Endovascular stent-graft placement for the treatment of acute aortic dissection. N Engl J Med. 1999;340(20):1546–52.
31. Marty-Ane CH, SerreCousine O, Laborde JC, Costes V, Mary H, Senac JP. Use of a balloon-expandable intravascular graft in the management of type B aortic dissection in an animal model. J Vasc Interv Radiol. 1995;6(1):97–103.
32. Trent MS, Parsonnet V, Shoenfeld R, et al. A balloon-expandable intravascular stent for obliterating experimental aortic dissection. J Vasc Surg. 1990;11(5):707–17.
33. Voitle E, Hofmann W, Cejna M. Aortic emergencies—diagnosis and treatment: a pictorial review. Insights Imaging. 2015;6(1):17–32.
34. Erbel R, Aboyans V, Boileau C, et al. 2014 ESC guidelines on the diagnosis and treatment of aortic diseases: document covering acute and chronic aortic diseases of the thoracic and abdominal aorta of the adult. The task force for the diagnosis and treatment of aortic diseases of the European. Eur Heart J. 2014;35(41):2873–926.
35. Nienaber CA, von Kodolitsch Y, Petersen B, et al. Intramural hemorrhage of the thoracic aorta. Diagnostic and therapeutic implications. Circulation. 1995;92(6):1465–72.
36. Eggebrecht H, Plicht B, Kahlert P, Erbel R. Intramural hematoma and penetrating ulcers: indications to endovascular treatment. Eur J Vasc Endovasc Surg. 2009;38(6):659–65.
37. Daily PO, Trueblood HW, Stinson EB, Wuerflein RD, Shumway NE. Management of acute aortic dissections. Ann Thorac Surg. 1970;10(3):237–47.
38. von Kodolitsch Y, Csosz SK, Koschyk DH, et al. Intramural hematoma of the aorta: predictors of progression to dissection and rupture. Circulation. 2003;107(8):1158–63.
39. Mussa FF, Horton JD, Moridzadeh R, Nicholson J, Trimarchi S, Eagle KA. Acute aortic dissection and intramural hematoma: a systematic review. JAMA. 2016;316(7):754–63.
40. Braverman AC, Harris KM. Management of aortic intramural hematoma. Curr Opin Cardiol. 1995;10(5):501–4.
41. Motoyoshi N, Moizumi Y, Komatsu T, Tabayashi K. Intramural hematoma and dissection involving ascending aorta: the clinical features and prognosis. Eur J Cardiothorac Surg. 2003;24(2):237–42. discussion 242
42. Aladham F, Sundaram B, Williams DM, Quint LE. Traumatic aortic injury: computerized tomographic findings at presentation and after conservative therapy. J Comput Assist Tomogr. 2010;34(3):388–94.
43. Holmes JH, Bloch RD, Hall RA, Carter YM, Karmy-Jones RC. Natural history of traumatic rupture of the thoracic aorta managed nonoperatively: a longitudinal analysis. Ann Thorac Surg. 2002;73(4):1149–54.
44. Hirose H, Gill IS, Malangoni MA. Nonoperative management of traumatic aortic injury. J Trauma. 2006;60(3):597–601.
45. Kepros J, Angood P, Jaffe CC, Rabinovici R. Aortic intimal injuries from blunt trauma: resolution profile in nonoperative management. J Trauma. 2002;52(3):475–8.
46. Zhang G, Feng Q, Zheng D, Ma L, Li R, Jiang J, Ni Y. Early aggressive medical treatment associated with selective prophylactic aortic stent-grafting for aortic intramural hematoma. Thorac Cardiovasc Surg. 2011;59(6):342–8.
47. Song JK, Kim HS, Song JM, et al. Outcomes of medically treated patients with aortic intramural hematoma. Am J Med. 2002;113(3):181–7.
48. Abed H, Ball WR, Stone T, Houghton A. Very late rupture of a post-traumatic abdominal aortic pseudoaneurysm. BMJ Case Rep. 2017;27:2017.
49. Hamilton JD, Kumaravel M, Censullo ML, Cohen AM, Kievlan DS, West OC, Multidetector CT. evaluation of active extravasation in blunt abdominal and pelvic trauma patients. Radiographics. 2008;28(6):1603–16.
50. Peterson AH, Williams DM, Rodriguez JL, Francis IR. Percutaneous treatment of a traumatic aortic dissection by balloon fenestration and stent placement. AJR. 1995;164(5):1274–6.
51. Garg L, Jain N, Agrawal S, Chauhan U, Goel V, Puri SK. Juxtarenal aortic pseudoaneurysm—right renal vein fistula with circumaortic renal collar-delayed manifestation of a gunshot injury—an uncommon entity diagnosed with CT angiography. Pol J Radiol. 2016;81:114–9.
52. Tucker S Jr, Rowe VL, Rao R, Hood DB, Harrell D, Weaver FA. Treatment options for traumatic pseudoaneurysms of the paravisceral abdominal aorta. Ann Vasc Surg. 2005;19(5):613–8.
53. Mattox KL. Red River anthology. J Trauma. 1997;42(3):353–68.

54. Mastracci TM, Greenberg RK. Complex aortic disease: changes in perception, evaluation and management. J Vasc Surg. 2008;48(6 Suppl):17S–23S. discussion 23S.
55. Saad NE, Saad WE, Davies MG, Waldman DL, Fultz PJ, Rubens DJ. Pseudoaneurysms and the role of minimally invasive techniques in their management. Radiographics. 2005;25(Suppl 1):S173–89.
56. Baltacioglu F, Cimsit NC, Cil B, Cekirge S, Ispir S. Endovascular stent-graft applications in iatrogenic vascular injuries. Cardiovasc Intervent Radiol. 2003;26(5):434–9.
57. Kapoor BS, Haddad HL, Saddekni S, Lockhart ME. Diagnosis and management of pseudoaneurysms: an update. Curr Probl Diagn Radiol. 2009;38(4):170–88.
58. Leyon JJ, Littlehales T, Rangarajan B, Hoey ET, Ganeshan A. Endovascular embolization: review of currently available embolization agents. Curr Probl Diagn Radiol. 2014;43(1):35–53.
59. Yamakado K, Nakatsuka A, Tanaka N, Takano K, Matsumura K, Takeda K. Transcatheter arterial embolization of ruptured pseudoaneurysms with coils and n-butyl cyanoacrylate. J Vasc Interv Radiol. 2000;11(1):66–72.
60. Morgan TA, Steenburg SD, Siegel EL, Mirvis SE. Acute traumatic aortic injuries: posttherapy multidetector CT findings. Radiographics. 2010;30(4):851–67.
61. McDermott VG, Shlansky-Goldberg R, Cope C. Endovascular management of splenic artery aneurysms and pseudoaneurysms. Cardiovasc Intervent Radiol. 1994;17(4):179–84.
62. Guillon R, Garcier JM, Abergel A, et al. Management of splenic artery aneurysms and false aneurysms with endovascular treatment in 12 patients. Cardiovasc Intervent Radiol. 2003;26(3):256–60.
63. Spencer TA, Smyth SH, Wittich G, Hunter GC. Delayed presentation of traumatic aortocaval fistula: a report of two cases and a review of the associated compensatory hemodynamic and structural changes. J Vasc Surg. 2006;43(4):836–40.
64. Kim H, Randolph S. Traumatic aortocaval fistula from gunshot wound, complicated by bullet embolization to the right ventricle. Radiol Case Rep. 2015;7(4):767.
65. Beton O, Kaplanoğlu H, Berkan Ö, Yılmaz MB. A case report of delayed diagnosed chronic aortocaval fistula: a rare complication of penetrating trauma to the abdomen. J Clin Imaging Sci. 2015;5:62.
66. Srisuwan T, Kanjanavanit R, Rerkasem K. Endovascular aortic stenting in patients with chronic traumatic aortocaval fistula. Ann Vasc Dis. 2013;6(4):741–4.
67. O'Brien GC, Murphy C, Martin Z, et al. Hybrid management of a spontaneous ilio-iliac arteriovenous fistula: a case report. J Med Case Reports. 2011;5:401.
68. Davis PM, Gloviczki P, Cherry KJ Jr, et al. Aortocaval and ilio-iliac arteriovenous fistulae. Am J Surg. 1998;176(2):115–8.
69. Brightwell RE, Pegna V, Boyne N. Aortocaval fistula: current management strategies. ANZ J Surg. 2013;83(1–2):31–5.
70. Boudghene F, Sapoval M, Bonneau M, Bigot JM. Aortocaval fistulae: a percutaneous model and treatment with stent grafts in sheep. Circulation. 1996;94(1):108–12.
71. Antoniou GA, Koutsias S, Karathanos C, Sfyroeras GS, Vretzakis G, Giannoukas AD. Endovascular stent-graft repair of major abdominal arteriovenous fistula: a systematic review. J Endovasc Ther. 2009;16(4):514–23.
72. Lau LL, O'Reilly MJ, Johnston LC, Lee B. Endovascular stent-graft repair of primary aortocaval fistula with an abdominal aortoiliac aneurysm. J Vasc Surg. 2001;33(2):425–8.
73. Siepe M, Koeppe S, Euringer W, Schlensak C. Aortocaval fistula from acute rupture of an abdominal aortic aneurysm treated with a hybrid approach. J Vasc Surg. 2009;49(6):1574–6.
74. Daly KP, Ho CP, Persson DL, Gay SB. Traumatic retroperitoneal injuries: review of multidetector CT findings. Radiographics. 2008;28(6):1571–90.
75. Akpinar E, Peynircioglu B, Turkbey B, Cil BE, Balkanci F. Endovascular management of life-threatening retroperitoneal bleeding. ANZ J Surg. 2008;78(8):683–7.
76. Marty B, Sanchez LA, Wain RA, et al. Endovascular treatment of a ruptured lumbar artery aneurysm: case report and review of the literature. Ann Vasc Surg. 1998;12(4):379–83.
77. Dondelinger RF, Trotteur G, Ghaye B, Szapiro D. Traumatic injuries: radiological hemostatic intervention at admission. Eur Radiol. 2002;12(5):979–93.
78. Scott AR, Gilani R, Tapia NM, Mattox KL, Wall MJ, Suliburk JW. Endovascular management of traumatic peripheral arterial injuries. J Surg Res. 2015;199(2):557–63.
79. Moore HM, List A, Holden A, Osborne TM. Therapeutic embolization for acute haemorrhage in the abdomen and pelvis. Australas Radiol. 2000;44(2):161–8.
80. Papakostidis C, Kanakaris N, Dimitriou R, Giannoudis PV. The role of arterial embolization in controlling pelvic fracture haemorrhage: a systematic review of the literature. Eur J Radiol. 2012;81(5):897–904.
81. Watarida S, Nishi T, Furukawa A, et al. Fenestrated stent-graft for traumatic juxtahepatic inferior vena cava injury. J Endovasc Ther. 2002;9(1):134–7.
82. Lindblad B, Brunkwall J, Lindh M, Nyman U, Malina M, Ivancev K. Traumatic aortic rupture and retroperitoneal haematoma—treatment including combined operative and endovascular approach. Eur J Vasc Endovasc Surg. 1999;17(5):451–5.
83. Fraga GP, Bansal V, Fortlage D, Coimbra R. A 20-year experience with portal and superior mesenteric venous injuries: has anything changed? Eur J Vasc Endovasc Surg. 2009;37:87e91.

84. Tsai R, Raptis C, Schuerer DJ, Mellnick VM. CT appearance of traumatic inferior vena cava injury. AJR. 2016;19:1–7.
85. Ierardi AM, Berselli M, Cuffari S, Castelli P, Cocozza E, Carrafiello G. Uncommon case of a post-traumatic portal vein pseudoaneurysm treated with percutaneous transhepatic stent grafting. Cardiovasc Intervent Radiol. 2016;39(10):1506–9.
86. Kunkala M, Jenkins DH, McEachen J, Stockland A, Zielinski MD. Nonoperative management of traumatic suprahepatic inferior vena cava pseudoaneurysms. J Vasc Surg. 2011;54(6 Suppl):80S–2S.
87. Chakroun A, Nakhli MS, Kahloul M, Harrathi MA, Naija W. Post traumatic inferior vena cava thrombosis: A case report and review of literature. Int J Surg Case Rep. 2017;15(36):59–63.
88. Cheaito A, Tillou A, Lewis C, Cryer H. Management of traumatic blunt IVC injury. Int J Surg Case Rep. 2016;28:26–30.
89. Valente T, Rossi G, Lassandro F, et al. MDCT evaluation of acute aortic syndrome (AAS). Br J Radiol. 2016;89(1061):20150825.
90. Erbel R, Alfonso F, Boileau C, et al. Task force on aortic dissection, European society of cardiology diagnosis and management of aortic dissection. Eur Heart J. 2001;22(18):1642–81.
91. Umana JP, Miller DC, Mitchell RS. What is the best treatment for patients with acute type B aortic dissections—medical, surgical, or endovascular stent-grafting? Ann Thorac Surg. 2002;74(5):S1840–3. discussion S1857-1863.
92. Brandt M, Hussel K, Walluscheck KP, et al. Stent-graft repair versus open surgery for the descending aorta: a case-control study. J Endovasc Ther. 2004;11(5):535–8.
93. Eggebrecht H, Nienaber CA, Neuhauser M, et al. Endovascular stent-graft placement in aortic dissection: a meta-analysis. Eur Heart J. 2006;27(4):489–98.
94. Nienaber CA, Erbel R, Ince H. Nihil nocere on the rocky road to endovascular stent-graft treatment. J Thorac Cardiovasc Surg. 2004;127(3):620–1.
95. Castelli P, Caronno R, Piffaretti G, et al. Endovascular repair for concomitant multilevel aortic disease. Eur J Cardiothorac Surg. 2005;28(3):478–82.
96. Fattori R, Montgomery D, Lovato L, et al. Survival after endovascular therapy in patients with type B aortic dissection: a report from the International Registry of Acute Aortic Dissection (IRAD). JACC Cardiovasc Interv. 2013;6(8):876–82.
97. Ganaha F, Miller DC, Sugimoto K, et al. Prognosis of aortic intramural hematoma with and without penetrating atherosclerotic ulcer: a clinical and radiological analysis. Circulation. 2002;106(3): 342–8.
98. Brinster DR, Wheatley GH 3rd, Williams J, Ramaiah VG, Diethrich EB, Rodriguez-Lopez JA. Are penetrating aortic ulcers best treated using an endovascular approach? Ann Thorac Surg. 2006;82(5):1688–91.
99. Brinster DR. Endovascular repair of the descending thoracic aorta for penetrating atherosclerotic ulcer disease. J Card Surg. 2009;24(2):203–8.
100. Kos X, Bouchard L, Otal P, et al. Stent-graft treatment of penetrating thoracic aortic ulcers. J Endovasc Ther. 2002;9(Suppl 2):II25–31.
101. Piffaretti G, Tozzi M, Lomazzi C, et al. Penetrating ulcers of the thoracic aorta: results from a single-centre experience. Am J Surg. 2007;193(4):443–7.
102. Demers P, Miller DC, Mitchell RS, Kee ST, Chagonjian L, Dake MD. Stent-graft repair of penetrating atherosclerotic ulcers in the descending thoracic aorta: mid-term results. Ann Thorac Surg. 2004;77(1):81–6.
103. Schwartz SA, Taljanovic MS, Smyth S, O'Brien MJ, Rogers LF. CT findings of rupture, impending rupture, and contained rupture of abdominal aortic aneurysms. AJR. 2007;188(1):W57–62.
104. Rakita D, Newatia A, Hines JJ, Siegel DN, Friedman B. Spectrum of CT findings in rupture and impending rupture of abdominal aortic aneurysms. Radiographics. 2007;27(2):497–507.
105. Williamson WK, Nicoloff AD, Taylor LM Jr, Moneta GL, Landry GJ, Porter JM. Functional outcome after open repair of abdominal aortic aneurysm. J Vasc Surg. 2001;33(5):913–20.
106. Kalman PG, Rappaport DC, Merchant N, Clarke K, Johnston KW. The value of late computed tomographic scanning in identification of vascular abnormalities after abdominal aortic aneurysm repair. J Vasc Surg. 1999;29(3):442–50.
107. Makaroun MS, Chaikof E, Naslund T, Matsumura JS. Efficacy of a bifurcated endograft versus open repair of abdominal aortic aneurysms: a reappraisal. J Vasc Surg. 2002;35(2):203–10.
108. Zarins CK, White RA, Schwarten D, et al. AneuRx stent graft versus open surgical repair of abdominal aortic aneurysms: multicenter prospective clinical trial. J Vasc Surg. 1999;29(2):292–305. discussion 306-298
109. Zarins CK, White RA, Moll FL, et al. The AneuRx stent graft: four-year results and worldwide experience 2000. J Vasc Surg. 2001;33(2 Suppl):S135–45.
110. May J, White GH, Yu W, et al. Concurrent comparison of endoluminal versus open repair in the treatment of abdominal aortic aneurysms: analysis of 303 patients by life table method. J Vasc Surg. 1998;27(2):213–20. discussion 220-211
111. White GH, May J, McGahan T, et al. Historic control comparison of outcome for matched groups of patients undergoing endoluminal versus open repair of abdominal aortic aneurysms. J Vasc Surg. 1996;23(2):201–11. discussion 211-202
112. Brewster DC, Geller SC, Kaufman JA, et al. Initial experience with endovascular aneurysm repair: comparison of early results with outcome of conventional open repair. J Vasc Surg. 1998;27(6):992–1003. discussion 1004-1005
113. Moore WS, Kashyap VS, Vescera CL, Quinones-Baldrich WJ. Abdominal aortic aneurysm: a 6-year

comparison of endovascular versus transabdominal repair. Ann Surg. 1999;230(3):298–306. discussion 306-298
114. Moore WS, Brewster DC, Bernhard VM. Aorto-uni-iliac endograft for complex aortoiliac aneurysms compared with tube/bifurcation endografts: results of the EVT/Guidant trials. J Vasc Surg. 2001;33(2 Suppl):S11–20.
115. Mastracci TM, Clase CM, Devereaux PJ, Cina CS. Open versus endovascular repair of abdominal aortic aneurysm: a survey of Canadian vascular surgeons. Can J Surg. 2008;51(2):142–8. quiz 149
116. Greenhalgh RM, Brown LC, Kwong GP, Powell JT, Thompson SG. EVAR trial participants. Comparison of endovascular aneurysm repair with open repair in patients with abdominal aortic aneurysm (EVAR trial 1), 30-day operative mortality results: randomised controlled trial. Lancet. 2004;364(9437):843–8.
117. Sadat U, Cooper DG, Cousins C, Boyle JR. Endovascular stenting of large popliteal artery aneurysm is feasible! Adv Med Sci. 2008;53(2):335–7.
118. Investigators IT, Powell JT, Sweeting MJ, et al. Endovascular or open repair strategy for ruptured abdominal aortic aneurysm: 30 day outcomes from IMPROVE randomised trial. BMJ. 2014;348:f7661.
119. Hinchliffe RJ, Bruijstens L, MacSweeney ST, Braithwaite BD. A randomised trial of endovascular and open surgery for ruptured abdominal aortic aneurysm—results of a pilot study and lessons learned for future studies. Eur J Vasc Endovasc Surg. 2006;32(5):506–13. discussion 514-505
120. Klocker J, Falkensammer J, Pellegrini L, Biebl M, Tauscher T, Fraedrich G. Repair of arterial injury after blunt trauma in the upper extremity—immediate and long-term outcome. Eur J Vasc Endovasc Surg. 2010;39(2):160–4.
121. Valente T, Rossi G, Rea G, et al. Multidetector CT findings of complications of surgical and endovascular treatment of aortic aneurysms. Radiol Clin North Am. 2014;52(5):961–89.
122. Wang T, Huang B, Zhao J, Yang Y, Yuan D. Aortocaval fistula resulting from rupture of abdominal aortic dissecting aneurysm treated by delayed endovascular repair: a case report. Medicine (Baltimore). 2016;95(18):e3570.
123. Saratzis N, Saratzis A, Melas N, Ktenidis K, Kiskinis D. Aortoduodenal fistulas after endovascular stent-graft repair of abdominal aortic aneurysms: single-center experience and review of the literature. J Endovasc Ther. 2008;15(4):441–8.
124. Oderich GS, Bower TC, Hofer J, et al. In situ rifampin-soaked grafts with omental coverage and antibiotic suppression are durable with low reinfection rates in patients with aortic graft enteric erosion or fistula. J Vasc Surg. 2011;53(1):99–106. 107 e101–107; discussion 106-107
125. Danneels MI, Verhagen HJ, Teijink JA, Cuypers P, Nevelsteen A, Vermassen FE. Endovascular repair for aorto-enteric fistula: a bridge too far or a bridge to surgery? Eur J Vasc Endovasc Surg. 2006;32(1):27–33.
126. Kakkos SK, Antoniadis PN, Klonaris CN, et al. Open or endovascular repair of aortoenteric fistulas? A multicentre comparative study. Eur J Vasc Endovasc Surg. 2011;41(5):625–34.
127. Valentine RJ, Timaran CH, Modrall GJ, Smith ST, Arko FR, Clagett GP. Secondary aortoenteric fistulas versus paraprosthetic erosions: is bleeding associated with a worse outcome? J Am Coll Surg. 2008;207(6):922–7.
128. Song Y, Liu Q, Shen H, Jia X, Zhang H, Qiao L. Diagnosis and management of primary aorto-enteric fistulas—experience learned from eighteen patients. Surgery. 2008;143(1):43–50.
129. Chuter TA, Lukaszewicz GC, Reilly LM, et al. Endovascular repair of a presumed aortoenteric fistula: late failure due to recurrent infection. J Endovasc Ther. 2000;7(3):240–4.
130. Kakkos SK, Bicknell CD, Tsolakis IA, Bergqvist D, Hellenic Co-operative Group on Aortic Surgery. Editor's choice—management of secondary aorto-enteric and other abdominal arterio-enteric fistulas: a review and pooled data analysis. Eur J Vasc Endovasc Surg. 2016;52(6):770–86.
131. Kakkos SK, Papadoulas S, Tsolakis IA. Endovascular management of arterioenteric fistulas: a systemic review and meta-analysis of the literature. J Endovasc Ther. 2011;18(1):66–77.
132. Bergqvist D, Bjorck M. Secondary arterioenteric fistulation—a systematic literature analysis. Eur J Vasc Endovasc Surg. 2009;37(1):31–42.
133. Bogie R, Willigendael EM, de Booij M, Meesters B, Teijink JA. Acute thrombosis of an abdominal aortic aneurysm: a short report. Eur J Vasc Endovasc Surg. 2008;35(5):590–2.
134. Prandoni P, Lensing AW, Piccioli A, et al. Recurrent venous thromboembolism and bleeding complications during anticoagulant treatment in patients with cancer and venous thrombosis. Blood. 2002;100(10):3484–8.
135. Nakao Y, Akagi H, Irie H, Sakaguchi S, Sakai K. Successful endovascular repair of a ruptured thoracoabdominal aortic aneurysm with severe mural thrombus. Kyobu Geka. 2014;67(12):1051–5.
136. Lozano P, Gomez FT, Julia J, MR E, Garcia F. Recurrent embolism caused by floating thrombus in the thoracic aorta. Ann Vasc Surg. 1998;12(6):609–11.
137. Dua A, Desai SS, Holcomb JB, Burgess AR, Freischlag JA. Clinical review of vascular trauma. Berlin Heidelberg: Springer; 2014. p. 191–9. ISBN 978-3-642-39100-2
138. Shames ML, Rubin BG, Sanchez LA, Thompson RW, Sicard GA. Treatment of embolizing arterial lesions with endoluminally placed stent grafts. Ann Vasc Surg. 2002;16(5):608–12.
139. Criado E, Wall P, Lucas P, Gasparis A, Proffit T, Ricotta J. Transesophageal echo-guided endovascular exclusion of thoracic aortic mobile thrombi. J Vasc Surg. 2004;39(1):238–42.

140. Fueglistaler P, Wolff T, Guerke L, Stierli P, Eugster T. Endovascular stent graft for symptomatic mobile thrombus of the thoracic aorta. J Vasc Surg. 2005;42(4):781–3.
141. Zhang WW, Abou-Zamzam AM, Hashisho M, Killeen JD, Bianchi C, Teruya TH. Staged endovascular stent grafts for concurrent mobile/ulcerated thrombi of thoracic and abdominal aorta causing recurrent spontaneous distal embolization. J Vasc Surg. 2008;47(1):193–6.
142. Alhan C, Karabulut H, Senay S, Cagil H, Toraman F. Endovascular treatment of occlusive abdominal aortic thrombosis. Heart Vessels. 2010;25(1):70–2.
143. Akagawa E, Ookawa K, Ohshima N. Endovascular stent configuration affects intraluminal flow dynamics and in vitro endothelialization. Biorheology. 2004;41(6):665–80.
144. Schoots IG, Levi MM, Reekers JA, Lameris JS, van Gulik TM. Thrombolytic therapy for acute superior mesenteric artery occlusion. J Vasc Interv Radiol. 2005;16(3):317–29.
145. Gonzalez C, Penado S, Llata L, Valero C, Riancho JA. The clinical spectrum of retroperitoneal hematoma in anticoagulated patients. Medicine (Baltimore). 2003;82(4):257–62.
146. Caleo O, Bocchini G, Paoletta S, et al. Spontaneous non-aortic retroperitoneal hemorrhage: etiology, imaging characterization and impact of MDCT on management. A multicentric study. Radiol Med. 2015;120(1):133–48.
147. Sunga KL, Bellolio MF, Gilmore RM, Cabrera D. Spontaneous retroperitoneal hematoma: etiology, characteristics, management, and outcome. J Emerg Med. 2012;43(2):e157–61.
148. Chan YC, Morales JP, Reidy JF, Taylor PR. Management of spontaneous and iatrogenic retroperitoneal haemorrhage: conservative management, endovascular intervention or open surgery? Int J Clin Pract. 2008;62(10):1604–13.
149. Kauppila LI. Prevalence of stenotic changes in arteries supplying the lumbar spine. A postmortem angiographic study on 140 subjects. Ann Rheum Dis. 1997;56(10):591–5.
150. Panetta T, Sclafani SJ, Goldstein AS, Phillips TF, Shaftan GW. Percutaneous transcatheter embolization for massive bleeding from pelvic fractures. J Trauma. 1985;25(11):1021–9.
151. Sharafuddin MJ, Andresen KJ, Sun S, Lang E, Stecker MS, Wibbenmeyer LA. Spontaneous extraperitoneal hemorrhage with hemodynamic collapse in patients undergoing anticoagulation: management with selective arterial embolization. J Vasc Interv Radiol. 2001;12(10):1231–4.
152. Pathi R, Voyvodic F, Thompson WR. Spontaneous extraperitoneal haemorrhage: computed tomography diagnosis and treatment by selective arterial embolization. Australas Radiol. 2004;48(2):123–8.
153. Shi W, Dowell JD. Etiology and treatment of acute inferior vena cava thrombosis. Thromb Res. 2017;149:9–16.
154. Kasirajan K, Gray B, Ouriel K. Percutaneous AngioJet thrombectomy in the management of extensive deep venous thrombosis. J Vasc Interv Radiol. 2001;12(2):179–85.
155. Meissner MH, Gloviczki P, Comerota AJ, et al. Society for Vascular Surgery; American Venous Forum. Early thrombus removal strategies for acute deep venous thrombosis: clinical practice guidelines of the Society for Vascular Surgery and the American Venous Forum. J Vasc Surg. 2012;55(5):1449–62.
156. Mewissen MW, Seabrook GR, Meissner MH, Cynamon J, Labropoulos N, Haughton SH. Catheter-directed thrombolysis for lower extremity deep venous thrombosis: report of a national multicenter registry. Radiology. 1999;211(1):39–49.
157. Alkhouli M, Zack CJ, Zhao H, Shafi I, Bashir R. Comparative outcomes of catheter-directed thrombolysis plus anticoagulation versus anticoagulation alone in the treatment of inferior vena caval thrombosis. Circ Cardiovasc Interv. 2015;8(2):e001882.
158. Enden T, Haig Y, Klow NE, et al. Long-term outcome after additional catheter-directed thrombolysis versus standard treatment for acute iliofemoral deep vein thrombosis (the CaVenT study): a randomised controlled trial. Lancet. 2012;379(9810):31–8.

10

Acute Abdominal Pain in Pregnant Patients

Gabriele Masselli, Martina Derme, and Gianfranco Gualdi

Abstract

Acute abdominal pain in pregnancy presents diagnostic and therapeutic challenges. Prompt diagnosis and treatment are crucial for the well-being of the mother and the fetus, and imaging is often required to clarify the clinical picture. Ultrasound (US) remains the primary imaging modality for the pregnant abdomen and pelvis because of its availability, portability, and absence of ionizing radiation. US can often be used to elucidate the cause of abdominal and pelvic pain, particularly if the pain is due to an obstetric or gynecologic abnormality. However, evaluation of the bowel, pancreas, ureters, and mesenteric vasculature may be limited on US because of patient body habitus, a small field of view, and the presence of overlying structures, especially in the later stages of pregnancy. Magnetic resonance imaging (MRI) has been shown to be highly useful in the diagnosis of acute gynecological and obstetric disorders, and particularly in the setting of an acute abdomen during pregnancy. MRI is often used when US is inconclusive. Computed tomography (CT) is the imaging examination of choice when there is a life-threatening situation, and in patients with trauma, when a rapid diagnosis is required, and US is not diagnostic.

Keywords

Acute abdominal pain · Pregnancy · Ultrasound Computed tomography · Magnetic resonance imaging

10.1 Obstetric Causes

10.1.1 Ectopic Pregnancy

An ectopic pregnancy (EP) occurs when a fertilized ovum implants outside the normal uterine cavity. The incidence of EP is approximately 11/1000 pregnancies, and it remains the main cause of maternal death during the first trimester [1]. Risk factors for EP include tubal damage following surgery or infection, smoking, in vitro fertilization, and advanced maternal age [2]. EP is most commonly located in the ampullary portion of the fallopian tube (80%), and less commonly in sites including the interstitial portion of the fallopian tube (2%), the cervix (<1%), a cesarean scar (6%), the anomalous rudimentary horn of the uterus (0.2–2%), and the peritoneal abdominal cavity (0.9–1.4%) [3].

G. Masselli, M.D., Ph.D. (✉) • G. Gualdi, M.D.
Radiology Department, Umberto I Hospital, Sapienza University, Rome, Italy
e-mail: gabriele.masselli@uniroma1.it

M. Derme, M.D.
Gynecology and Obstetrics Department, Umberto I Hospital, Sapienza University, Rome, Italy

M. Patlas et al. (eds.), *MDCT and MR Imaging of Acute Abdomen*,
https://doi.org/10.1007/978-3-319-70778-5_10

EP should be suspected in any woman of reproductive age when a positive blood pregnancy test is associated with acute abdominal/pelvic pain, vaginal bleeding, and a tender adnexal mass.

Early diagnosis and treatment of EP are crucial in order to reduce maternal mortality and to preserve future fertility. The initial evaluation includes a quantitative measurement of serum human chorionic gonadotropin (hCG), and transvaginal ultrasound (US).

Transvaginal US has reported sensitivities of 87.0–99.0% and specificities of 94.0–99.9% for the diagnosis of EP [1]. In 15–20% of patients, US provides a definitive diagnosis, showing an extrauterine gestational sac (GS) containing a yolk sac and/or embryo which may or may not have cardiac activity [1]. More frequently, it is only suggestive of an EP, showing an adnexal mass and pelvic free fluid. The adnexal mass may appear as a sac-like ring, solid, or complex [4].

MRI is an excellent problem-solving imaging modality when US is equivocal or inconclusive before intervention or therapy. MRI provides additional information for complicated forms of EP, when the diagnosis is unclear and US is equivocal, in particular for unusual implantation sites [5, 6]. MRI offers the benefits of multiplanar imaging, absence of ionizing radiation, excellent soft-tissue contrast, and more specific characterization of tissues and fluids. MRI can be performed only in hemodynamically stable patients. Reported MRI findings of EP include a GS-like structure which typically appears sac-like, an adnexal or abdominal hematoma, tubal dilatation due to hemosalpinx, and tubal wall enhancement (Fig. 10.1) [7].

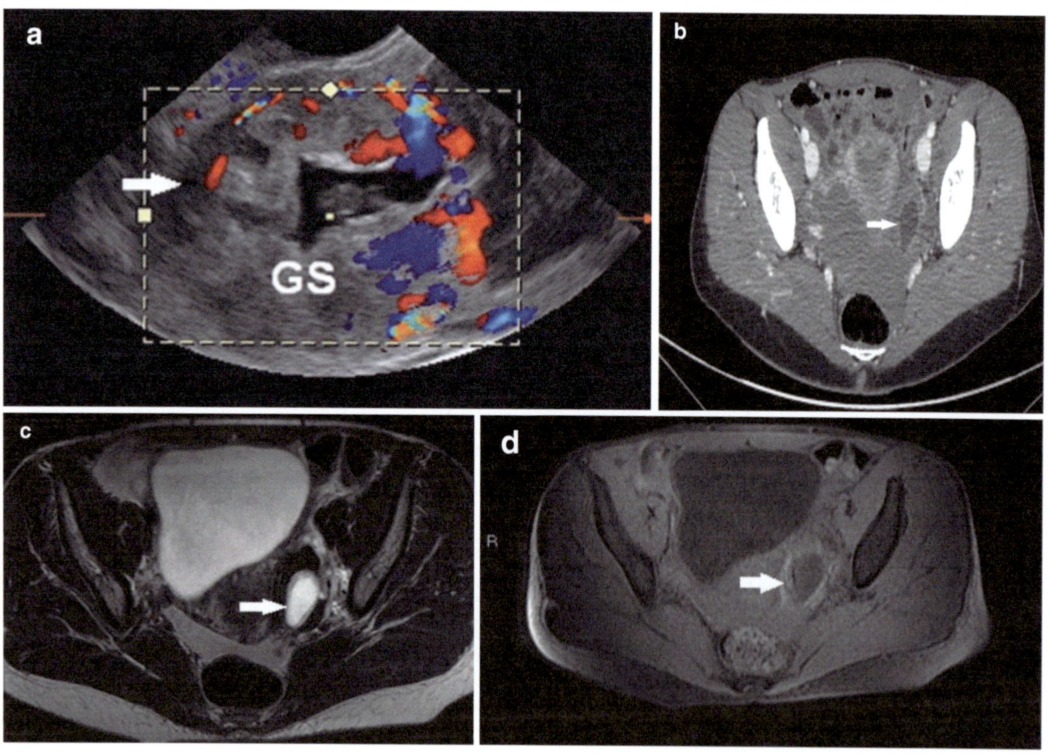

Fig. 10.1 A 29-year-old woman presented with amenorrhea for 7 weeks, abdominal pain, and vaginal bleeding; serum hCG level was elevated. Transvaginal 3D sonogram (**a**) in sagittal plane shows a GS at the level of the tube (arrow). CT of the pelvis (**b**) shows a GS (arrow). Axial (**c**) T2-weighted MR image and axial contrast T1-weighted image (**d**) of the pelvis show a left GS measuring 10 mm in diameter, surrounded by a thick wall, which is a tubal pregnancy associated with hemoperitoneum (arrow)

Expectant management is an option for clinically stable asymptomatic women with an US diagnosis of EP and a decreasing serum hCG value, initially lower than 1500 mIU/mL. Medical therapy, using methotrexate (MTX), should be offered to women with a serum hCG value lower than 5000 mIU/mL and minimal symptoms. Surgery is usually needed when EP causes severe symptoms, bleeding, or when high hCG levels are present. Laparoscopic surgery is typically used. For a ruptured EP, emergency laparotomy is needed [1].

10.1.2 Placental Abruption

Placental abruption (PA) is defined as the premature separation of the implanted placenta before the delivery of the fetus. It complicates approximately 1% of all pregnancies, and is a major obstetrical complication associated with an increased risk of substantial fetal and maternal morbidity and mortality [8]. Several risk factors have been associated with PA, including young or advanced maternal age, previous history of PA and/or cesarean section, multiparity, cigarette smoking, multiple gestations, hypertensive and thrombophilic disorders, abdominal trauma, and polyhydramnios [9]. The main clinical features are vaginal bleeding, abdominal pain, uterine contractions or uterine tenderness, and signs of fetal distress. The most important US criteria for PA (sensitivity 80%, specificity 92%) are the detection of pre-/retroplacental fluid collections, evidence of marginal subchorionic or intra-amniotic hematomas, increased placental thickness (>5 cm), and jelly-like movements of the chorionic plate [10, 11]. However, 25–50% of hematomas, mostly retroplacental, are undetectable using US [11–13], because the echotexture of recent hemorrhage is similar to that of the placenta [14], or because of small dimensions. Moreover, clots resulting from chronic abruption may drain through the cervix. MRI is superior to US for the evaluation of placenta hemorrhage, because it improves soft-tissue contrast and has a wider field of view [15]. Diffusion- and T1-weighted MR sequences (sensitivity, respectively of 100% and 94%; diagnostic accuracy, respectively of 100% and 97%) are more accurate than T2-weighted half-Fourier RARE (sensitivity 94%; diagnostic accuracy 87%) and true FISP sequences (sensitivity 79%; diagnostic accuracy 90%) for the detection of PA [15]. Moreover, MRI can be used to date hemorrhage on the basis of the paramagnetic effects of methemoglobin and to classify intrauterine hematomas as hyperacute (first few hours, intracellular oxyhemoglobin), acute (1–3 days, intracellular deoxyhemoglobin), early subacute (3–7 days, intracellular methemoglobin), late subacute (≥14 days, extracellular methemoglobin), and chronic (>4 weeks, intracellular hemosiderin and ferritin) [16].

Due to abruption may rapidly worsen, requiring rapid surgical delivery to prevent adverse maternal and fetal outcomes, an accurate diagnosis of PA and, possibly, the prediction of its worsening are extremely important when considering initial conservative treatment. The presence of a hematoma with hyperacute or acute MR signal intensity characteristics may correlate with progression of the abruption to higher grades. Because of the possible rapid and unpredictable worsening of abruption, it is important to avoid any delay in performing MRI (Fig. 10.2).

In summary, MRI is an extremely accurate modality able to identify placental abruptions, even in patients with negative US findings. It is important to note that signs of acute or recent bleeding within a hematoma are indicative of a potentially unstable abruption, whereas hematomas with late subacute bleeding are stable [8].

10.1.3 Placental Adhesive Disorders

Placental adhesive disorders (PAD) include placenta accreta (placental villi attached to the myometrium), placenta increta (placental villi invading the myometrium), and placenta percreta (placental villi penetrating up to the uterine serosa). The incidence of PAD is 1 in 2000

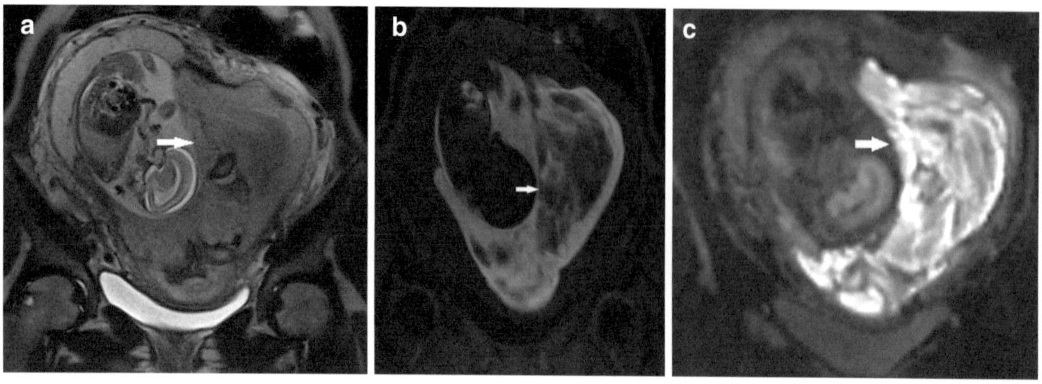

Fig. 10.2 A 25-year-old woman at 28 weeks gestation, with acute pelvic pain and vaginal bleeding. Coronal T2-weighted MR image (**a**) shows intrauterine clot, with hypointense areas along the left side of the uterine cavity, and extending inferiorly to cover the uterine ostium (arrow). Coronal T1-weighted fat-saturated gradient-echo (**b**) and diffusion-weighted images (**c**) show a large subchorionic hematoma with heterogeneous signal due to acute and subacute bleeding (arrow)

pregnancies, with a rapid increase in recent years, reflecting the rising number of cesarean sections and other uterine surgery [17]. The presence of acute abdominal pain is generally related to placenta percreta.

US is the first imaging modality used to diagnose PAD. Sonographic features include loss of the normal hypoechoic retroplacental myometrium zone, thinning or disruption of the hyperechoic uterine serosa-bladder interface, focal exophytic masses, and lacunae in the placenta (this latter finding is the most predictive sonographic sign, with a sensitivity of 79%, and a positive predictive value of 92%) [18]. Color Doppler can add information and, when three dimensions are available, can often help to distinguish placenta accreta from placenta percreta, highlighting areas of increased vascularity with dilated blood vessels that cross the placenta and the uterine wall [19].

MRI is not used as the first imaging modality to diagnose PAD, but can provide additional information in equivocal patients, especially those with a posterior placenta and previous myomectomy [20, 21].

Intravenous (iv) contrast-enhanced MR images can improve the confidence in the diagnosis of PAD, but their use is limited in pregnancy since gadolinium-based contrast agents, classified as category C drugs by the Food and Drug Administration (FDA), cross the placenta, and are excreted by the fetal kidneys into the amniotic fluid [5]. Lim et al. [22] found that the volume of dark placental bands (first described by Lax) was the most predictive MRI finding in true PAD. Derman et al. confirmed that the most reliable MR sign is a larger dark band on T2 HASTE images [23]. They added an additional finding: vessels of 6 mm or larger which presumably correspond to lacunae. Moreover, when there is placenta percreta, MRI is able to depict infiltration of adjacent organs by showing tenting of the bladder, interruption of the myometrial line, and direct infiltration of pelvic organs [18].

In conclusion, if US findings suggest possible percreta or are inconclusive or negative in an at-risk woman, MRI can be very useful. Invasion of adjacent organs can be seen better on MRI than on US. Situations in which MRI may also contribute additional information include women with placenta previa with a posterior or lateral implantation, a posterior scar from a myomectomy, a history of difficult placental removal in the past with a posterior or lateral placenta in the present pregnancy, or a history of endometrial ablation (Fig. 10.3) [18].

The correct and prompt diagnosis of placenta percreta is important because this condition may cause uterine rupture, requiring an emergency cesarean section.

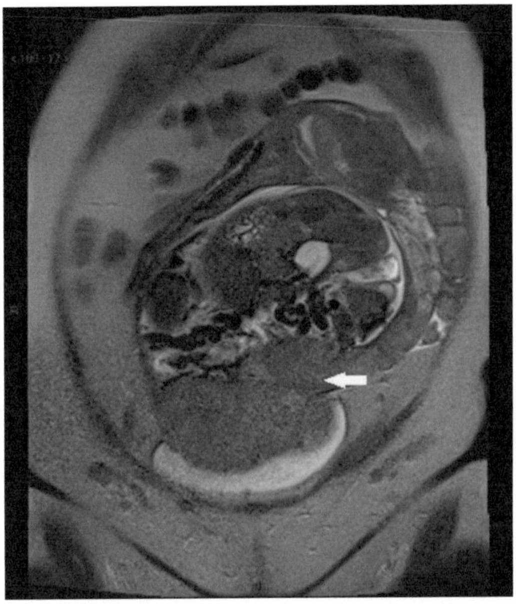

Fig. 10.3 A 29-year-old woman at 32 weeks gestation, with acute pelvic pain and vaginal bleeding. Coronal T2 HASTE image shows multiple irregular areas of the placenta bulging into the myometrium, with marked invasion of the bladder, and a bicornuate uterus (arrow). These findings indicate placenta percreta. A hysterectomy was performed at delivery, which confirmed the MR findings

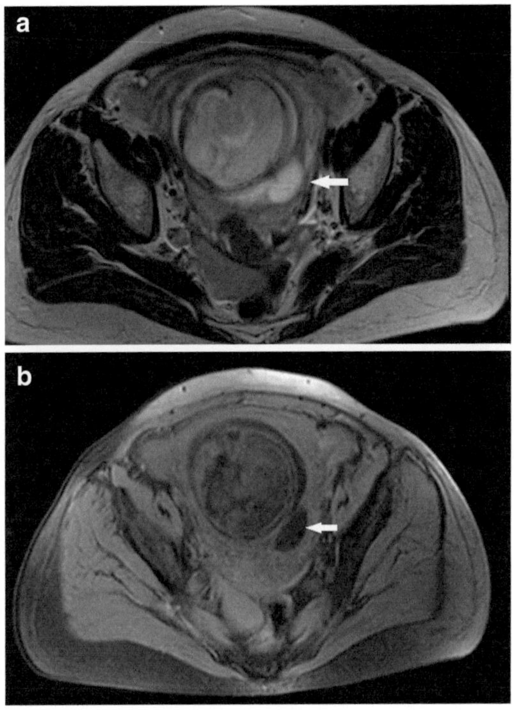

Fig. 10.4 A 38-year-old woman was admitted at 26 weeks gestation, with vomiting and acute abdominal pain. Axial T2-weighted HASTE (**a**) and T1-weighted fat-saturated MR images (**b**) show posterior extravasation of amniotic fluid into a hernia sac which contains a small fluid level (arrow). These findings are consistent with a partially sealed uterine rupture. Note the presence of hemoperitoneum

10.1.4 Uterine Rupture

Uterine rupture is a rare obstetrical complication and frequently results in life-threatening maternal and fetal compromise. It occurs when a full-thickness disruption of the uterine wall, which also involves the uterine serosa, is present. A 10-year study by Gardeil et al. showed that the overall rate of unscarred uterine rupture during pregnancy was 1 per 30,764 deliveries (0.0033%) [24]. Congenital uterine anomalies, multiparity, uterine myomectomy and/or cesarean deliveries, fetal macrosomia, labor induction, and uterine trauma all increased the risk of uterine rupture. The classic signs and symptoms of uterine rupture are fetal distress, loss of uterine contractility, abdominal pain, hemorrhage, and shock. Diagnosis of uterine rupture by US relies on nonspecific and secondary signs, including free fluid or hematoma formation. In comparison to US, MRI is less operator-dependent and provides a more comprehensive examination with a larger field of view. MRI allows for better evaluation of soft tissues than both CT and US. Finally, MRI allows clear visualization of the uterine wall; therefore, it helps to diagnose both antepartum uterine rupture when US is indeterminate, showing the tear itself, as well as other uterine wall defects, including uterine dehiscence and uterine sacculation (Fig. 10.4) [11, 25].

A correct differential diagnosis between complete uterine rupture and uterine dehiscence is important to choose the most appropriate management. When a diagnosis of complete uterine rupture is established, the immediate stabilization of the mother and the surgical delivery of the fetus are imperative. In contrast, expectant management can be used after the diagnosis of uterine dehiscence [24].

10.2 Gynecological Causes

10.2.1 Adnexal Masses

The incidence of adnexal masses during pregnancy is approximately 1% [26]. Common adnexal cystic masses include simple cysts, hemorrhagic cysts, and hyperstimulated ovaries in patients who have undergone assisted fertility. Lower abdominal and pelvic pain is the most common symptom. Although ovarian cyst torsion or rupture is uncommon in pregnancy, some women may require emergency surgery for these complications. US is the imaging examination of choice for the primary evaluation of adnexal masses, but is less accurate for the assessment of complex or indeterminate masses, even when combined with color Doppler. Further evaluation with MRI may be indicated for diagnosis, especially when the findings are not clear on US. MRI has been shown to be more specific and accurate than US and Doppler assessment, with an accuracy ranging from 83% to 89%, compared with 63% for US [27]. MRI can be used to determine, using frequency-selective fat saturation, whether a mass contains fat, which can be highly useful in the diagnosis of a teratoma. MRI can be used to help distinguish benign ovarian cysts from ovarian neoplasms, because of the presence of papillary projections and nodular septae in neoplasms (Fig. 10.5) [28].

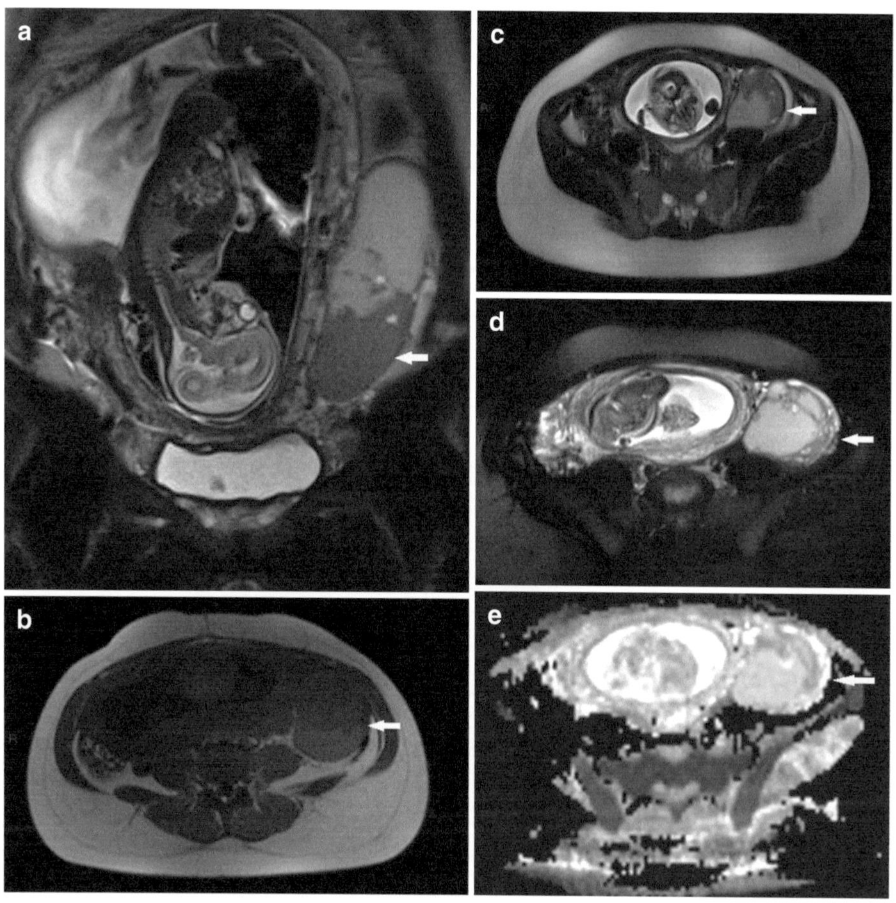

Fig. 10.5 A 35-year-old woman at 30 weeks gestation, with acute pelvic pain. Coronal (**a**) and axial (**b** and **c**) T2-weighted MR images show a complex mass, with fluid and solid components in the left ovary (arrow). Hemorrhagic areas are seen on an axial T1-weighted sequence (**d**). Axial DWI image shows reduction of diffusion in relationship to the high cellularity of the solid component of the mass (**e**). Cystoadenocarcinoma was confirmed at surgery

Most ovarian masses diagnosed in pregnancy are benign and resolve spontaneously. Surgical management is warranted when masses are suspicious for malignancy, are at high risk for torsion, or are clinically symptomatic. With increasing numbers of successful laparoscopic procedures reported in pregnancy, laparoscopy appears to be a safe option with trained and experienced providers [28].

10.2.2 Adnexal Torsion

Adnexal torsion (AT) is the fifth most common gynecologic surgical emergency. The incidence of AT among women of reproductive age is estimated at 9.9 per 100,000 women [29]. Pregnancy is a risk factor for AT. According to previous studies, 13.7% of patients with AT were pregnant [29]. The most common causes of AT during pregnancy appear to be corpus luteum cysts, and ovarian hyperstimulation syndrome (OHSS) associated with assisted reproductive technologies (ART).The clinical signs and symptoms are often confused with those of other abdominal conditions, and the imaging features are sometimes nonspecific. US is the first imaging modality used to evaluate suspected AT in pregnancy. US findings include an enlarged ovary with multiple peripherally located follicles, a twisted vascular pedicle (the "whirlpool sign"), and free pelvic fluid. Normal Doppler flow can be observed in 45–61% of all patients with AT [30, 31]. MRI should be performed after inconclusive US. Asymmetric enlargement of the ovary and stromal edema are well demonstrated by MRI, especially using T2-weighted sequences (Fig. 10.6). A twisted vascular pedicle can also be observed by MRI. Ovarian hemorrhage, a frequent consequence of torsion, can be identified on MRI, especially using T1-weighted MR images, where blood products are hyperintense [30].

It may be necessary to perform a CT in emergency situations, for example, when there is substantial associated hemoperitoneum.

The missed diagnosis of AT can lead not only to ovarian necrosis and sepsis, but also threaten the pregnancy. An early diagnosis and subsequent laparoscopic management are needed, and they are related to favorable maternal and fetal outcomes.

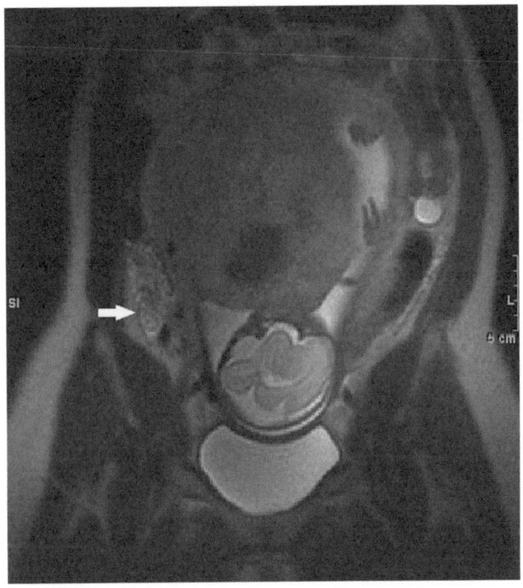

Fig. 10.6 Ovarian torsion in a 29-year-old woman at 34 weeks gestation, who presented with acute pelvic pain. Coronal T2-weighted MR image shows an enlarged, edematous right ovary (arrow), with peripheral follicles

10.2.3 Uterine Leiomyoma

Leiomyomas have a prevalence during pregnancy of up to 20%. They have been associated with an increased obstetrical complication rate, including an increased incidence of spontaneous abortion, fetal malpresentation, intrauterine growth restriction, placenta previa, labor dystocia, placental abruption, retained placenta, preterm labor, premature rupture of membranes, postpartum hemorrhage, and an increased frequency of cesarean sections [32]. Leiomyomas are usually asymptomatic during pregnancy. However, abdominal pain and uterine contractions can result from their degeneration and necrosis. The Muram criteria have been used to evaluate the presence of a leiomyoma by US. They included visualization of a spherical mass with a diameter ≥3 cm; distortion of the adjacent myometrium by the mass; and a distinctive echogenicity, differentiating the mass from myometrium [33]. In acute hemorrhagic infarction (red degeneration), US shows heterogeneous or hyperechoic mass, and later anechoic components resulting from cystic necrosis [5]. MRI is the most accurate imaging technique for the detection and localization of leiomyomas. On T2-weighted MR images, nondegenerated leiomyomas appear as well-circumscribed masses of decreased signal intensity. Leiomyomas with hemorrhagic degeneration often exhibit diffuse or peripheral high signal intensity on T1-weighted MR imaging and variable signal intensity on T2-weighted MR imaging [34, 35].

There is no consensus, to our knowledge, regarding the best approach to the treatment of symptomatic leiomyomas during pregnancy. Conservative therapy is the first option to be considered. Myomectomy may be performed in selected patients, with low perioperative and postoperative morbidity, in symptomatic, subserosal, or pedunculated leiomyomas with signs of degeneration, after the failure of conservative treatment [35].

10.3 Non-obstetric and Gynecological Causes

10.3.1 Urolithiasis

Renal colic is the most frequent non-obstetric and gynecological cause for abdominal pain and subsequent hospitalization during pregnancy. Symptomatic nephrolithiasis complicates 1 in 3300 pregnancies, with an incidence ranging from 1:200 to 1:1500 [36]. Renal colic has been associated with several pregnancy complications, including preterm labor and delivery, recurrent abortions, hypertensive disorders, gestational diabetes, and cesarean sections [37]. US is the first investigation when there is a suspicion of urinary tract calculus disease during pregnancy. It is operator dependent, and its sensitivity for the depiction of nephrolithiasis during pregnancy ranges from 34% to 92.5%. Moreover, it is highly nonspecific, and ureteral obstruction secondary to calculi and physiological hydronephrosis may not be distinguishable. Transvaginal US can be helpful to evaluate the distal ureter and to help distinguish obstruction from physiological hydronephrosis, the latter of which can occur in up to 90% of pregnant patients in this situation. Doppler-assisted measurement of the resistive index (RI) (peak systolic velocity of intrarenal blood flow minus the end-diastolic velocity, divided by the peak systolic velocity) has shown some promise in pregnancy. The RI does not appear to be affected by the physiologic hydronephrosis of pregnancy. An elevated RI (>0.70) should not therefore be attributed to pregnancy. Absence of a "ureteral jet" (passage of urine at the ureterovesical junction) on the suspected side of an obstruction has been reported to have a sensitivity of 100% and a specificity of 91%. Patients should be imaged in the contralateral decubitus position to decrease false-positive results [38, 39].

When results are equivocal, half-Fourier single-shot turbo spin-echo (HASTE) magnetic resonance urography (MRU) without IV contrast is safe and effective. It is comparable to CT accuracy and is now considered second-line during pregnancy when available. Calculi appear as signal voids within the high signal of urine of a dilated ureter. The presence of a standing column of urine below the level of the pelvic brim, in addition to proximal ureteral dilation, is strongly suggestive of an obstructing distal ureteral calculus ("double kink sign"). Other MRI features which suggest pathologic rather than physiologic hydronephrosis include an unusual site of obstruction (including the ureteropelvic junction or ureterovesical junction), an abrupt ending of the ureter (rather than a smooth tapering at the level of the pelvic brim), and perinephric or periureteral edema (Fig. 10.7) [6, 36]. MRI is helpful in demonstrating complications including pyelonephritis, which are visualized as an enlarged, edematous and heterogeneous kidney. Areas of focal pyelonephritis have lower signal intensity on T2-weighted MR images and restricted diffusion on diffusion-weighted MR images. In unresolved patients, low radiation dose noncontrast CT remains a reliable technique for depicting obstructing urinary tract calculi in pregnant women.

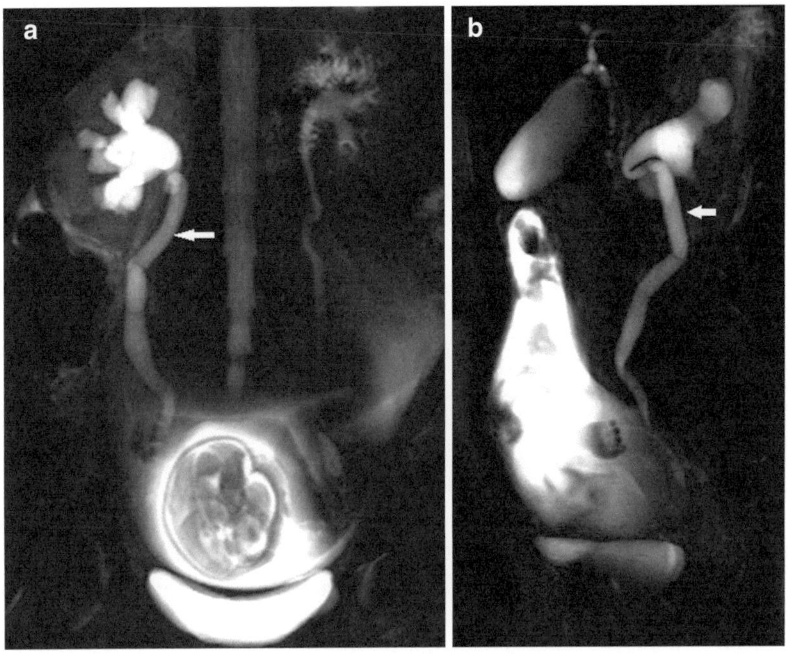

Fig. 10.7 A 32-year-old woman was admitted at 30 weeks of gestation with acute abdominal pain. A standing column of urine below the level of the pelvic brim, in addition to proximal right ureteral dilation (arrow), is strongly suggestive of an obstructing distal ureteral calculus ("double kink sign") on these maximal intensity projection MR urography images (**a**, **b**). Other MRI features which suggest pathologic rather than physiologic hydronephrosis include an unusual site of obstruction (such as the ureteropelvic junction or ureterovesical junction), an abrupt ending of the ureteral dilatation (rather than a smooth tapering at the level of the pelvic brim), and perinephric and periureteric edema

A conservative approach should be the initial management in all pregnant patients with symptomatic ureteral calculi. Conservative treatment, which requires close communication between the urologist and obstetrician, includes hydration (oral or intravenous), analgesia, antibiotics (if infection is present), antiemetics, rest, and routine sieving of the urine. If conservative approach fails, stenting with ureteral double-J stent placement may be performed as an initial procedure in patients who have fever and/or proximal ureteral calculi. Percutaneous nephrostomy (PCN) should be reserved for patients with urosepsis or pyonephrosis if a stent cannot be placed. Ureteroscopy with a Holmium laser has become the procedure of choice in pregnancy for symptomatic calculi less than 1 cm, and in those patients without evidence of sepsis or a history of renal transplant [36].

Anti-inflammatory agents and iv antibiotics are required in the treatment of pyelonephritis. Rarely, rapid spread of infection may result in a perinephric abscess. This may occur due to a delay in diagnosis, incorrect treatment, diabetes mellitus, or an immunocompromised state. Aggressive treatment with intravenous antibiotics and surgical drainage of the abscess are indicated [36].

10.3.2 Gastrointestinal Causes

10.3.2.1 Acute Appendicitis

Acute appendicitis occurs in approximately 1:2000 pregnancies and is the most common non-obstetric surgical emergency in pregnancy. Fetal mortality is as high as 37% if the appendix perforates. Thus, early and accurate diagnosis of appendicitis in pregnant patients is critical to prevent adverse outcomes to both mother and fetus.

Clinical examination and laboratory tests are often altered during pregnancy, potentially leading to a delay in diagnosis. US is the first investigation used to diagnose acute appendicitis, with the same parameters as for nonpregnant patients, including visualization of a blind-ending, dilated (>6–7 mm in diameter), aperistaltic and noncompressible tubular structure arising from the cecum [40]. US of the appendix, with reported sensitivity and specificity values ranging from 50% to 100% and from 33% to 92% respectively, is a highly operator-dependent examination and can be limited by the pregnant body habitus, especially in the later stages of gestation [41]. If the appendix is not visualized by US, the multiplanar capacity and the excellent soft-tissue contrast of MRI make it an optimal test for suspected acute appendicitis. MR features of a normal appendix include a diameter less than 6 mm, an appendiceal wall thickness less than 2 mm, low luminal signal intensity on T1- and T2-weighted images, and no periappendiceal fat stranding or fluid. MRI features of appendicitis include an appendiceal diameter greater than 7 mm, an appendiceal wall thickness greater than 2 mm, high-signal-intensity luminal contents on T2-weighted images due to fluid or edema, and hyperintense periappendiceal fat stranding and fluid [37, 42]. MRI has been described as an effective modality for the diagnosis as well as exclusion of appendicitis during pregnancy, with 100% sensitivity and 94% specificity reported [37]. If MRI cannot be performed, because of absolute contraindications or it is not available, CT is an alternative.

If appendicitis is strongly suspected clinically, surgical management is indicated, even in the face of indeterminate imaging findings. This is justified in view of increased maternal and perinatal morbidity and mortality if the diagnosis is delayed or missed. Laparoscopic appendicectomy has also been reported as a successful procedure during pregnancy [40].

10.3.2.2 Intestinal Obstruction

Intestinal obstruction in pregnancy is relatively rare. It is the second most common non-obstetric reason for abdominal surgical intervention during pregnancy. The incidence ranges from 1 in 1500 to 1 in 66,000 deliveries [43]. Adhesions from previous abdominal surgery are the most common etiology of this condition (60–70%). An additional 25% result from volvulus, while intussusception causes approximately 5% [44]. The common symptoms of intestinal obstruction in pregnancy include abdominal pain (98%), vomiting (82%), and constipation (30%). US may show dilated loops of bowel with fluid levels and aperistalsis, but the point and the cause of bowel obstruction usually remain undetermined. CT is the mainstay imaging modality which is used in the management of small bowel obstruction in nonpregnant patients. In pregnant patients, however, CT exposes the fetus to ionizing radiation. MRI is capable of providing large field-of-view images of maternal abnormalities with excellent soft-tissue contrast. Furthermore, the images obtained with MRI do not expose the fetus to ionizing radiation and are often diagnostic without the need for iv administration of contrast. MRI, using multiplanar T2-weighted single-shot fast spin-echo (SSFSE) sequences, confirmed the presence and identified the site of bowel obstruction in approximately 70% of patients [10, 45].

If undiagnosed, intestinal obstruction is associated with increased maternal and perinatal mortality. Correction of electrolyte disturbances, emergency laparotomy (midline), and resection and anastomosis or decompression of the bowel are the mainstay of management [43].

10.3.3 Hepatobiliary Causes

10.3.3.1 Acute Cholecystitis

The prevalence of gallstones in pregnant women is 5–12% [6]. A right upper quadrant US is the most appropriate initial imaging examination for the evaluation of suspected acute cholecystitis in pregnancy. US findings of acute cholecystitis include gallbladder distension (>5 cm in diameter), wall thickening (>3 mm), pericholecystic fluid, and wall hyperemia, as in nonpregnant individuals. A sonographic Murphy's sign is defined as the presence of maximal tenderness elicited by direct pressure of the transducer over a sonographically localized gallbladder. This sign was present in 99% of 497 non-pregnant patients with suspected acute cholecystitis [46, 47]. MRI is the most appropriate second-line imaging examination to evaluate known or suspected biliary tract disease during pregnancy. MRI findings include gallbladder wall thickening of greater than 3 mm, increased signal intensity in the gallbladder wall (edema) on T2-weighted images, increased signal intensity surrounding the gallbladder (pericholecystic fluid) on T2-weighted images, and a signal void in the cystic duct or gallbladder neck due to an obstructing calculus. Complications include perforation and pericholecystic abscess. MRI has a positive predictive value of up to 100% for accurate diagnosis of acute cholecystitis in pregnant and nonpregnant patients [37].

Management involves iv fluids to correct electrolyte imbalance, analgesics and anti-inflammatory agents, nasogastric suction, and intravenous antibiotics. Recurrent attacks of cholecystitis and complications including empyema or perforation warrant surgery. Percutaneous drainage of an associated abscess may be warranted. Laparoscopic cholecystectomy has been performed successfully during pregnancy [46].

10.3.3.2 Acute Pancreatitis

Acute pancreatitis is relatively rare in pregnancy, with an estimated incidence of approximately 1 in 1000 to 1 in 10,000 pregnancies. The incidence increases with gestational age; 53–79% of patients are diagnosed in the third trimester. More than 65% of such patients have acute pancreatitis during pregnancy from gallstones [48]. Patients typically present with abdominal pain, nausea, vomiting, and elevated serum amylase and/or lipase levels. US of the right upper quadrant is a safe and relatively inexpensive test; although it has low diagnostic value for acute pancreatitis, it can reliably depict the gallstones and biliary dilatation. The value of US is limited by intestinal gas and by patient body habitus. Magnetic resonance cholangiopancreatography (MRCP) without iv contrast (gadolinium) should be considered when the US findings are indeterminate. It enables the evaluation of the pancreatic parenchyma, and the diagnosis or exclusion of common bile duct calculi with a sensitivity of over 90%, without exposing the mother or the fetus to ionizing radiation [49]. At MR, the peripancreatic fluid and edema associated with pancreatitis appear as high signal intensity surrounding the pancreas on T2-weighted MR images. Biliary and pancreatic ductal dilatation can also be seen. Complications of acute pancreatitis which can be identified on MR include abscess, pseudocyst, pancreatic necrosis, and splenic vein thrombosis [37].

Although unrecognized and untreated pancreatitis may be associated with increased maternal and perinatal morbidity and mortality, it is generally a self-limiting illness. Supportive treatment with iv fluids, correction of electrolyte imbalance, glucose levels, serum calcium levels, and keeping the patient nil by mouth are the mainstay of treatment. In severe disease, nasogastric tube suction and total parenteral nutrition may need to be considered. Rarely, if the patient's condition deteriorates, emergency surgery may be indicated to remove the etiologic gallstones [49].

10.3.4 HELLP Syndrome

The incidence of HELLP syndrome is reported as 0.2–0.6% of all pregnancies and 10–20% of women with comorbid pre-eclampsia [50]. HELLP syndrome is characterized by three diagnostic lab criteria: hemolysis (H), elevated liver function tests (EL), and low platelet count (LP). In some patients, elevated liver function tests are associated with right upper quadrant or epigastric pain. The main US findings are hepatic edema, ascites, and hepatomegaly. Acute complications of HELLP syndrome which are more readily identified at MR imaging include intra- and extra-hepatic hematomas, hepatic edema due to early ischemia, and hepatic necrosis [37].

Management includes control of blood pressure, prevention of seizures, and correction of coagulation abnormality, and delivery. The role of corticosteroids is controversial, to our knowledge. Distension of Glisson's capsule of the liver may lead to hepatic rupture. Patients may present with acute upper abdominal pain and hemorrhagic shock. Emergency laparotomy with repair of liver laceration, packing to control bleeding, and correction of coagulation abnormalities with recombinant factor VII need to be considered. Very rarely, hepatic resection or hepatic artery ligation may need to be undertaken as potentially life-saving measures [50].

10.3.5 Vascular Causes

10.3.5.1 Venous Thromboembolic Disease

During pregnancy, venous stasis and hypercoagulability increase the risk of venous thrombosis. Venous stasis is due to a combination of progesterone-induced venodilation, pelvic venous compression by the gravid uterus, and pulsatile compression of the left iliac vein by the right iliac artery. Most venous thromboembolic events occur in the lower extremities. However, pregnant patients are also at increased risk for pelvic, hepatic (Budd-Chiari syndrome), mesenteric, and gonadal venous thrombosis. Prompt diagnosis and treatment of venous thrombosis during pregnancy are essential to avoid potential complications including thrombophlebitis, occlusion of the inferior vena cava and renal veins, and pulmonary embolus. Mesenteric venous thrombosis, a possible cause of bowel infarction, is difficult to diagnose, as patients typically present with nonspecific and poorly localized abdominal pain [41].

Although the preferred imaging examination for evaluating venous disease is iv contrast-enhanced CT or MR, venous disease during pregnancy can be detected with the same MR sequences performed for suspected appendicitis in pregnancy. For example, a true FISP sequence can demonstrate the presence (high signal intensity) or absence (low signal intensity) of flow within veins. It can also demonstrate a luminal thrombus as a low-signal-intensity filling defect in an otherwise high-signal-intensity patent abdominal or pelvic vein. In contrast, thrombosis or absence of flow in a vein on T2-weighted MR images appears as absence of the normal low-signal-intensity flow void of a patent vessel. On T1-weighted images, a venous thrombus can be of variable signal intensity, depending on the age of luminal blood products [36]. However, images from these nonenhanced MR imaging sequences should be interpreted with caution, as nonenhanced sequences can be limited by flow signal artifacts [51].

Low-molecular-weight heparin (LMWH) is frequently recommended for the treatment of pregnancy associated venous thromboembolism. When acute episodes occur, LMWH should be continued throughout pregnancy [41].

10.3.6 Gonadal Vein Dilatation

Unenhanced true FISP, T2-weighted, and T1-weighted MR sequences can also demonstrate the caliber of abdominal and pelvic vessels. In particular, the MR images from an examination performed for possible appendicitis should also be reviewed for enlargement of the gonadal veins as a potential cause of abdominal pain.

Although gonadal vein dilatation is a common and typically normal finding in pregnancy as the veins dilate to accommodate increased blood flow, dilatation of the gonadal vein itself or resulting extrinsic compression of the ureter by the enlarged gonadal vein has been referred to as right ovarian vein syndrome [52]. Very rarely, rupture of the dilated right ovarian vein during pregnancy has been described [53]. However, ovarian vein dilatation is a diagnosis of exclusion when it is the only finding at MR imaging to account for a pregnant patient's abdominal pain.

Conclusion

Determining the cause of acute abdominal and pelvic pain in pregnant women can be difficult because of the multiple confounding factors found in normal pregnancy. Pelvic US is the preferred primary imaging investigation, but may be of limited value due to the altered body habitus, a small field of view, and the presence of interfering overlying structures. MR imaging is extremely accurate for the identification of both obstetric and non-obstetric causes, and should be used when US findings are nondiagnostic or equivocal. In unresolved patients, CT remains a reliable technique for depicting obstructing urinary tract calculi in pregnant women.

References

1. The Royal College of Obstetricians and Gynaecologists (RCOG). Diagnosis and management of ectopic pregnancy (Green-top Guideline No. 21). https://www.rcog.org.uk/en/guidelines-research-services/guidelines/gtg21/. Published: 04/11/2016
2. Moini A, Hosseini R, Jahangiri N, Shiva M, Akhoond MR. Risk factors for ectopic pregnancy: a case-control study. J Res Med Sci. 2014;19:844–9.
3. Parker VL, Srinivas M. Non-tubal ectopic pregnancy. Arch Gynecol Obstet. 2016;294:19–27.
4. Brown DL, Doubilet PM. Transvaginal sonography for diagnosing ectopic pregnancy: positivity criteria and performance characteristics. J Ultrasound Med. 1994;13:259–66.
5. Masselli G, Brunelli R, Monti R, et al. Imaging for acute pelvic pain in pregnancy. Insights Imaging. 2014;5:165–81.
6. Masselli G, Derme M, Laghi F, Framarino-dei-Malatesta M, Gualdi G. Evaluating the acute abdomen in the pregnant patient. Radiol Clin North Am. 2015;53:1309–25.
7. Takahashi A, Takahama J, Marugami N, et al. Ectopic pregnancy: MRI findings and clinical utility. Abdom Imaging. 2013;38:844–50.
8. Leunen K, Hall DR, Odendaal HJ, Grove D. The profile and complications of women with placental abruption and intrauterine death. J Trop Pediatr. 2003;49:231–4.
9. Hruska KM, Coughlin BF, Coggins AA, Wiczyk HP. MRI diagnosis of spontaneous uterine rupture of an unscarred uterus. Emerg Radiol. 2006;12:186–8.
10. Juglard R, Rimbot A, Marty A, et al. Bowel obstruction in pregnancy: value of Single Shot Fast Spin Echo MR sequence (SS-FSE). J Radiol. 2003;84(12 Pt 1):1986–8.
11. Harris RD, Cho C, Wells WA. Sonography of the placenta with emphasis on pathological correlation. Semin Ultrasound CT MR. 1996;17:66–89.
12. Jaffe MH, Schoen WC, Silver TM, Bowerman RA, Stuck KJ. Sonography of abruptio placentae. Am J Roentgenol. 1981;137:1049–54.
13. Yeo L, Ananth C, Vintzileos A. Placenta abruption. In: Sciarra J, editor. Gynecology and obstetrics. Hagerstown: Lippincott Williams & Wilkins; 2014.
14. Nyberg DA, Cyr DR, Mack LA, Wilson DA, Shuman WP. Sonographic spectrum of placental abruption. AJR Am J Roentgenol. 1987;148:161–4.
15. Masselli G, Brunelli R, Di Tola M, Anceschi M, Gualdi G. MR imaging in the evaluation of placental abruption: correlation with sonographic findings. Radiology. 2011;259:222–30.
16. Atlas SW, Thulborn KR. Intracranial hemorrhage. In: Atlas SW, editor. Magnetic resonance imaging of the brain and of the spine. 4th ed. Lippincott Williams & Wilkins: Philadelphia; 2009. p. 644–94.
17. Wu S, Kocherginsky M, Hibbard JU. Abnormal placentation: twenty-year analysis. Am J Obstet Gynecol. 2005;192:1458–61.
18. Comstock CH, Love JJ Jr, Bronsteen RA, et al. Sonographic detection of placenta accrete in the second and third trimesters of pregnancy. Am J Obstet Gynecol. 2004;190:1135–40.
19. Comstock CH, Bronsteen RA. The antenatal diagnosis of placenta accreta. BJOG. 2014;121:171–81.
20. Masselli G, Brunelli R, Casciani E, et al. Magnetic resonance imaging in the evaluation of placental adhesive disorders: correlation with color Doppler ultrasound. Eur Radiol. 2008;18:1292–9.
21. Masselli G, Gualdi G. MR imaging of the placenta: what a radiologist should know. Abdom Imaging. 2013;38:573–87.
22. Lim PS, Greenberg M, Edelson MI, Bell KA, Edmonds PR, Mackey AM. Utility of ultrasound and MRI in prenatal diagnosis of placenta accreta: a pilot study. Am J Roentgenol. 2011;197:1506–13.
23. Derman AY, Nikac V, Haberman S, Zelenko N, Ophsa O, Flyer M. MRI of placenta accreta: a new imaging perspective. Am J Roentgenol. 2011;197:1514–21.
24. Gardeil F, Daly S, Turner MJ. Uterine rupture in pregnancy reviewed. Eur J Obstet Gynecol Reprod Biol. 1994;56:107–10.
25. Masselli G, Brunelli R, Casciani E, et al. Acute abdominal and pelvic pain in pregnancy: MR imaging as a valuable adjunct to ultrasound? Abdom Imaging. 2011;36:596–603.
26. Cengiz H, Kaya C, Ekin M, Yeşil A, Yaşar L. Management of incidental adnexal masses on caesarean section. Niger Med J. 2012;53:132–4.
27. Anthoulakis C, Nikoloudis N. Pelvic MRI as the "gold standard" in the subsequent evaluation of ultrasound-indeterminate adnexal lesions: a systematic review. Gynecol Oncol. 2014;132:661–8.
28. Yacobozzi M, Nguyen D, Rakita D. Adnexal masses in pregnancy. Semin Ultrasound CT MR. 2012;33:55–64.
29. Yuk JS, Shin JY, Park WI, Kim DW, Shin JW, Lee JH. Association between pregnancy and adnexal torsion: a population-based, matched case-control study. Medicine (Baltimore). 2016;95:e3861.
30. Lourenco AP, Swenson D, Tubbs RJ, Lazarus E. Ovarian and tubal torsion: imaging findings on US, CT, and MRI. Emerg Radiol. 2014;21:179–87.
31. Chiou SY, Lev-Toaff AS, Masuda E, Feld RI, Bergin D. Adnexal torsion: new clinical and imaging observations by sonography, computed tomography, and magnetic resonance imaging. J Ultrasound Med. 2007;26:1289–301.
32. Rothmund R, Taran FA, Boeer B, et al. Surgical and conservative management of symptomatic

leiomyomas during pregnancy: a retrospective pilot study. Geburtshilfe Frauenheilkd. 2013;73:330–4.
33. Muram D, Gillieson M, Walters JH. Myomas of the uterus in pregnancy: ultrasonographic follow-up. Am J Obstet Gynecol. 1980;138:16–9.
34. Masselli G, Brunelli R, Parasassi T, Perrone G, Gualdi G. Magnetic resonance imaging of clinically stable late pregnancy bleeding: beyond ultrasound. Eur Radiol. 2011;21:1841–9.
35. Murase E, Siegelman ES, Outwater EK, Perez-Jaffe LA, Tureck RW. Uterine leiomyomas: histopathologic features, MR imaging findings, differential diagnosis, and treatment. Radiographics. 1999;19:1179–97.
36. Semins MJ, Matlaga BR. Management of urolithiasis in pregnancy. Int J Womens Health. 2013;5: 599–604.
37. Spalluto LB, Woodfield CA, DeBenedectis CM, Lazarus E. MRI imaging evaluation of abdominal pain during pregnancy: appendicitis and other nonobstetric causes. Radiographics. 2012;32:317–34.
38. Masselli G, Derme M, Laghi F, et al. Imaging of stone disease in pregnancy. Abdom Imaging. 2013;38:1409–14.
39. Masselli G, Derme M, Bernieri MG, et al. Stone disease in pregnancy: imaging-guided therapy. Insights Imaging. 2014;5:691–6.
40. Gilo NB, Amini D, Landy HJ. Appendicitis and cholecystitis in pregnancy. Clin Obstet Gynecol. 2009;52:586–96.
41. Masselli G, Derchi L, McHugo J, et al. Acute abdominal and pelvic pain in pregnancy: ESUR recommendations. Eur Radiol. 2013;23:3485–500.
42. Dewhurst C, Beddy P, Pedrosa I. MRI evaluation of acute appendicitis in pregnancy. J Magn Reson Imaging. 2013;37:566–75.
43. Zachariah SK, Fenn MG. Acute intestinal obstruction complicating pregnancy: diagnosis and surgical management. BMJ Case Rep. 2014;2014:bcr2013203235.
44. Daimon A, Terai Y, Nagayasu Y, et al. A case of intestinal obstruction in pregnancy diagnosed by MRI and treated by intravenous hyperalimentation. Case Rep Obstet Gynecol. 2016;2016:8704035.
45. Masselli G, Gualdi G. MR imaging of the small bowel. Radiology. 2012;264:333–48.
46. Ellington SR, Flowers L, Legardy-Williams JK, Jamieson DJ, Kourtis AP. Recent trends in hepatic diseases during pregnancy in the United States, 2002–2010. Am J Obstet Gynecol. 2015;212(4):524.e1–7.
47. Ralls PW, Halls J, lapin SA, et al. Prospective evaluation of the sonographic Murphy sign in suspected acute cholecystitis. JCU. 1982;10:113–5.
48. Hara T, Kanasaki H, Oride A, Ishihara T, Kyo SA. Case of idiopathic acute pancreatitis in the first trimester of pregnancy. Case Rep Obstet Gynecol. 2015;2015:469527.
49. Papadakis EP, Sarigianni M, Mikhailidis DP, Mamopoulos A, Karagiannis V. Acute pancreatitis in pregnancy: an overview. Eur J Obstet Gynecol Reprod Biol. 2011;159:261–6.
50. Bennett M. Do not forget about HELLP! BMJ Case Rep. 2011;28:2011.
51. Pedrosa I, Morrin M, Oleaga L, Baptista J, Rofsky NMI. true FISP imaging reliable in the evaluation of venous thrombosis? Am J Roentgenol. 2005;185:1632–40.
52. Pedrosa I, Zeikus EA, Levine D, Rofsky NM. Is true MR imaging of acute right lower quadrant pain in pregnant and nonpregnant patients. Radiographics. 2007;27:721–43.
53. Munir SI, Lo T, Seaton J. Spontaneous rupture of utero-ovarian vessels in pregnancy. BMJ Case Rep. 2012;30:2012.

MRI of the Acute Female Pelvis

11

Joseph W. Owen and Christine O. Menias

Abstract

Magnetic resonance (MR) imaging can be used as a primary or secondary modality in the evaluation of acute pelvic pain in women. MR avoids the ionizing radiation exposure of computed tomography (CT) and provides a larger field of view with greater detail than ultrasound. This chapter first addresses practical considerations including scanner strength, intravenous gadolinium contrast use, and essential MR sequences. Then pelvic inflammatory disease, ectopic pregnancy, and ovarian torsion are reviewed with an emphasis on the MR imaging findings. At the end of this chapter, the reader should be able to structure an MR protocol, implement it in an emergency department setting, and recognize the common causes of acute pelvic pain on MR.

J. W. Owen, M.D.
Department of Radiology, University of Kentucky, Lexington, KY, USA

C. O. Menias, M.D. (✉)
Department of Radiology, Mayo Clinic, Phoenix, AZ, USA
e-mail: Menias.Christine@mayo.edu

11.1 Introduction

Magnetic resonance (MR) imaging has sufficient spatial resolution and soft-tissue contrast to accurately diagnose most disease processes presenting as acute pelvic pain. Ultrasound (US) is the preferred initial modality used for the evaluation of pelvic pain due to its low cost and absence of ionizing radiation, but US has limitations, and additional cross-sectional imaging is often needed in women presenting with acute pelvic pain. In a study of pregnant women presenting with acute pain, 30% of CT scans performed after a normal US showed acute pathology [1]. CT is widely available, but growing societal concern over ionizing radiation has led to increased use of MR in place of CT, particularly in children, women of reproductive age, and pregnant women.

MR imaging is now available 24/7 in many hospitals with busy emergencies departments, driven in part by neuroimaging, and can be an effective tool for body imagers. Radiologists can facilitate adoption of MR in the emergency department by streamlining patient screening/scheduling, developing efficient MR protocols, and ensuring that the radiologists responsible for covering the emergency department are familiar with acute MR findings. Most gynecologic emergencies are traditionally characterized with ultrasound, and many radiologists in the past have not been exposed to MR imaging of acute pelvic pain

M. Patlas et al. (eds.), *MDCT and MR Imaging of Acute Abdomen*,
https://doi.org/10.1007/978-3-319-70778-5_11

during training. The classic US findings are often translatable to MR, however, and much of the literature promoting the use of MR for acute body imaging is descriptive [2–7]. Peer-reviewed scientific publications are more limited, but have revealed instances when MR can be prognostic or affect patient management.

This chapter will address the practical aspects of implementing MR imaging for acute pelvic pain in the ER, and then will review the MR features of the most common gynecologic emergencies.

11.2 MR Protocol

11.2.1 Magnetic Strength

Both 1.5 Tesla and 3 Tesla MR scanners can be used to image the female pelvis, with minor trade-offs in image quality, acquisition time, and availability. A comparison of 1.5 T and 3 T MR imaging of the female pelvis showed similar overall image quality [8], with increased motion artifacts on 1.5 T images, and increased inhomogeneity on 3 T images. Qualitative evaluation of the cervix, vagina, and ovaries was better at 3 T than at 1.5 T. The improved spatial resolution of 3 T may be necessary for staging gynecological malignancy [9], but the minor differences in image quality are unlikely to impact the diagnosis of acute pathology. An optimized 3 T protocol just can permit fast acquisitions (less than 10 min) which are motion insensitive and high resolution [10], but 1.5 T scanners are more widely available and have less competition with acute neuroimaging examinations for MR scanner time. 3 T scanners are preferable for pelvic imaging, but quality diagnostic imaging can be achieved with either field strength with optimized protocols.

In pregnant women there are theoretical risks of fetal heating and fetal hearing damage from MR scanning. No adverse effects have been reported in any trimester at 1.5 T or 3 T, to our knowledge; however, the American College of Radiology guidelines on MR safety recommend screening of reproductive age women for pregnancy before MR, but there is no contraindication to MR imaging at 3 T or 1.5 T during the first trimester, or at any other point during pregnancy. Some institutions may choose to obtain written informed consent prior to MR scanning in known pregnant patients, but this is not a universal practice [11]. The radiologist ideally should monitor these examinations and use only the necessary sequences in pregnant patients.

11.2.2 Gadolinium Contrast

Gadolinium-based intravenous contrast agents are routinely used when imaging the female pelvis, if not contraindicated due to allergy, impaired renal function, or pregnancy. Intravenous contrast is not as essential for MR imaging of the pelvis as it is for CT, since enhancement patterns are often less important than anatomic and morphologic changes evident on noncontrast imaging.

Gadolinium-based intravenous contrast agents have a good safety profile in properly selected nonpregnant patients. Mild nonallergic adverse reactions are much more common than allergic reactions, and fatal reactions are rarely reported [12]. There is little evidence to support premedication with corticosteroids and diphenhydramine, but premedication is still recommended in the rare person with a prior allergic reaction to gadolinium-based intravenous contrast agents. Where the reaction was mild/relatively mild, and the repeat use of IV gadolinium contrast material is otherwise indicated. Premedication prior to intravenous gadolinium is not recommended in those with documented allergy to iodinated contrast agents or "shellfish."

Patients with impaired renal function are at risk for the development of systemic nephrogenic fibrosis, and gadolinium-based intravenous contrast agents should be restricted in patients with a glomerular filtration rate of 15–30 mL/min/1.73 m^2, and should be avoided in patients with a glomerular filtration rate of <15 mL/min/1.73 m^2. If gadolinium is to be administered to a patient with impaired renal function, lower-risk gadolinium-based agents including gadobutrol (Gadovist®, Gadavist®), gadoterate meglumine (Dotarem®, Magnescope®), or gadoteridol (Prohance®) should be used when available [13].

GBCAs are not routinely administered to pregnant patients or to patients with suspected pregnancy. No adverse outcome to the mother or fetus in humans has been reported after GBCA administration to our knowledge, but no large trial has assessed its safety. GBCAs have been shown to cross the placenta and to accumulate in amniotic fluid. This creates the potential for prolonged gadolinium exposure to the fetus and mother, and a theoretical risk of connective tissue disease. The limited potential benefit of GBCAs administration in pregnant women outweighs potential risks in most patients [12]. GBCAs administration can be considered selectively in patients with nonviable pregnancy, known extrauterine gestation, or pregnancy of unknown location.

11.2.3 Essential MR Sequences

T2-weighted sequences are the foundation of pelvic MR imaging, with T1-weighted in- and opposed-phase, post-contrast T1-weighted, diffusion-weighted, and balance steady-state free-precession sequences adding complementary information. A basic examination should start with partial Fourier single-shot turbo spin-echo sequences (HASTE, SS-TSE, SS-FSE) in the coronal, axial, and sagittal planes, a T2-weighted fast spin-echo sequence with fat suppression in the axial plane, and T1-weighted in- and opposed-phase sequences in the axial plane.

The single-shot turbo spin-echo sequences are preferably breath-hold acquisitions, but can be performed with free breathing. They are relatively motion insensitive and often provide sufficient anatomic detail for initial differential diagnosis. The axial T2-weighted turbo spin-echo (TSE) sequence with fat suppression (FS) complements the single-shot technique by increasing the conspicuity of cysts, free fluid, edema, and inflammation. The axial gradient-recalled echo (GRE) T1-weighted in- and opposed-phase sequence helps with the identification of blood products, fat-containing masses - particularly dermoid cysts - and can accentuate pathologic gas.

If gadolinium-based intravenous contrast agents are used, an axial pre-contrast T1-weighted gradient-recalled echo (GRE) sequence with fat suppression (VIBE, LAVA, or THRIVE) precedes a post-contrast sequence, with the same imaging parameters. Sagittal and coronal post-contrast images are often helpful and may be added if the examination is not time constrained. Post-contrast imaging permits characterization of focal abnormalities, hyperemic or inflamed tissue, demonstrates vessel patency, and may show nonenhancement of a torsed ovary. If intravenous gadolinium is not administered, a steady-state free-precession sequence (TrueFISP, Balanced FFE, or FIESTA) can be added to characterize the patency of the pelvic vasculature.

Diffusion-weighted imaging (DWI) should be considered in all patients undergoing pelvic MR and is increasingly seen as an essential sequence with a growing body of evidence supporting its use. Abscesses, masses, lymphadenopathy, and inflammation are made more conspicuous on DWI. Small studies have shown improved characterization of pelvic inflammatory disease [14], ovarian vein thrombophlebitis, and hemorrhagic infarction of a torsed ovary [15, 16] when DWI is employed. If high-quality DWI is routinely obtained, the low *B*-value sequence may function in place of the axial T2 fast spin-echo fat-suppressed sequence, to save time, as low *B*-value DWI is essentially a heavily T2-weighted fat-suppressed sequence.

11.3 Pelvic Inflammatory Disease

11.3.1 Background

Pelvic inflammatory disease (PID) is classified into three distinct subtypes: acute, subacute, and chronic. Acute PID manifests in less than 30 days and often presents with acute pelvic pain, vaginal discharge, abnormal vaginal bleeding, dyspareunia, and dysuria. It is caused by ascending infection of sexually transmitted diseases, bacterial vaginosis, or gastrointestinal or respiratory flora colonized in the vagina [17, 18]. The ascending infection progresses along a continuum from cervicitis to endometritis, salpingitis, tubo-ovarian abscess, and peritonitis [19, 20]. Acute PID occasionally presents as right upper quadrant abdominal pain due to peritoneal spread of infection resulting in perihepatitis, also known as Fitz-Hugh-Curtis syndrome [21, 22], with recent reports showing perihepatitis in upwards of 50% of patients with PID [23]. Subclinical PID is a low-grade infection, typically caused by chlamydia or gonorrhea, and often manifests as tubal occlusion-related infertility. It may be incidentally detected as an asymptomatic hydrosalpinx on MR, but rarely presents as acute pain. Chronic PID is relatively rare and is associated with *Mycobacterium tuberculosis* and actinomycosis infection. The sensitivity of MR for revealing subtle inflammation makes it a useful tool to reinforce the clinical and laboratory signs of pelvic inflammatory disease and can impact treatment planning [18].

11.3.2 Epidemiology

The U.S. Centers for Disease Control estimate the lifetime prevalence of pelvic inflammatory disease (PID) to be 4.4%, with approximately 2.5 million American women age 14–44 experiencing at least 1 episode [24]. The incidence of PID has been decreasing in North America and Europe over the past 30 years [25, 26], possibly due to improved screening for chlamydia and gonorrhea in asymptomatic sexually active women [27].

Risk factors for pelvic inflammatory disease include prior incidence of sexually transmitted infection, early first sexual encounter, increasing number of partners, and homosexual or bisexual orientation. No difference in prevalence was found with age, race, ethnicity, or socio-economic status [24].

11.3.3 MR Findings

Cervicitis commonly presents as mucopurulent endocervicitis, with approximately 40% of cases due to gonorrhea, chlamydia, or trichinosis, and 60% of cases due to unknown pathogens [28, 29]. Visual inspection demonstrates mucopurulent discharge from the cervix, with easily inducible bleeding, and >10 white blood cells on gram stain. Isolated cervical infection is often asymptomatic and is diagnosed on routine physical examination or on sexually transmitted disease screening.

MR imaging of isolated cervicitis may be normal, but a spectrum of nonspecific findings may increase the suspicion for infection. The normal cervix has three defined layers on T2-weighted sequences, with a T2 hyperintense endocervical inner layer, a T2 hypointense fibrous stroma, and a T2 intermediate signal cervical myometrium [30–32] (Fig. 11.1). When infection is present, the cervix may enlarge, and the endocervical tissue may thicken. The thickened endocervix can show hyperenhancement on post-contrast images. Parametrial fat stranding related to inflammation may cause the outer margin of the cervix to become indistinct [33, 34] on T2- and T1-weighted MR images (Fig. 11.2). In subacute and chronic infection, focal T2 hyperintense, and T1 intermediate to hyperintense cysts can develop in the endocervix [31]. The endocervical cysts can be indistinguishable from nabothian cysts, and it is believed that nabothian cysts may be the result of chronic or healed inflammation related to cervicitis [35, 36].

Endometritis can result from ascending infection from the cervix along the PID continuum [20], but is more commonly seen in the postpartum period after prolonged rupture of membranes, intra-partum fever, chorioamnionitic, or cesarean section [37, 38]. As with other forms of PID, endometritis presents along a spectrum of acuity, with chronic colonization of the endometrium often manifesting as infertility due to poor implantation [39], and acute infections, often related to gonorrhea and chlamydia, presenting with pelvic pain. PID related acute endometritis may present as nonspecific pelvic pain, with abnormal vaginal discharge, but no fever or leukocytosis. Bimanual examination may reveal cervical motion tenderness or uterine tenderness, but routine abdominal palpation may be normal

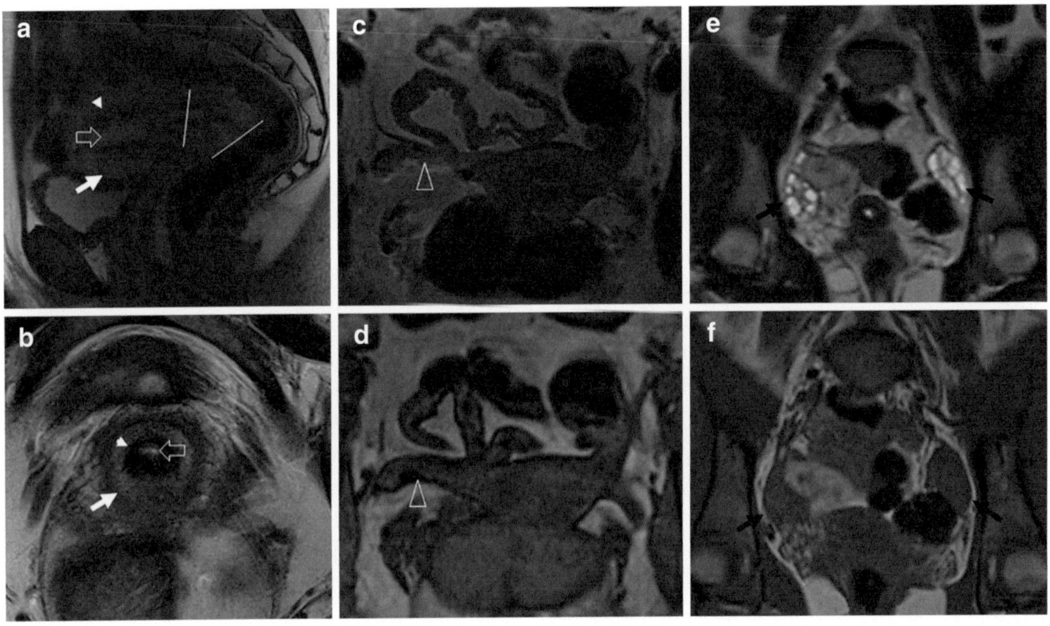

Fig. 11.1 Normal pelvic anatomy—(**a**) Sagittal and axial (**b**) T2-weighted MR images demonstrating the three layers of the uterus and cervix. Hyperintense endometrium/endocervix (open arrow), hypointense junctional zone/cervical fibrous stroma (arrowhead), and intermediate intensity uterine/cervical myometrium (white arrow). The cervix is demarcated by white lines. (**c**) Axial T2-weighted and (**d**) opposed-phase T1-weighted MR images demonstrating a normal fallopian tube (open arrowhead). (**e**) Coronal T2-weighted and (**f**) T1-weighted MR images demonstrating normal ovaries with physiologic follicles

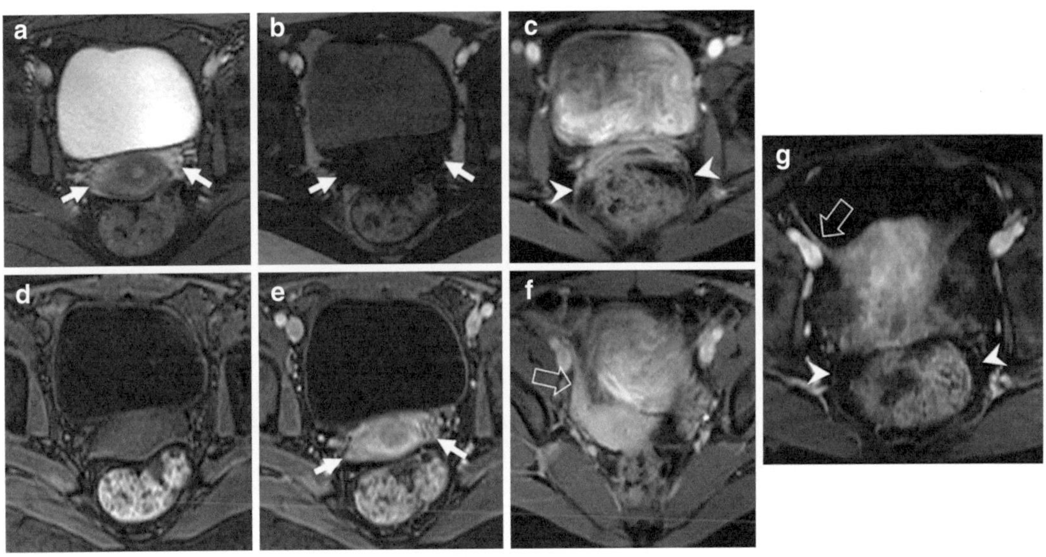

Fig. 11.2 Cervicitis—(**a**) T2-weighted and (**b**) opposed-phase T1-weighted MR images showing indistinct margins of the cervix due to parametrial stranding and edema in a patient with cervicitis. (**c**) Pre-contrast T1-weighted and (**d**) post-contrast T1-weighted MR images demonstrating enhancement of the parametrial fat. (**e** and **f**) Post-contrast T1-weighted MR images demonstrating uterosacral ligament thickening (open arrow) and round ligament thickening (arrowheads). (**g**) Post-contrast T1-weighted MR images demonstrating normal uterosacral ligaments (arrowheads), and a normal round ligament (open arrow) for comparison

in the absence of salpingitis, tubo-ovarian abscess, or peritonitis [20].

The normal uterus has three distinct layers on MR: the well-defined T2 hyperintense endometrium, the T2 hypointense poorly marginated junctional zone, and the T2 intermediate intensity myometrium (Fig. 11.1). MR may be normal in isolated endometritis, but when abnormal, endometritis manifests as thickened heterogeneous endometrium, with hyperenhancement. T1 intermediate fluid may fill the endometrial canal. Intra-cavitary gas can be seen as multifocal signal voids on the T1-weighted in-phase MR images, and is more common in post-partum endometritis. As with cervicitis, parametrial fat stranding may be present, is most evident on T2-weighted fat-suppressed MR imaging, and may result in indistinct outer margins of the myometrium. Round ligament and uterosacral ligament thickening are sensitive signs for PID [33, 40–43] and should trigger close inspection for more specific signs of infection (Fig. 11.2).

Salpingitis results in degeneration of the tubal epithelium, deciliation, decreased mucosal fold density, peritubal adhesions, partial or complete tubal occlusion, and hydrosalpinx [44]. Salpingitis may present with acute symptoms or can be clinically asymptomatic, but acute and silent cases have similar histology, and both result in decreased fertility and increased risk of ectopic pregnancy. In addition to the signs and symptoms of cervicitis and endometritis, salpingitis may manifest as pelvic tenderness to palpation and adnexal tenderness on bimanual examination [20].

On MR, the normal fallopian tubes are barely perceptible, 1–4 mm thick, serpentine, T2 intermediate intensity structures extending from the uterine cornua to the ovary [45] (Fig. 11.1). MR of salpingitis reveals a mildly dilated, tortuous fallopian tube, with a thin or slightly thickened wall. There may be perceptible enhancement of the wall, and peritubal fat stranding. The fallopian tube will have T1 hypointense, T2 hyperintense, and simple fluid without diffusion restriction. Acute or subacute salpingitis may not be distinguishable from chronic hydrosalpinx related to prior salpingitis. Incomplete longitudinal folds from mucosal plicae may be seen, but with more severe dilation, the plicae become effaced [14, 45]. Mild thickening of the round ligament and uterosacral ligaments, in this setting, are associated with acute infection. Isolated tubular torsion is a rare, but reported cause of acute pelvic pain, which may be indistinguishable from salpingitis, hematosalpinx, or hydrosalpinx [14], but which is often associated with "beaking" or a closed-loop appearance of the torsed fallopian tube [46, 47] (Fig. 11.3).

Pyosalpinx and tubo-ovarian abscess constitute severe forms of PID and often require hospitalization for inpatient therapy or intervention. Up to one-third of patients hospitalized with severe PID will have a tubo-ovarian abscess [48]. Women hospitalized for PID should undergo cross-sectional imaging [20] to assess for abscesses greater than 5 cm, as these may require drainage. Most patients present with infectious symptoms including fever, leukocytosis, and acute pelvic pain; however, a subset of patients with tubo-ovarian abscess have low-grade symptoms including chronic fever of unknown origin or have a remote history of sexually transmitted infection treated with antibiotics [49]. Physical examination reveals tenderness to palpation, and tender adnexal fullness or masses on bimanual examination. While ultrasound remains the first-line imaging modality, MR or IV contrast-enhanced CT are often required to fully characterize pyosalpinx and tubo-ovarian abscess.

MR of pyosalpinx shows a dilated tortuous tubular structure, with a thick enhancing wall, surrounding fat stranding, and thickening of the adjacent fascial planes [14, 33, 45, 50, 51]. The dilated fallopian tube is filled with T2 hyperintense or heterogeneous fluid which has variable T1 intensity related to the presence of pus, blood, or protein. The fluid is hyperintense on diffusion-weighted imaging and hypointense on ADC maps [14]. The morphology of the tube is often described as sausage-like, c-shaped, or s-shaped. The thickened wall is T1 hypointense, T2 intermediate to hyperintense, and markedly enhances. Pyosalpinx is not always distinguishable from

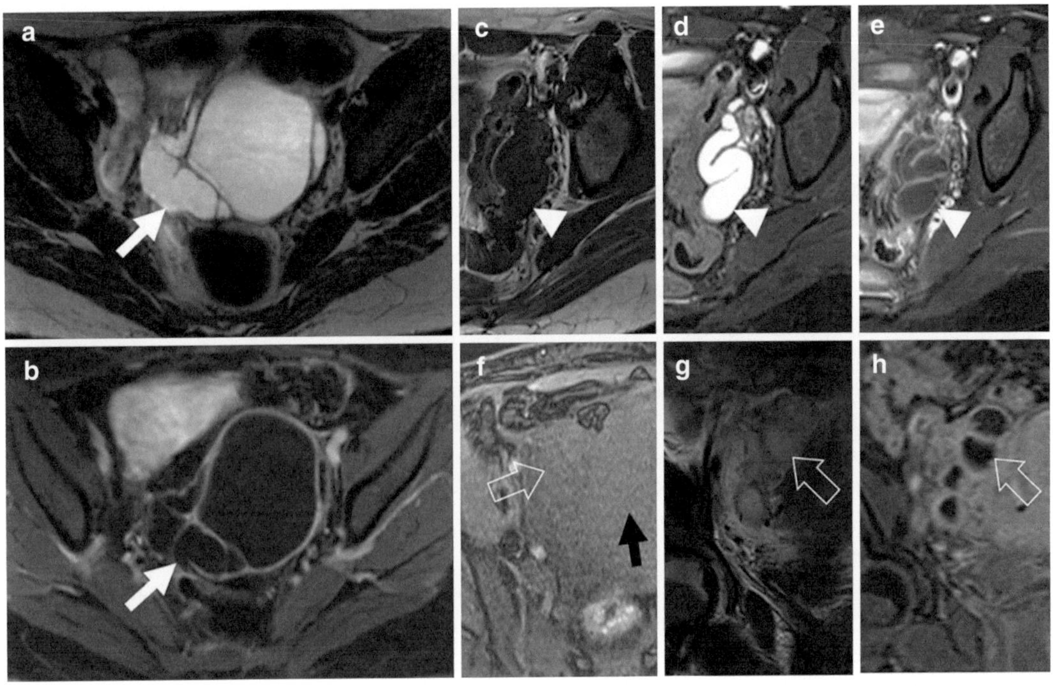

Fig. 11.3 Hydrosalpinx, salpingitis, and pyosalpinx—(**a**) T2-weighted and (**b**) post-contrast T1-weighted MR images demonstrating chronic hydrosalpinx with a dilated fallopian tube, a thin enhancing wall and simple fluid (white arrow). (**c**) T1-weighted, (**d**) T2-weighted FS, and (**e**) post-contrast T1-weighted MR images demonstrating salpingitis with an s-shaped, dilated fallopian tube (arrowhead), simple fluid, a mildly thickened enhancing wall, and mild peritubal stranding. (**f**) Opposed-phase T1-weighted, (**g**) T2-weighted, and (**h**) post-contrast T1-weighted MR images demonstrating pyosalpinx (open arrow), with a dilated fallopian tube, T1 and T2 intermediate intensity complex fluid, thick enhancing walls, and marked adnexal inflammation. Note the T1 signal intensity within the tube is similar to myometrium (black arrow)

hydrosalpinx, but tends to have more wall thickening and T2 heterogeneous fluid than expected with the simple fluid of hydrosalpinx, or salpingitis. Pyosalpinx can mimic inflamed or obstructed bowel, and is distinguished by its location in the adnexa, continuity with the uterine cornua, and lack of continuity with bowel. Concomitant bowel inflammation and obstruction can occur, especially if peritonitis or tubo-ovarian abscess is present. At times, the diagnosis of TOA on MR may be challenging in patients with inflammatory bowel disease, as these patients may present with active bowel inflammation which may also involve the adnexa, resulting in inflammation and tubo-ovarian abscesses. Careful review of the bowel and epicenter of the inflammation can be useful to help distinguish between these two diagnoses (Fig. 11.3).

Tubo-ovarian abscesses are complex cystic adnexal masses, which often result in severe surrounding inflammation. Mild forms of ovarian inflammation associated with PID are described as oophoritis and manifest as periovarian stranding and ovarian enlargement. Progression of inflammation beyond oophoritis may lead to tubo-ovarian abscess. Tubo-ovarian abscesses have T2 hyperintense or heterogeneous cystic spaces with variable T1 intensity and may demonstrate a thin inner rim of T1 hyperintensity [52]. Enhancing internal septations often create a multiloculated appearance. The margins of tubo-ovarian abscesses are indistinct on T2- and T1-weighted imaging due to adjacent edema and exudate. Diffusion-weighted images show hyperintense fluid with low signal on ADC [14]. Dense surrounding adhesions result in distortion of the local anatomy. Adhesions are T2 hypointense and T1 hypointense, with mild enhancement. Free fluid, periovarian stranding, thickening of the pelvic fascial plains, round ligaments and uterosacral ligaments, smooth peritoneal enhancement, adjacent bowel wall thickening, and lymphadenopathy are all common features [23, 42, 49, 52]. Rupture of a tubo-ovarian abscess may lead to severe peritonitis, sepsis, and if treatment is delayed, rarely death (Figs. 11.4 and 11.5).

Distinguishing features of tubo-ovarian abscess from cystic ovarian neoplasm include associated fallopian tube dilation [52], a T2 hyperintense peri-cystic "halo" of edema [49], smooth peritoneal enhancement as opposed to nodular enhancement, and absence of enhancing soft-tissue nodules. Pus can appear "pseudo-solid" with T1 intermediate intensity, variable T2 intensity, and restricted diffusion, but the "pseudo-solid" areas of diffusion restriction in tubo-ovarian abscess should not enhance [14]. Necrotic and/or cystic components of an ovarian neoplasm do not typically restrict diffusion.

Thrombophlebitis of the ovarian vein can be a complication of PID, but is more common in post-partum women or women with recent pelvic surgery, and is rarely life threatening. It is often asymptomatic, detected incidentally, and can be treated with anticoagulation. MR is highly sensitive for the demonstration of ovarian vein thrombophlebitis [53], with improved characterization when MR venography sequences are employed [54]. Partial Fourier single-shot turbo spin-echo images are susceptible to flow artifacts within the veins, but loss of signal void within the vein and venous enlargement should prompt closer inspection. Thrombus is often T2 intermediate to hyperintense and is associated with perivascular stranding. Stranding may be more evident on T2-weighted fat-suppressed images or on low *B*-value diffusion-weighted images. On T1-weighted images, thrombus can appear with T1 hypointensity or hyperintensity within the vessel [55]. Post-contrast images or balanced steady-state free-precession MR images will demonstrate loss of signal with the lumen of the dilated ovarian vein. Thrombus is hyperintense on DWI and hypointense on ADC images [56].

Actinomycosis is a rare form of severe pelvic inflammatory disease which is associated with the protracted presence of intrauterine devices or pessaries. Women with IUDs have reported colonization rates of 1–14% [57, 58]. Actinomycosis infection is often mistaken as malignancy, and the presence of an IUD should raise suspicion for infection when a complex adnexal mass is detected [59, 60].

Pelvic actinomycosis often presents with abdominal pain, vaginal bleeding, fever, anemia, and leukocytosis, although in approximately one-fifth of patients the findings are detected incidentally on imaging [61]. On CT and MR, pelvic actinomycosis presents as an invasive heterogeneous mass [60, 62] which obliterates the tissue planes of the pelvis. It tends to invade the rectum and the bladder [61], sometimes extending through the abdominal and pelvic wall. Compared with malignancy, the soft-tissue components tend to be T2 hypointense [60], and extend in thick linear bands throughout the pelvis without respecting tissue planes [63]. Scatter cystic spaces are common and may represent small abscesses [63]. There is marked enhancement of the soft-tissue components, and on FDG-PET the soft-tissue components may demonstrate FDG avidity [64].

11.3.4 Management

Pelvic inflammatory disease has a broad range of severity, which impacts treatment strategies. Mild to moderate pelvic inflammatory disease can be managed with outpatient therapy, typically a combination of intramuscular cephalosporin and oral doxycycline with or without metronidazole [65]. Lack of symptomatic improvement with 72 h of outpatient therapy may require parenteral therapy, repeat imaging, and hospitalization. Patients who are clinically unstable, have refractory nausea and vomiting or high fever, cannot tolerate oral antibiotics, are pregnant, or have a tubo-ovarian abscess require hospitalization, imaging, and parenteral antibiotics. Typical regimes include oral/IV doxycycline and an IV cephalosporin, or IV clindamycin and gentamycin. Inpatients can be transitioned to oral antibiotics with 24 h of clinical improvement [18, 66].

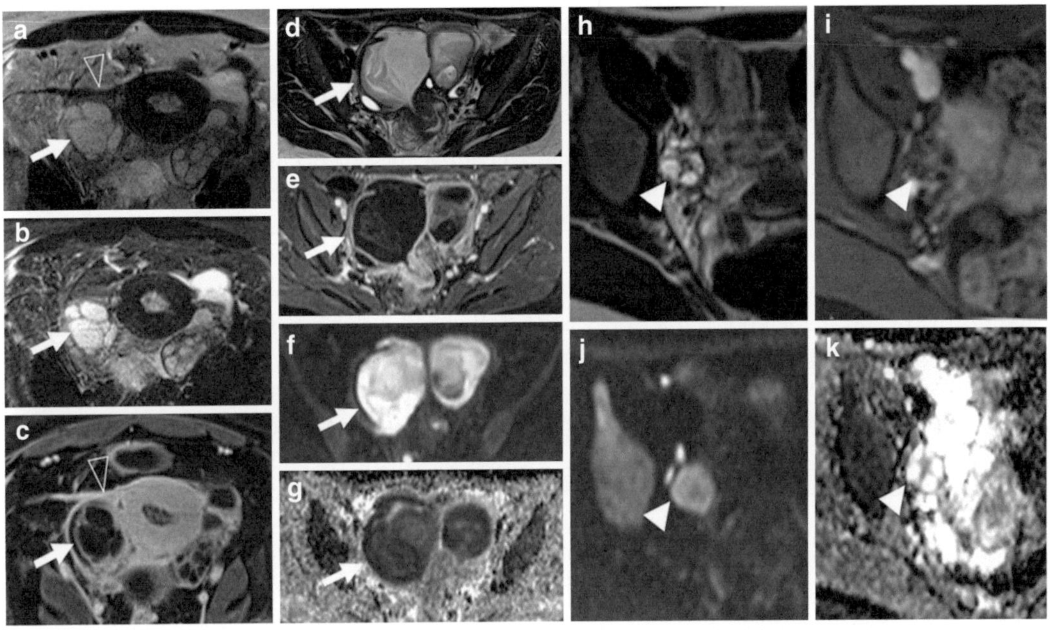

Fig. 11.4 Tubo-ovarian abscesses—(**a**) T2-weighted, (**b**) T2-weighted FS, and (**c**) post-contrast T1-weighted MR images demonstrating a tubo-ovarian abscess with a multiloculated cystic mass (white arrow), with enhancing septations, adnexal stranding, and round ligament thickening (open arrowhead). (**d**) T2-weighted, (**e**) T2-weighted FS, (**f**) DWI, and (**g**) ADC MR images showing a different tubo-ovarian abscess (white arrow) with complex fluid that restricts diffusion. (**h**) T2-weighted, (**i**) post-contrast T1-weighted, (**j**) DWI, and (**k**) ADC MR images showing a normal ovary with physiologic follicles for comparison

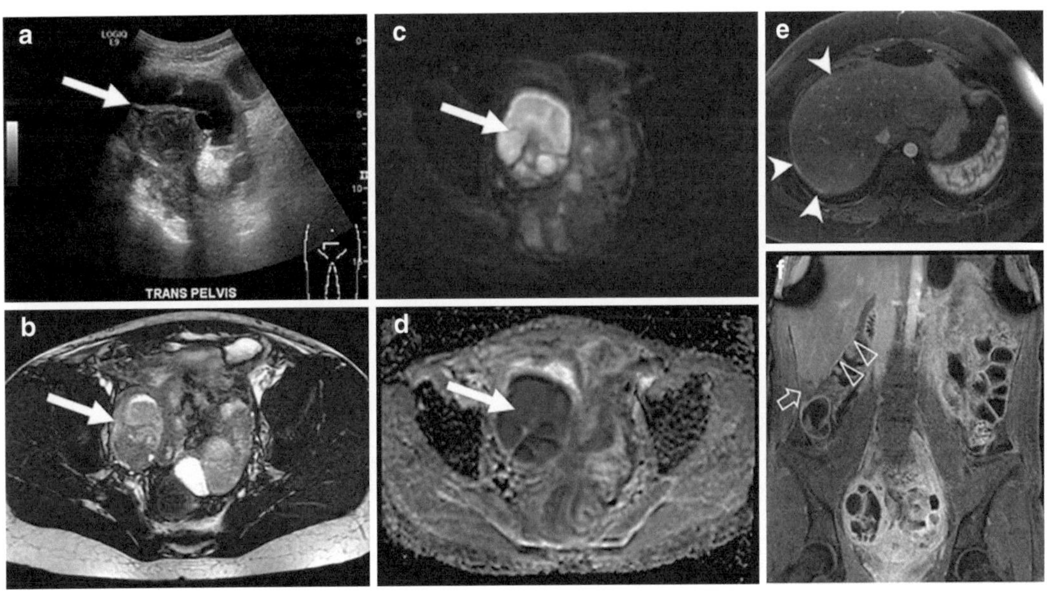

Fig. 11.5 Tubo-ovarian abscess with perihepatitis—(**a**) ultrasound demonstrating a complex adnexal mass (white arrow). (**b**) T2-weighted MR image confirming the complex cystic mass (white arrow) in the right adnexa. (**c**) DWI and (**d**) ADC MR images showing diffusion restriction in the cystic portions of the mass, compatible with abscess. (**e**) T2-weighted FS image showing T2 hyperintensity along the liver capsule (arrowhead) and (**f**) coronal post-contrast T1-weighted MR image showing pericapsular enhancement (open arrowhead) and a small complex fluid collection (open arrow), representing the perihepatitis of Fitz-Hugh-Curtis syndrome

Stable patients with tubo-ovarian abscess may be initially treated with parenteral antibiotics. Patients without resolution of pain and fever in 48–72 h may require repeat imaging and imaged-guided percutaneous drainage. Tubo-ovarian abscesses over 5 cm have a high rate of antibiotic therapy failure and often require percutaneous drainage [67]. Multiple reports advocate primary percutaneous drainage and antibiotics as a safe and effective treatment for tubo-ovarian abscesses larger than 5 cm. Surgical intervention is often unnecessary with the widespread availability of image-guided minimally invasive techniques, but laparoscopic drainage may be necessary if an abscess cannot be safely accessed percutaneously or if interventional radiology services are unavailable [67–70].

Detection of ovarian vein thrombophlebitis warrants treatment with anticoagulation to prevent pulmonary embolism. Patients failing anticoagulation with breakthrough pulmonary embolus may need a suprarenal inferior vena cava filter. The majority of patients will recanalize their ovarian vein with anticoagulation, but may experience long-term sequelae, including recurrent deep venous thrombosis and pelvic venous congestion syndrome from ovarian vein valvular incompetence [71]. Work-up for hypercoagulability disorders should be considered after the diagnosis of ovarian vein thrombophlebitis, in the absence of a predisposing condition such as recent surgery or infection.

If actinomycosis infection is suspected, due a locally invasive inflammatory process and an IUD, aspiration is recommended to confirm the diagnosis. Unfortunately, actinomycosis is a gram-positive anaerobic bacteria, which is difficult to culture, and many patients with surgically confirmed actinomycosis infection are culture negative [72]. Proper anaerobic sampling technique [73] combined with gram stain and hematoxylin and eosin stain can improve sensitivity [74]. Primary resection is difficult and initial treatment with long-term high-dose antibiotics is recommended [75]. Resection may be done secondarily to remove or divert portions of the genital, urinary, or gastrointestinal tract, due to fistula or obstruction.

11.4 Ovarian Torsion

11.4.1 Background

Ovarian torsion occurs due to rotation of the ovary around the vascular pedicle, resulting in ischemia of the ovarian tissue. With progressive rotation of the ovary around the pedicle, there is first compromise of the venous outflow, followed by compromise of the arterial supply. This results in enlargement of the ovary with subsequent ischemia. Ischemia may progress to hemorrhagic infarction and necrosis if not quickly diagnosed and treated. The diagnosis of ovarian torsion is often delayed due to a nonspecific clinical presentation [76], and the potential for intermittent torsion adds to the diagnostic challenge.

Ovarian torsion classically presents with sudden onset, moderate to severe, sharp stabbing, lower quadrant pain, which may radiate to the back, flank, or groin [77]. The pain can be subacute or chronic in a substantial subset of patients [78], particularly those with intermittent or partial torsion. A palpable mass may be evident on physical examination; however, one-third of patients have no mass or tenderness. Presentation after onset of pain is reportedly as short as 4 h in 80% of patients [79], but can be considerably longer with intermittent or partial torsion.

Ovarian torsion has been extensively characterized with ultrasound in the literature, but due to its nonspecific presentation and because of this initial imaging is often performed with CT. Even when ultrasound is performed first, Doppler US demonstrates adnexal blood flow in 20–50% patients with confirmed ovarian torsion [77, 78, 80], likely due to the ovary's dual blood supply. When US or CT demonstrates an adnexal mass in the setting of acute or subacute pelvic pain, or when ultrasound is equivocal, MR may be performed for additional characterization of the abnormal adnexa [81]. MR is highly sensitive and specific for torsion when used as a primary modality, or after indeterminate US or CT [79, 82] (Fig. 11.6).

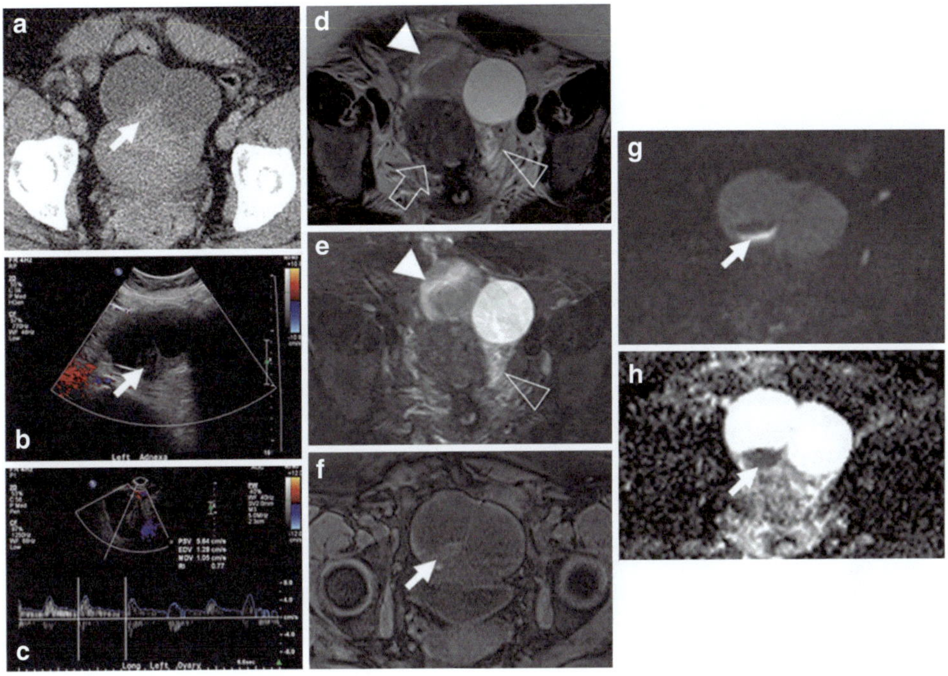

Fig. 11.6 Ovarian torsion—(**a**) CT image showing an enlarged torsed ovary (black arrow) eccentrically positioned anterior to the uterus with 2 cysts. (**b**) Color Doppler and (**c**) spectral wave Doppler US showing an enlarged hypovascular ovary, but detectable arterial flow. (**d**) T2-weighted and (**e**) T2-weighted FS MR images showing the eccentric anteriorly positioned torsed ovary, with a hemorrhagic cyst (white arrowhead), thickened and edematous pedicle (open arrowhead), and deviated uterus (open arrow). (**f**) T1-weighted FS, (**g**) DWI, and (**h**) ADC MR images demonstrating layering hemorrhage and an adjacent rim of diffusion restriction (white arrow) at the interface of the cyst and the ovarian tissue

11.4.2 Epidemiology

Ovarian torsion is an uncommon condition, predominately described with single institutional experience, and few large epidemiologic studies characterize its incidence to our knowledge. Early reports estimate that 2.7% of acute gynecologic emergencies are due to ovarian torsion [76], which is similar to a recent report by Petkovska et al. [83]. One population-based epidemiologic study from South Korea showed an incidence of 5.9/100,000 in women of all ages, and 9.9/100,000 in reproductive age women [84].

Multiple conditions have been implicated as risk factors for ovarian torsion. Ovarian cysts and ovarian neoplasms are well-recognized risk factors for torsion, with 25–80% [77, 78] associated with a cyst (Fig. 11.7). Prior pelvic surgery, specifically prior tubal ligation, is an important risk factor for ovarian torsion, with 40–50% of patients having a history of surgery [77, 80]. Adhesions from tubal ligation, or other procedures, may serve as a pivot point for rotation of the ovary around the vascular pedicle. Prior PID is a risk factor, presumably for a similar reason, with peritubal adhesions a common sequela of salpingitis. Treatment for infertility, specifically hormonal stimulation, is an increasingly important etiology for ovarian torsion, especially when infertility treatment results in pregnancy [85, 86] (Fig. 11.8).

11.4.3 MR Findings

Thickening of the twisted vascular pedicle and fallopian tube is frequently evident on MR in the

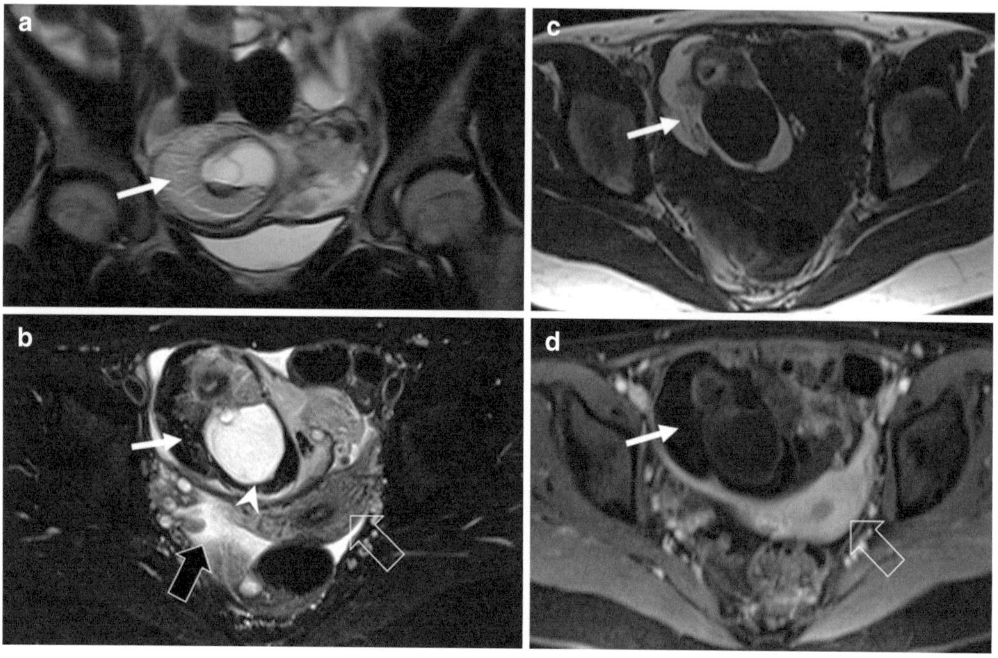

Fig. 11.7 Ovarian torsion with teratoma—(**a**) Coronal T2-weighted and (**b**) axial T2-weighted FS MR images demonstrating a complex cystic right adnexal mass with T2 hyperintense soft-tissue which becomes hypointense with fat suppression, representing a cystic teratoma (white arrow). The same soft tissue shows T1 hyperintensity with fat suppression and no enhancement on (**c**) pre-contrast T1-weighted and (**d**) post-contrast T1-weighted FS MR images. There is associated uterine deviation (open arrow), wall thickening of the cystic lesion (arrowhead), free fluid, edema (black arrow), and anterior positioning of the torsed ovary

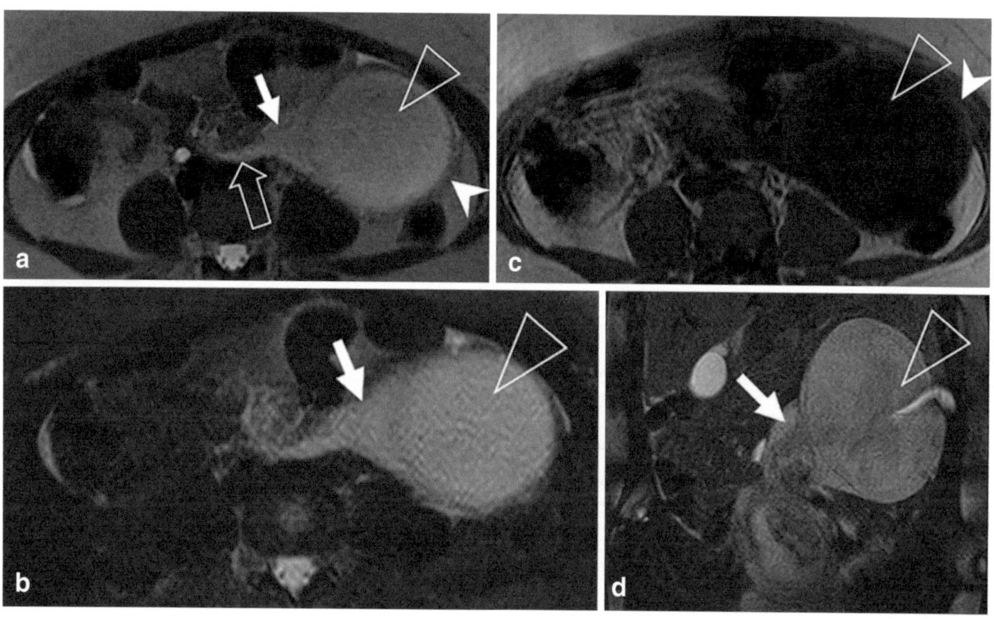

Fig. 11.8 Ovarian torsion in pregnancy—(**a**) T2-weighted, (**b**) T2-weighted FS, (**c**) T1-weighted, and (**d**) coronal T2-weighted FS MR images demonstrating a thickened and edematous vascular pedicle (white arrow), and a large simple cyst (open arrowhead) with mild wall thickening (arrowhead). Note the beaking and subtle swirled appearance of the vascular pedicle (open arrow)

setting of torsion [87]. Rotation of the pedicle results in vascular compromise, edema, and/or hemorrhage in the tube and the pedicle. The twist can be seen on US [88] and MR [79] and is described as the "whirlpool sign." Edema and hemorrhage cause enlargement of the tube and pedicle. The normal fallopian tube is less than 3 mm in diameter at its narrowest point [78], and up to 10 mm at the cornua or fimbriae. Asymmetric thickening of a fallopian tube should prompt close evaluation of the ipsilateral adnexa for additional signs of torsion. Tubal thickening is evident on T2-weighted images [15, 89] and may be more conspicuous on low *B*-value DWI because of its high T2 contrast [16]. Simple hydrosalpinx can look similar to a torsed tube, but identifying twisting or beaking [89] of the tube increases confidence in the diagnosis of torsion. A torsed fallopian tube may appear T1 hyperintense, due to development of hematosalpinx. Hemorrhagic infarction of the pedicle results in restricted diffusion, with curvilinear high DWI signal and low ADC signal [87, 90] extending from the uterine cornua to the ovary. Isolated tubal torsion can occur, but is extremely rare, and should be a diagnosis of exclusion. Tubal thickening and the "whirlpool" sign are the most specific and reliable signs of ovarian torsion, with diffusion restriction and tubal hemorrhage highly specific for hemorrhagic infarction [79] (Fig. 11.9).

Abnormal positioning of the ovary may indicate torsion, as rotation of the ovary around the pedicle causes deviation of the pelvic structures. The normal ovary tends to reside along the pelvic sidewall, near the iliac vessels, lateral and just superior to the uterine cornua. It can be located by following the gonadal veins inferiorly from the renal vein on the left or from the infrarenal inferior vena cava on the right. A torsed ovary commonly rotates to lie on top of the uterus or within the rectouterine pouch. Less commonly, a torsed ovary is located anterior to the uterus or in the contralateral pelvis [78, 80]. The uterus also deviates in torsion, with early reports of deviation ipsilateral to the torsed ovary [91, 92], but later reports showing ipsilateral and contralateral deviation [80, 87, 89]. In the majority of patients, the

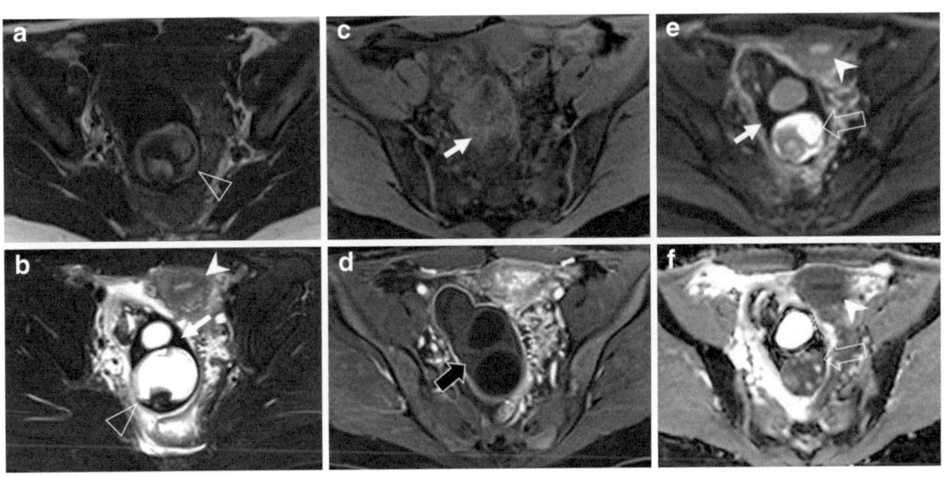

Fig. 11.9 Ovarian torsion with hemorrhagic infarction—(**a**) T2-weighted MR image demonstrating a cystic teratoma (open arrowhead) in an enlarged, eccentric, posteriorly positioned torsed ovary. (**b**) T2-weighted FS and (**c**) pre-contrast T1-weighted MR images showing thickened ovarian stroma (white arrow), with loss of T2 signal intensity and T1 signal hyperintensity compatible with hemorrhagic infarction of the stroma. (**d**) Post-contrast T1-weighted MR image shows no enhancement of the stroma (black arrow). (**e**) DWI and (**f**) ADC MR images show signal voids in the ovarian stroma (white arrow) indicating dephasing from blood products, and diffusion restriction within the teratoma (open arrow). Note the uterine deviation on multiple images (arrowhead)

ovary is in an atypical location, and the uterus is deviated from midline.

Asymmetric ovarian enlargement should prompt consideration of ovarian torsion. The measured ovary should include cysts or solid masses, and be compared to the contralateral ovary. Four centimeters is the upper limit of normal for maximum long-axis diameter of the ovary, although reproductive age women may have normal cysts measuring 5–7 cm, which can result in asymmetry of normal ovaries. The range of ovarian diameter in confirmed patients with torsion is 1–30 cm, with reported mean/median sizes of 8.7–13.5 cm [77, 78, 80]. Some investigators describe increased cross-sectional area or volume in torsion, with reported mean areas of 11.3–19 cm^2, and a range 3.8–50 cm^2 [79, 89].

Edema or hemorrhage in the ovarian stroma partially accounts for the enlargement of a torsed ovary. On T2-weighted MR imaging, normal ovarian stroma is isointense to skeletal muscle, with the stroma of torsed ovaries described as T2 hyperintense and T1 hypointense [89, 93] due to edema. Later investigations have suggested that stromal T2 signal is not sensitive or specific [79] for torsion, since malignancy and infection can result in T2 hyperintensity. Focal or diffuse T1 hyperintensity, DWI hyperintensity, and ADC hypointensity within the ovarian stroma have a poor prognosis and correlate with hemorrhagic infarction [15, 79, 87, 89, 90]. If the ADC values of ovarian stroma are below 1.8×10^{-3} mm^2/s, the sensitivity and specificity for hemorrhagic infarction is reportedly 88% and 100%, respectively [15]. The vast majority of torsed ovaries will demonstrate enhancement after intravenous gadolinium administration; however, a nonenhancing ovary has a poor prognosis, and hemorrhagic infarction and nonviability are common [87].

Cysts are present in up to 80% of torsed ovaries [78], and the walls of cysts within an ovary may develop abnormalities in the setting of torsion. The wall thickness of a normal ovarian follicle or hemorrhagic cyst is less than 3 mm, and has signal intensity similar to ovarian stroma. Edema or hemorrhage resulting from torsion results in wall thickening [78, 87, 91]. A thin T2 hypointense rim in the wall correlates with hemorrhagic infarction on histology and may carry a poor prognosis for the viability of the ovary [83]. Subacute hemorrhagic infarction results in a thin rim of T1 hyperintensity due to the presence of methemoglobin, but hyperacute and acute hemorrhage can be T1 iso- to hypointense, as oxy- and deoxyhemoglobin predominate in the early stages of hematoma formation [15]. Blood products with the wall of a cyst also result in DWI hyperintensity, and ADC hypointensity, and may indicate hemorrhage [87].

Ascites and periovarian fat stranding are common findings in torsion, but are often present in other acute processes presenting with abdominal or pelvic pain. Ascites is reported on CT and MR in most patients with ovarian torsion [78, 80, 87, 92], and while it has high sensitivity, its lack of specificity diminishes its usefulness in the diagnosis of torsion. Periovarian fat stranding is not present in most patients with ovarian torsion, but when present correlates with a nonviable ovary and the development of hemorrhagic infarction [78, 80].

11.4.4 Management

In the past, ovarian torsion was managed with salpingo-oophorectomy due to concerns that a necrotic ovary might lead to infection, that detorsion of the ovary could result in thromboembolism, and concern for underlying malignancy. Adnexal sparing surgery is now the preferred treatment option. Patients treated with detorsion do not have an increased incidence of pulmonary embolism, or increased morbidity and mortality, compared to those treated with oophorectomy [94, 95]. Even patients with "black-bluish" appearing ovaries at surgery had recovery of ovarian function and no increased morbidity when treated with detorsion [96, 97]. However, if an ovary is frankly necrotic due to delayed diagnosis of torsion, oophorectomy should be considered. When an ovarian cyst or benign ovarian neoplasm is present, cystectomy or cyst aspiration can be performed to reduce the potential for retorsion. Oophoropexy may also reduce the risk of retorsion and may be considered for prophylactic treatment of the contralateral ovary [98, 99].

Identification of hemorrhagic infarction in torsed ovaries is a focus in the radiology literature. It is not clear that the presence of hemorrhagic infarction indicates the ovary is nonviable, and additional studies are required before management decisions are made based on the MR findings of hemorrhage.

11.5 Ectopic Pregnancy

11.5.1 Background

Ectopic pregnancy refers to the implantation of an embryo outside of the uterine canal, which if untreated can result in maternal hemorrhage and death. The treatment and presentation of ectopic pregnancy differs based on the site of implantation. Ectopic pregnancy is most common in the fallopian tube [100], and as the gestational sac enlarges and increases in vascularity, there is increasing risk of tubal rupture, hemorrhage, and death. Less common sites of ectopic pregnancy include interstitial, abdominal, cervical, ovarian, and cesarean scar-related presentation [101]. The increased use of transvaginal sonography to confirm intrauterine pregnancy has led to earlier diagnosis of ectopic pregnancy [102]. Nonruptured ectopic pregnancy often presents with mild vaginal bleeding, crampy abdominal and pelvic pain, and positive HCG levels [103]. Ruptured ectopic pregnancy presents with hypotension, tachycardia, and rebound tenderness and may rapidly progress to death.

Transvaginal sonography should demonstrate a gestational sac when the estimated gestational age is 5.5 weeks, and when quantitative HCG is 1500–2500 mIU/mL. The absence of a gestational sac on ultrasound should be described as a pregnancy of unknown location [103, 104]. Transvaginal ultrasound is sensitive for ectopic pregnancy [105–107], but ectopic pregnancies can be mistaken for corpus luteal cysts, hemorrhagic cysts, ovarian neoplasms, pedunculated fibroids, bowel, and endometriomas. Sonographic diagnosis of pregnancy of unknown location is often managed with serial HCG levels and follow-up US in 2–7 days. If there is persistent pain and/or vaginal bleeding, MRI may be warranted to further characterize the etiology of pelvic pain, without additional delay in diagnosis.

11.5.2 Epidemiology

The incidence of ectopic pregnancy has been increasing over the past 4 decades, with the last comprehensive review by the U.S. Centers for Disease Control estimating that 2% of pregnancies are ectopic [108, 109]. As the incidence has risen, death related to ectopic pregnancy has fallen over 90%, now accounting for only 6% of maternal deaths [110–112]. Ectopic pregnancy requiring hospitalization has also fallen, with more than 50% of ectopic pregnancy treated in outpatient settings [109].

The predominant risk factors for ectopic pregnancy are related to abnormalities of the fallopian tube. Women with prior ectopic pregnancy, prior tubal surgery, or known tubal abnormality are at highest risk for ectopic pregnancy. Women with prior pelvic inflammatory disease, sexually transmitted infection, IUD, or subfertility/infertility have an intermediate risk for ectopic pregnancy. Ectopic pregnancy has a mild association with prior abdominal or pelvic surgery, smoking, early age of sexual intercourse, and multiple sexual partners. When the HCG level is positive, ultrasound fails to demonstrate an intrauterine gestation, and ectopic pregnancy is suspected, an MR can be used to distinguish ectopic pregnancy from other acute conditions including ovarian torsion, appendicitis, and pelvic inflammatory disease [113, 114].

11.5.3 MR Findings

Tubal ectopic pregnancy occurs most frequently in the ampulla of the fallopian tube. The ectopic gestational sac has been described on MR as a sac-like cystic structure in the adnexa but outside of the ovary [114]. The gestational sac tends to have a thick wall, and MR may demonstrate three distinct layers, described as a “3-ring” appearance [115]. The wall may have focal hemorrhage or rim-like hemorrhage, evident by T1 intermediate to hyperintense signal, and corresponding T2 hypointensity. The wall will show marked enhancement, which is sometime "dot-like" or stippled [116]. The central portion of the gestational sac is often heterogeneous, with solid enhancing nodules, internal hemorrhage, fluid-fluid levels, or less likely simple fluid [115]. Hemorrhage within the sac is most commonly T1 intermediate to hyperintense and T2 hypointense, and may show loss of signal on T2*-weighted MR imaging [117]. The gestational sac size increases with increasing gestational age. Tubal ectopics present with a mean sac diameter of 4 cm [118]. Hematosalpinx is often present with tubal ectopic pregnancy. The fallopian tube will be dilated and contain T1 intermediate to hyperintense signal. There may be T2 heterogeneity and a fluid-fluid level in the tube. The wall of the fallopian tube may be slightly thickened and will show marked enhancement [8, 115–117] (Figs. 11.10 and 11.11).

Differentiation of a tubal ectopic pregnancy from a corpus luteal cyst can be challenging. A corpus luteal cyst is present in early pregnancy and has imaging features similar to an ectopic gestational sac. On MR, a corpus luteal cyst should have a smooth, convex, or mildly wavy thick wall. The wall is T1 intermediate to hyperintense and uniformly T2 hypointense, with uniform enhancement [116]. Intra- or extra-ovarian location is the best distinguishing factor. Corpus luteal cysts are always located within the ovary, and ovarian ectopic pregnancy is rare [100] (Fig. 11.12).

Nontubal ectopic pregnancy accounts for fewer than 5% of ectopic pregnancies [119], often present later than tubal ectopics, and have higher morbidity and mortality due to higher rate of rupture and delayed presentation. The gestational sac of nontubal ectopics has similar MR features, with a thick-walled, sac-like, hemorrhagic mass, and is distinguished from tubal ectopics by their rarity, location, and management.

Interstitial ectopics present when the gestational sac implants in the intrauterine portion of the

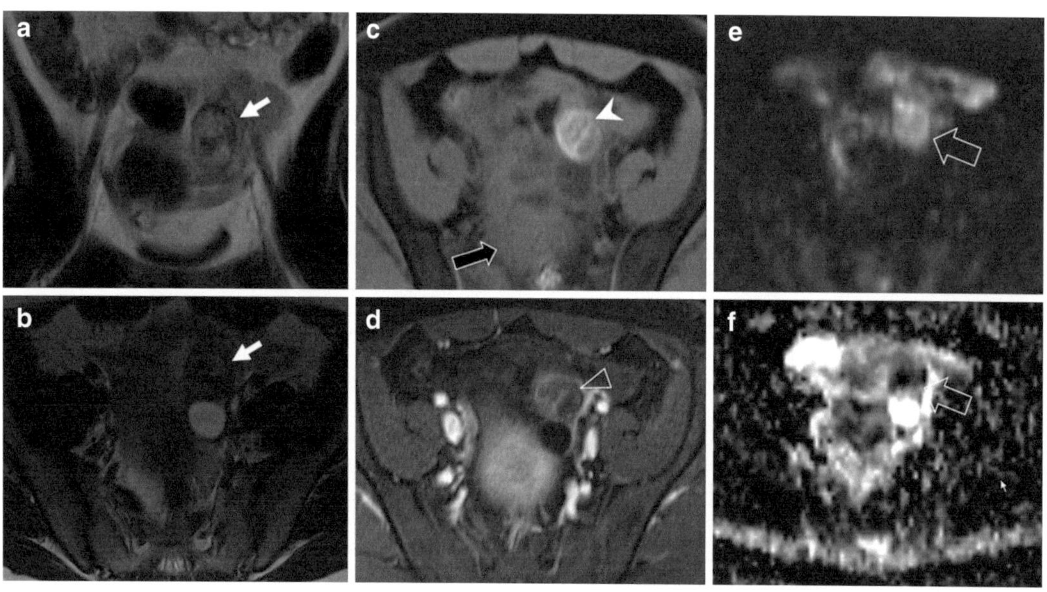

Fig. 11.10 Tubal ectopic pregnancy—(**a**) T2-weighted and (**b**) T2-weighted FS MR images demonstrating a complex adnexal mass (white arrow) in a woman with positive HCG level and no intrauterine gestation. (**c**) Pre-contrast T1-weighted MR image showing a hemorrhagic mass (arrowhead) and intraperitoneal hemorrhage (black arrow). (**d**) Post-contrast T1-weighted MR image showing mild stippled enhancement. (**e**) DWI and (**f**) ADC MR images showing diffusion restriction of the adnexal mass (open arrow). Surgery confirmed a ruptured tubal ectopic pregnancy

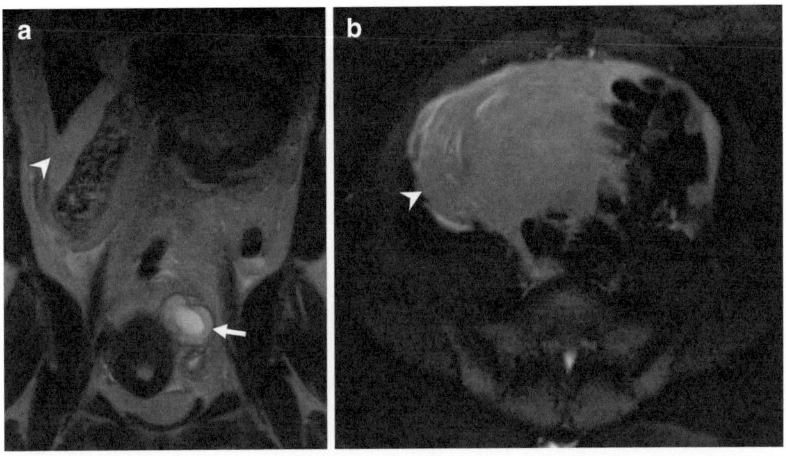

Fig. 11.11 Three-ring sign of tubal ectopic pregnancy—(**a**) coronal and (**b**) axial T2-weighted MR images demonstrate a tubal ectopic gestational sac (white arrow), with a thin hypointense outer ring, a thick hyperintense middle ring, and a thin hypointense inner ring. Note the large volume hemoperitoneum on both images (arrowhead)

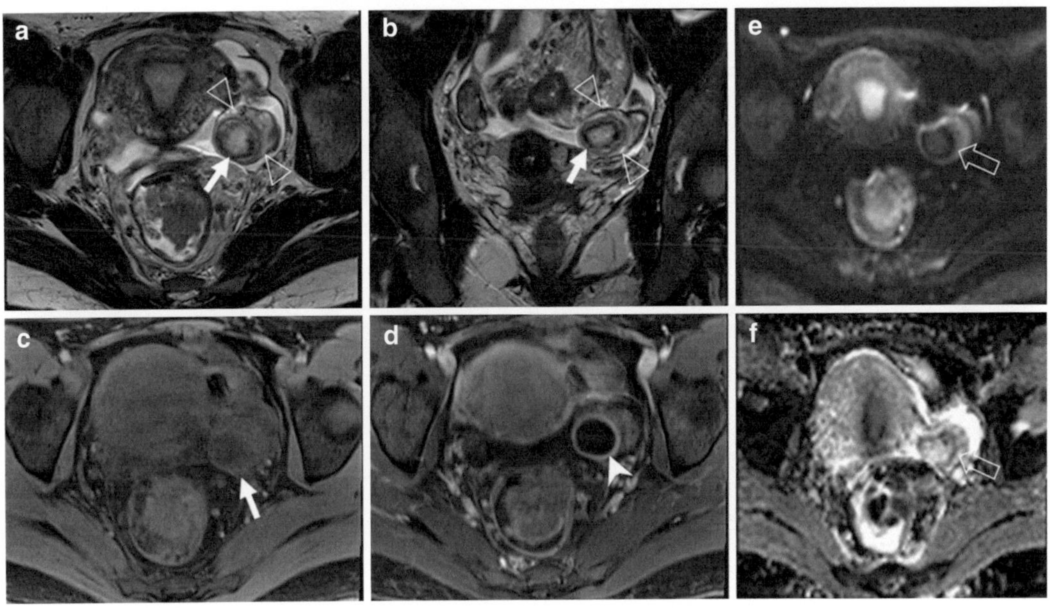

Fig. 11.12 Corpus luteal cyst—(**a**) axial and (**b**) coronal T2-weighted MR images demonstrate a corpus luteal cyst in the left ovary. Its location in the ovary is evident by a "claw sign" (open arrowheads) with ovarian stroma partially encompassing the cyst. Note the wavy hypointense rim (white arrow). (**c**) Pre-contrast T1 and (**d**) post-contrast T1-weighted MR images demonstrate smooth circumferential enhancement (arrowhead). The rim is hypointense on (**e**) DWI and (**f**) ADC (open arrow) indicating dephasing from blood products

fallopian tube, and is characterized by a gestational sac eccentrically located in or at the margin of the uterine cornua with less than 5 mm of surrounding myometrium [120, 121]. A closely related entity is cornual implantation, which is defined by implantation in the horn of a bicornuate uterus, and is similarly managed [122]. Cornual pregnancy may also refer to an eccentric implantation onto endometrium within the uterine cornua, and can be distinguished by a surrounding myometrial thickness of >5 mm (Figs. 11.13 and 11.14).

Abdominal ectopics are defined by implantation of the gestational sac on a peritoneal surface and can occur anywhere in the abdomen or pelvis. Abdominal pregnancy can be carried to term, but is at high risk for fetal demise from poor placental blood supply, and high risk for maternal demise from rupture [123–129].

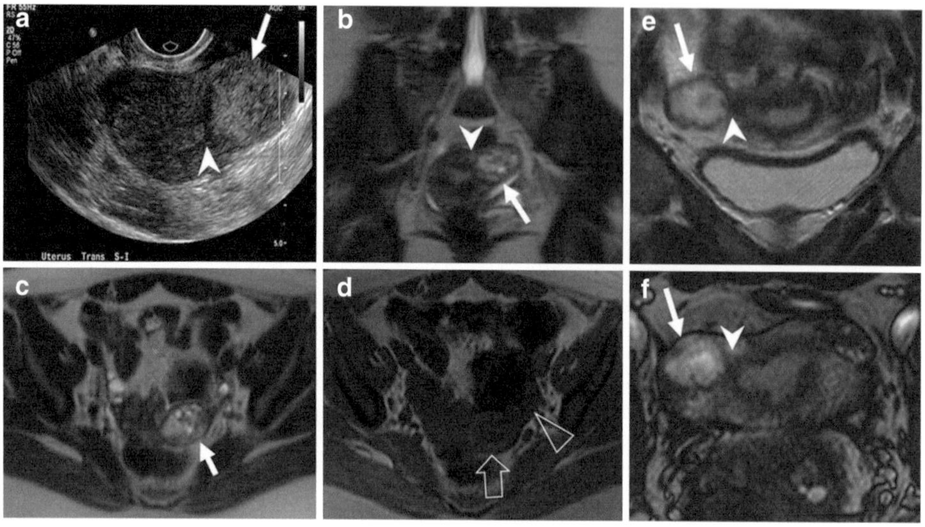

Fig. 11.13 Interstitial pregnancy—(**a**) US demonstrating a hyperechoic, heterogeneous ectopic pregnancy (white arrow) at the cornua (arrowhead) of the uterus in a women with positive HCG. (**b**) Coronal and (**c**) trans axial T2-weighted MR images demonstrate a heterogeneously T2 hyperintense ectopic (white arrow) at the junction of the uterine cornua and the fallopian tube (arrowhead). (**d**) T1-weighted MR image shows a hyperintense rim of hemorrhage (open arrow) along the margin of the ectopic and T1 hyperintense hemorrhage within the contiguous fallopian tube (open arrowhead). (**e**) Coronal T2-weighted and (**f**) axial SSFP MR images in a different patient with interstitial pregnancy demonstrate a heterogeneously T2 hyperintense ectopic (white arrow) at the uterine cornua (arrowhead). Both ectopic pregnancies were successfully treated with methotrexate

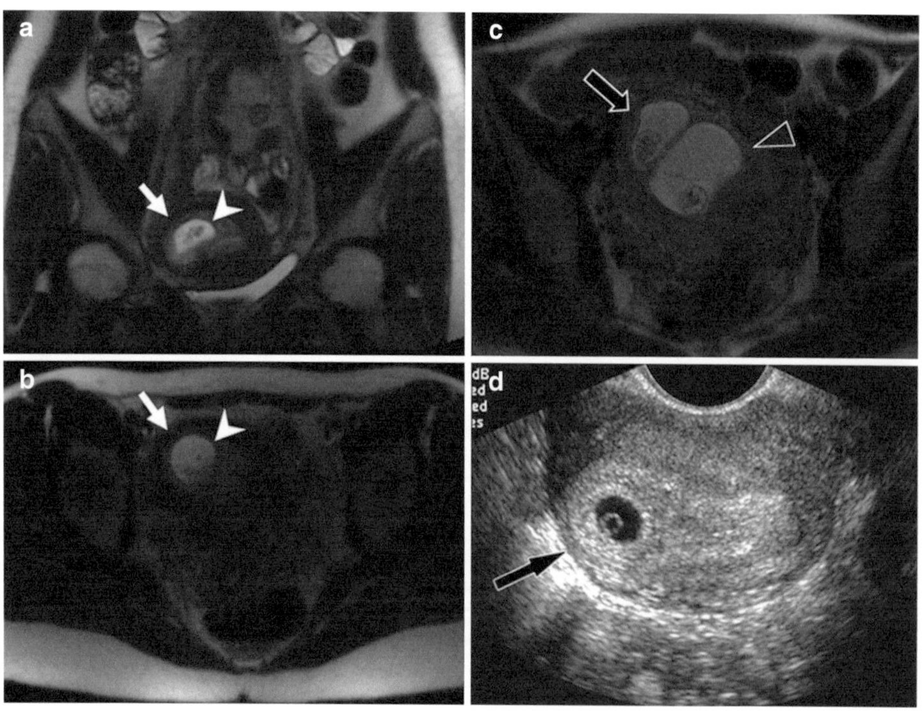

Fig. 11.14 Cornual pregnancy—(**a**) coronal and (**b**) axial T2-weighted MR images demonstrate an eccentric gestational sac in the uterine cornua with >5 mm of surrounding myometrium. (**c**) Axial T2 image in a different patient demonstrates a twin gestation, with one gestational sac located in the cornua of the uterus (black arrow), and one in the uterine body (open arrowhead). (**d**) US image shows the gestational sac in the uterine cornua. The cornual gestation was treated with selective reduction

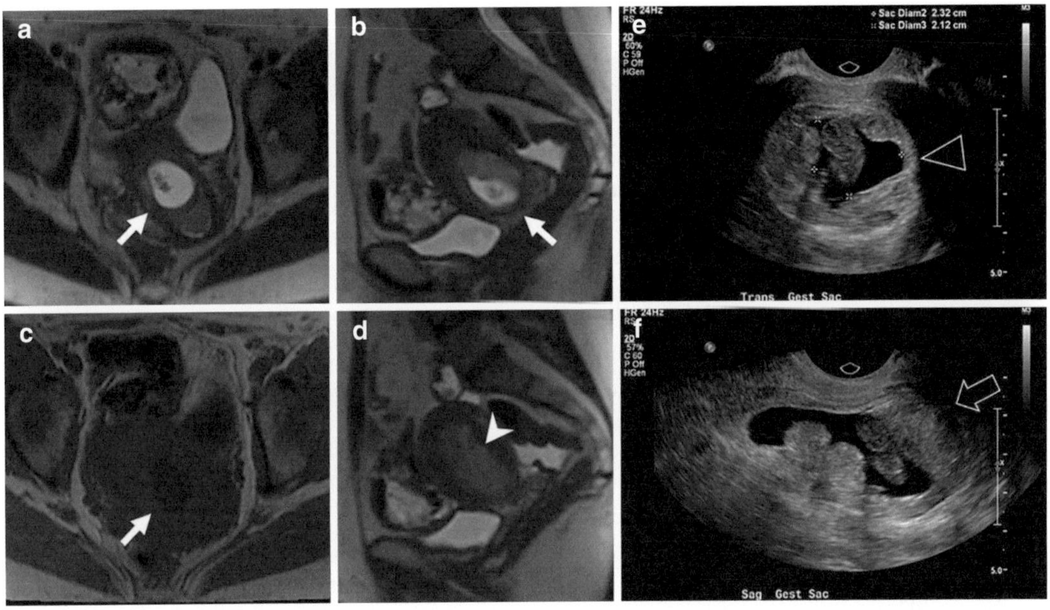

Fig. 11.15 Cervical pregnancy—(**a**) axial and (**b**) sagittal T2-weighted, and (**b**) T1-weighted MR images show a gestational sac located low in the endocervical canal (white arrow). (**d**) Sagittal T2-weighted MR image shows no gestational sac in the endouterine canal (arrowhead). (**e**) Transverse and (**f**) long axis transvaginal ultrasound images show a gestational sac and a fetal pole

Cervical pregnancy accounts for fewer than 1% of ectopic pregnancies and is predominately described in case reports and small case series. Cervical pregnancy typically presents with vaginal bleeding and can mimic spontaneous abortion or a cervical polyp, with the gestational sac located between the internal and external cervical os [130–133] (Fig. 11.15).

Ovarian ectopic pregnancies present a unique diagnostic challenge, as the gestation sac and a hemorrhagic corpus luteal cyst can be difficult to distinguish. Ovarian ectopic pregnancies have an association with an IUD [134]. The features of corpus luteal cyst and ectopic gestational sac described above may help distinguish an ovarian ectopic from a corpus luteal cyst.

Cesarean scar pregnancies have an increasing incidence in certain parts of the World, which is related to the increasing rate of cesarean section in North America. Diagnosis is made when a gestational sac is identified in the anterior lower uterine myometrium in a woman with prior cesarean section. Termination is recommended, although there are case reports of expectant management and early cesarean section [135–137].

11.5.4 Management

Ectopic pregnancy is preferably treated with single dose of systemic methotrexate, with greater than 90% success rate in select patient populations [138]. Methotrexate therapy is commonly offered to hemodynamically stable women, with an HCG level less than 5000 mIU/mL, a gestational sac smaller than 4 cm, no contraindication to methotrexate, and a willingness to follow-up for serial evaluation [139]. Failure of systemic therapy occurs more often in patients with high HCG levels (5000–10,000) and fetal cardiac activity [140].

Multidose therapy, local methotrexate injection, and local KCl injection have been proposed after single dose failure or in patients with fetal cardiac activity, high HCG levels, or late presentation [139, 141]. Surgical therapy is required for unstable patients, patients with evidence of rupture, or those who fail medical therapy. The presence of a small volume of hemorrhage confined to the pelvis is not a contraindication to medical therapy, as small volume hemorrhage is commonly seen with nonruptured tubal ectopics

[140, 142, 143]. Hemorrhage which extends into the paracolic gutters and abdomen may indicate tubal rupture and require emergent surgery.

Imaging follow-up after medical treatment is not routinely indicated. If follow-up imaging is obtained, the ectopic pregnancy often enlarges, prior to normalization of HCG levels. Mean ectopic enlargement on US is reportedly 6 cm. Sixty-nine percent of residual ectopics resolved with HCG normalization, but many patients will have residual complex masses after HCG normalization. Mean time to resolution of the ectopic is reportedly 44 days (range 25–63), when it persists beyond HCG normalization [118].

Conclusion

MR imaging can function as a primary or secondary imaging modality for the evaluation of acute pelvic pain. Most often, acute pelvic pain is evaluated with ultrasound or CT, and indeterminate or complex findings prompt MR imaging. Pelvic MR can be performed at 1.5 T or 3 T, with or without intravenous gadolinium, and with optimal sequence selection should take 30 min or less. Single-shot T2-weighted imaging is the foundation of any pelvic MR examination and should be done in multiple planes. Infection is often evident by parametrial stranding, thickening of the round ligament and uterosacral ligament, tubal enlargement and wall thickening, and inflammatory cystic adnexal masses. Ovarian torsion should be suspected when the ovary is asymmetrically enlarged, abnormally positioned, and is accompanied by thickening of the vascular pedicle. Ectopic pregnancies are circumscribed hypervascular masses with internal heterogeneity, which are most commonly located in the fallopian tube. MR utilization continues to rise, and familiarity with acute MR findings is an increasingly important part of effective emergency radiology and body imaging.

References

1. Lazarus E, Mayo-Smith WW, Mainiero MB, Spencer PK. CT in the evaluation of nontraumatic abdominal pain in pregnant women. Radiology. 2007;244(3):784–90.
2. Nagayama M, Watanabe Y, Okumura A, Amoh Y, Nakashita S, Dodo Y, Fast MR. Imaging in obstetrics. Radiographics. 2002;22(3):563–80.
3. Leyendecker JR, Gorengaut V, Brown JJ. MR imaging of maternal diseases of the abdomen and pelvis during pregnancy and the immediate postpartum period. Radiographics. 2004;24(5):1301–16.
4. Singh A, Danrad R, Hahn PF, Blake MA, Mueller PR, Novelline R. MR imaging of the acute abdomen and pelvis: acute appendicitis and beyond. Radiographics. 2007;27(5):1419–31.
5. Heverhagen JT, Klose KJ. MR imaging for acute lower abdominal and pelvic pain. Radiographics. 2009;29(6):1781–96.
6. Qayyum A. Diffusion-weighted imaging in the abdomen and pelvis: concepts and applications. Radiographics. 2009;29(6):1797–810.
7. Lubarsky M, Kalb B, Sharma P, Keim SM, Martin DR. MR imaging for acute nontraumatic abdominopelvic pain: rationale and practical considerations. Radiographics. 2013;33(2):313–37.
8. Kataoka M, Kido A, Koyama T, Isoda H, Umeoka S, Tamai K, et al. MRI of the female pelvis at 3T compared to 1.5T: evaluation on high-resolution T2-weighted and HASTE images. J Magn Reson Imaging. 2007;25(3):527–34.
9. Choi SH, Kim SH, Choi HJ, Park BK, Lee HJ. Preoperative magnetic resonance imaging staging of uterine cervical carcinoma: results of prospective study. J Comput Assist Tomogr. 2004;28(5):620–7.
10. Johnson AK, Filippi CG, Andrews T, Higgins T, Tam J, Keating D, et al. Ultrafast 3-T MRI in the evaluation of children with acute lower abdominal pain for the detection of appendicitis. Am J Roentgenol. 2012;198(6):1424–30.
11. Expert Panel on MR Safety, Kanal E, Barkovich AJ, Bell C, Borgstede JP, Bradley WG, et al. ACR guidance document on MR safe practices: 2013. J Magn Reson Imaging. 2013;37(3):501–30.
12. ACR Manual on Contrast Media v10.2. American College of Radiology; 2016
13. Thomsen HS, Morcos SK, Almén T, Bellin M, Bertolotto M, Bongartz G, et al. Nephrogenic systemic fibrosis and gadolinium-based contrast media: updated ESUR Contrast Medium Safety Committee guidelines. Eur Radiol. 2013;23(2): 307–18.
14. Li W, Zhang Y, Cui Y, Zhang P, Wu X. Pelvic inflammatory disease: evaluation of diagnostic accuracy with conventional MR with added diffusion-weighted imaging. Abdom Imaging. 2013;38(1):193–200.
15. Kato H, Kanematsu M, Uchiyama M, Yano R, Furui T, Morishige K. Diffusion-weighted imaging of ovarian torsion: usefulness of apparent diffusion coefficient (ADC) values for the detection of hemorrhagic infarction. Magn Reson Med Sci. 2014;13(1):39–44.

16. Fujii S. Diffusion-weighted imaging findings of adnexal torsion: initial results. Eur J Radiol. 2011;77:330–4.
17. Eschenbach DA, Wölner-Hanssen P, Hawes SE, Pavletic A, Paavonen J, Holmes KK. Acute pelvic inflammatory disease: associations of clinical and laboratory findings with laparoscopic findings. Obstet Gynecol. 1997;89(2):184–92.
18. Brunham RC, Gottlieb SL, Paavonen J. Pelvic inflammatory disease. N Engl J Med. 2015;372(21): 2039–48.
19. Monif GR. Clinical staging of acute bacterial salpingitis and its therapeutic ramifications. Am J Obstet Gynecol. 1982;143(5):489–95.
20. Soper DE. Pelvic inflammatory disease. Obstet Gynecol. 2010;116(2 Part 1):419–28.
21. Fitz-Hugh T. Acute gonococcic perihepatitis, a new syndrome of right upper quadrant abdominal pain in young women. Rev Gastroenterol. 1936;3:125–31.
22. Pickhardt PJ, Fleishman MJ, Fisher AJ. Fitz-Hugh–Curtis syndrome: multidetector CT Findings of transient hepatic attenuation difference and gallbladder wall thickening. Am J Roentgenol. 2003;180(6):1605–6.
23. Lee MH, Moon MH, Sung CK, Woo H, Oh S. CT findings of acute pelvic inflammatory disease. Abdom Imaging. 2014;39(6):1350–5.
24. Kreisel K. Prevalence of pelvic inflammatory disease in sexually experienced women of reproductive age—United States, 2013–2014. MMWR Morb Mortal Wkly Rep [Internet]. 2017 [cited 2017 May 16];66. http://www.cdc.gov/mmwr/volumes/66/wr/mm6603a3.htm
25. Sutton MY, Sternberg M, Zaidi A, St Louis ME, Markowitz LE. Trends in pelvic inflammatory disease hospital discharges and ambulatory visits, United States, 1985–2001. Sex Transm Dis. 2005;32(12):778–84.
26. Bohm MK, Newman L, Satterwhite CL, Tao G, Weinstock HS. Pelvic inflammatory disease among privately insured women, United States, 2001–2005. Sex Transm Dis. 2010;37(3):131–6.
27. Scholes D, Stergachis A, Heidrich FE, Andrilla H, Holmes KK, Stamm WE. Prevention of pelvic inflammatory disease by screening for cervical chlamydial infection. N Engl J Med. 1996;334(21):1362–6.
28. Brunham RC, Paavonen J, Stevens CE, Kiviat N, Kuo C-C, Critchlow CW, et al. Mucopurulent cervicitis—the ignored counterpart in women of urethritis in men. N Engl J Med. 1984;311(1):1–6.
29. Taylor SN, Lensing S, Schwebke J, Lillis R, Mena LA, Nelson AL, et al. Prevalence and treatment outcome of cervicitis of unknown etiology. Sex Transm Dis. 2013;40(5):379–85.
30. Imaoka I, Wada A, Matsuo M, Yoshida M, Kitagaki H, Sugimura K. MR imaging of disorders associated with female infertility: use in diagnosis, treatment, and management. Radiographics. 2003;23(6):1401–21.
31. Okamoto Y, Tanaka YO, Nishida M, Tsunoda H, Yoshikawa H, Itai YMR. Imaging of the uterine cervix: imaging-pathologic correlation. Radiographics. 2003;23(2):425–45.
32. Yitta S, Hecht EM, Mausner EV, Bennett GL. Normal or abnormal? Demystifying uterine and cervical contrast enhancement at multidetector CT. Radiographics. 2011;31(3):647–61.
33. Dohke M, Watanabe Y, Okumura A, Amoh Y, Hayashi T, Yoshizako T, et al. Comprehensive MR imaging of acute gynecologic diseases. Radiographics. 2000;20(6):1551–66.
34. Siddall KA, Rubens DJ. Multidetector CT of the female pelvis. Radiol Clin North Am. 2005;43(6): 1097–118.
35. Paavonen J, Critchlow CW, DeRouen T, Stevens CE, Kiviat N, Brunham RC, et al. Etiology of cervical inflammation. Am J Obstet Gynecol. 1986;154(3): 556–64.
36. Saini S, Kanetkar SR. Histopathol study lesions uterine cervix [Internet]. 2016 Dec 26 [cited 2017 May 17];(95463). http://www.jebmh.com/latest-articles.php?at_id=95463
37. Wager GP, Martin DH, Koutsky L, Eschenbach DA, Daling JR, Chiang WT, et al. Puerperal infectious morbidity: relationship to route of delivery and to antepartum Chlamydia trachomatis infection. Am J Obstet Gynecol. 1980;138(7):1028–33.
38. Watts DH, Eschenbach DA, Kenny GE. Early postpartum endometritis: the role of bacteria, genital mycoplasmas, and chlamydia trachomatis. Obstet Gynecol. 1989;73(1):52–60.
39. Cicinelli E, Matteo M, Tinelli R, Lepera A, Alfonso R, Indraccolo U, et al. Prevalence of chronic endometritis in repeated unexplained implantation failure and the IVF success rate after antibiotic therapy. Hum Reprod. 2015;30(2):323–30.
40. Nalaboff KM, Pellerito JS, Ben-Levi E. Imaging the endometrium: disease and normal variants. Radiographics. 2001;21(6):1409–24.
41. Sudderuddin S, Helbren E, Telesca M, Williamson R, Rockall A. MRI appearances of benign uterine disease. Clin Radiol. 2014;69(11):1095–104.
42. Jung SI, Kim YJ, Park HS, Jeon HJ, Jeong KA. Acute pelvic inflammatory disease: diagnostic performance of CT. J Obstet Gynaecol Res. 2011;37(3):228–35.
43. Revzin MV, Mathur M, Dave HB, Macer ML, Spektor M. Pelvic inflammatory disease: multimodality imaging approach with clinical-pathologic correlation. Radiographics. 2016;36(5):1579–96.
44. Patton DL, Moore DE, Spadoni LR, Soules MR, Halbert SA, Wang SP. A comparison of the fallopian tube's response to overt and silent salpingitis. Obstet Gynecol. 1989;73(4):622–30.
45. Kim MY, Rha SE, Soon Nam O, Jung SE, Lee YJ, Kim YS, et al. MR imaging findings of hydrosalpinx: a comprehensive review. Radiographics. 2009;29(2):495–507.
46. Propeck PA, Scanlan KA. Isolated fallopian tube torsion. Am J Roentgenol. 1998;170(4):1112–3.
47. Gross M, Blumstein SL, Chow LC. Isolated fallopian tube torsion: a rare twist on a common theme. Am J Roentgenol. 2005;185(6):1590–2.

48. Landers DV, Sweet RL. Current trends in the diagnosis and treatment of tuboovarian abscess. Am J Obstet Gynecol. 1985;151(8):1098–110.
49. Ueda H, Togashi K, Kataoka ML, Koyama T, Fujiwara T, Fujii S, et al. Adnexal masses caused by pelvic inflammatory disease: MR appearance. Magn Reson Med Sci. 2002;1(4):207–15.
50. Tukeva TA, Aronen HJ, Karjalainen PT, Molander P, Paavonen T, Paavonen J. MR imaging in pelvic inflammatory disease: comparison with laparoscopy and US. Radiology. 1999;210(1):209–16.
51. Rezvani M, Shaaban AM. Fallopian tube disease in the nonpregnant patient. Radiographics. 2011;31(2):527–48.
52. Ha HK, Lim GY, Cha ES, Lee HG, Ro HJ, Kim HS, et al. MR imaging of tubo-ovarian abscess. Acta Radiol 1987. 1995;36(5):510–4.
53. Twickler DM, Setiawan AT, Evans RS, Erdman WA, Stettler RW, Brown CE, et al. Imaging of puerperal septic thrombophlebitis: prospective comparison of MR imaging, CT, and sonography. Am J Roentgenol. 1997;169(4):1039–43.
54. Kubik-Huch RA, Hebisch G, Huch R, Hilfiker P, Debatin JF, Krestin GP. Role of duplex color Doppler ultrasound, computed tomography, and MR angiography in the diagnosis of septic puerperal ovarian vein thrombosis. Abdom Imaging. 1999;24(1):85–91.
55. Sharma P, Abdi S. Ovarian vein thrombosis. Clin Radiol. 2012;67(9):893–8.
56. Cuyper K, Eyselbergs M, Bernard P, Clabout L, Vanhoenacker FM. Added value of diffusion weighted MRI in the diagnosis of postpartum ovarian vein thrombosis. J Belg Soc Radiol [Internet]. 2014 [cited 2017 May 23];97(4). http://www.jbsr.be/articles/abstract/10.5334/jbr-btr.86/
57. Valicenti JF, Pappas AA, Graber CD, Williamson HO, Willis NF. Detection and prevalence of IUD-associated Actinomyces colonization and related morbidity. A prospective study of 69,925 cervical smears. JAMA. 1982;247(8):1149–52.
58. Chatwani A, Amin-Hanjani S. Incidence of actinomycosis associated with intrauterine devices. J Reprod Med. 1994;39(8):585–7.
59. Perlow JH, Wigton T, Yordan EL, Graham J, Wool N, Wilbanks GD. Disseminated pelvic actinomycosis presenting as metastatic carcinoma: association with the progestasert intrauterine device. Rev Infect Dis. 1991;13(6):1115–9.
60. Hawnaur JM, Reynolds K, McGettigan C. Magnetic resonance imaging of actinomycosis presenting as pelvic malignancy. Br J Radiol. 1999;72(862):1006–11.
61. Bae JH, Song R, Lee A, Park JS, Kim MR. Computed tomography for the preoperative diagnosis of pelvic actinomycosis. J Obstet Gynaecol Res. 2011;37(4):300–4.
62. O'Connor KF, Bagg MN, Croley MR, Schabel SI. Pelvic actinomycosis associated with intrauterine devices. Radiology. 1989;170(2):559–60.
63. Kim SH, Kim SH, Yang DM, Kim KA. Unusual causes of tubo-ovarian abscess: CT and MR imaging findings. Radiographics. 2004;24(6):1575–89.
64. Dejanović D, Ahnlide JA, Nilsson C, Berthelsen AK, Loft A. Pelvic actinomycosis associated with an intrauterine contraceptive device demonstrated on F-18 FDG PET/CT. Diagnostics. 2015;5(3):369–71.
65. Ness RB, Soper DE, Holley RL, Peipert J, Randall H, Sweet RL, et al. Effectiveness of inpatient and outpatient treatment strategies for women with pelvic inflammatory disease: results from the pelvic inflammatory disease evaluation and clinical health (peach) randomized trial. Am J Obstet Gynecol. 2002;186(5):929–37.
66. Pelvic Inflammatory Disease (PID)—2015 STD Treatment Guidelines [Internet]. [cited 2017 May 23]. https://www.cdc.gov/std/tg2015/pid.htm
67. Farid H, Lau TC, Karmon AE, Styer AK. Clinical characteristics associated with antibiotic treatment failure for tuboovarian abscesses. Infect Dis Obstet Gynecol. 2016;2016:e5120293.
68. Perez-Medina T, Huertas MA, Bajo JM. Early ultrasound-guided transvaginal drainage of tuba-ovarian abscesses: a randomized study. Ultrasound Obstet Gynecol. 1996;7(6):435–8.
69. Goharkhay N, Verma U, Maggiorotto F.Comparison of CT- or ultrasound-guided drainage with concomitant intravenous antibiotics vs. intravenous antibiotics alone in the management of tubo-ovarian abscesses. Ultrasound Obstet Gynecol. 2007;29(1):65–9.
70. Gjelland K, Ekerhovd E, Granberg S. Transvaginal ultrasound-guided aspiration for treatment of tubo-ovarian abscess: a study of 302 cases. Am J Obstet Gynecol. 2005;193(4):1323–30.
71. Labropoulos N, Malgor RD, Comito M, Gasparis AP, Pappas PJ, Tassiopoulos AK. The natural history and treatment outcomes of symptomatic ovarian vein thrombosis. J Vasc Surg Venous Lymphat Disord. 2015;3(1):42–7.
72. Taga S. Diagnosis and therapy of pelvic actinomycosis. J Obstet Gynaecol Res. 2007;33(6):882–5.
73. Smego RA, Foglia G. Actinomycosis. Clin Infect Dis. 1998;26(6):1255–61.
74. Lippes J. Pelvic actinomycosis: a review and preliminary look at prevalence. Am J Obstet Gynecol. 1999;180(2):265–9.
75. Garner JP, Macdonald M, Kumar PK. Abdominal actinomycosis. Int J Surg. 2007;5(6):441–8.
76. Hibbard LT. Adnexal torsion. Am J Obstet Gynecol. 1985;152(4):456–61.
77. Houry D, Abbott JT. Ovarian torsion: a fifteen-year review. Ann Emerg Med. 2001;38(2):156–9.
78. Hiller N, Appelbaum L, Simanovsky N, Lev-Sagi A, Aharoni D, Sella TCT. Features of adnexal torsion. Am J Roentgenol. 2007;189(1):124–9.
79. Béranger-Gibert S, Sakly H, Ballester M, Rockall A, Bornes M, Bazot M, et al. Diagnostic value of MR imaging in the diagnosis of adnexal torsion. Radiology. 2015;279(2):461–70.

80. Chiou S-Y, Lev-Toaff AS, Masuda E, Feld RI, Bergin D. Adnexal torsion. J Ultrasound Med. 2007;26(10):1289–301.
81. Duigenan S, Oliva E, Lee SI. Ovarian torsion: diagnostic features on CT and MRI with pathologic correlation. Am J Roentgenol. 2012;198(2):W122–31.
82. Fahmy HS, Swamy N, Elshahat HM. Revisiting the role of MRI in gynecological emergencies: an institutional experience. Egypt J Radiol Nucl Med. 2015;46(3):769–79.
83. Petkovska I, Duke E, Martin DR, Irani Z, Geffre CP, Cragun JM, et al. MRI of ovarian torsion: correlation of imaging features with the presence of perifollicular hemorrhage and ovarian viability. Eur J Radiol. 2016;85(11):2064–71.
84. Yuk J-S, Kim LY, Shin J-Y, Choi DY, Kim TY, Lee JHA. national population-based study of the incidence of adnexal torsion in the Republic of Korea. Int J Gynecol Obstet. 2015;129(2):169–70.
85. Mashiach S, Bider D, Moran O, Goldenberg M, Ben-Rafael Z. Adnexal torsion of hyperstimulated ovaries in pregnancies after gonadotropin therapy. Fertil Steril. 1990;53(1):76–80.
86. Ginath S, Shalev A, Keidar R, Kerner R, Condrea A, Golan A, et al. Differences between adnexal torsion in pregnant and nonpregnant women. J Minim Invasive Gynecol. 2012;19(6):708–14.
87. Moribata Y, Kido A, Yamaoka T, Mikami Y, Himoto Y, Kataoka M, et al. MR imaging findings of ovarian torsion correlate with pathological hemorrhagic infarction. J Obstet Gynaecol Res. 2015;41(9):1433–9.
88. Lee EJ, Kwon HC, Joo HJ, Suh JH, Fleischer AC. Diagnosis of ovarian torsion with color Doppler sonography: depiction of twisted vascular pedicle. J Ultrasound Med. 1998;17(2):83–9.
89. Ghossain MA, Hachem K, Buy J-N, Hourany-Rizk RG, Aoun NJ, Haddad-Zebouni S, et al. Adnexal torsion: magnetic resonance findings in the viable adnexa with emphasis on stromal ovarian appearance. J Magn Reson Imaging. 2004;20(3):451–62.
90. Fujii S, Kaneda S, Kakite S, Kanasaki Y, Matsusue E, Harada T, et al. Diffusion-weighted imaging findings of adnexal torsion: initial results. Eur J Radiol. 2011;77(2):330–4.
91. Rha SE, Byun JY, Jung SE, Jung JI, Choi BG, Kim BS, et al. CT and MR imaging features of adnexal torsion. Radiographics. 2002;22(2):283–94.
92. Kimura I, Togashi K, Kawakami S, Takakura K, Mori T, Konishi J. Ovarian torsion: CT and MR imaging appearances. Radiology. 1994;190(2):337–41.
93. Haque TL, Togashi K, Kobayashi H, Fujii S, Konishi J. Adnexal torsion: MR imaging findings of viable ovary. Eur Radiol. 2000;10(12):1954–7.
94. Zweizig S, Perron J, Grubb D, Mishell DR. Conservative management of adnexal torsion. Am J Obstet Gynecol. 1993;168(6):1791–5.
95. McGovern PG, Noah R, Koenigsberg R, Little AB. Adnexal torsion and pulmonary embolism: case report and review of the literature. Obstet Gynecol Surv. 1999;54(9):601–8.
96. Oelsner G, Bider D, Goldenberg M, Admon D, Mashiach S. Long-term follow-up of the twisted ischemic adnexa managed by detorsion. Fertil Steril. 1993;60(6):976–9.
97. Galinier P, Carfagna L, Delsol M, Ballouhey Q, Lemasson F, Le Mandat A, et al. Ovarian torsion. Management and ovarian prognosis: a report of 45 cases. J Pediatr Surg. 2009;44(9):1759–65.
98. Germain M, Rarick T, Robins E. Management of intermittent ovarian torsion by laparoscopic oophoropexy. Obstet Gynecol. 1996;88(4):715–7.
99. Grunewald B, Keating J, Brown S. Asynchronous ovarian torsion: the case for prophylactic oophoropexy. Postgrad Med J. 1993;69(810):318–9.
100. Breen JL. A 21 year survey of 654 ectopic pregnancies. Am J Obstet Gynecol. 1970;106(7):1004–19.
101. Körolu M, Kayhan A, Soylu FN, Erol B, Schmidtannwald C, Gürses C, et al. MR imaging of ectopic pregnancy with an emphasis on unusual implantation sites. Jpn J Radiol. 2013;31(2):75–80.
102. Cacciatore B, Stenman U-H, Ylostalo P. Early screening for ectopic pregnancy in high-risk symptom-free women. Lancet. 1994;343(8896):517–8.
103. Barnhart KT. Ectopic pregnancy. N Engl J Med. 2009;361(4):379–87.
104. Kirk E, Bottomley C, Bourne T. Diagnosing ectopic pregnancy and current concepts in the management of pregnancy of unknown location. Hum Reprod Update. 2014;20(2):250–61.
105. Barnhart K, Mennuti MT, Benjamin I, Jacobson S, Goodman D, Coutifaris C. Prompt diagnosis of ectopic pregnancy in an emergency department setting. Obstet Gynecol. 1994;84(6):1010–5.
106. Condous G, Lu C, Van Huffel SV, Timmerman D, Bourne T. Human chorionic gonadotrophin and progesterone levels in pregnancies of unknown location. Int J Gynecol Obstet. 2004;86(3):351–7.
107. Shalev E, Yarom I, Bustan M, Weiner E, Ben-Shlomo I. Transvaginal sonography as the ultimate diagnostic tool for the management of ectopic pregnancy: experience with 840 cases. Fertil Steril. 1998;69(1):62–5.
108. Goldner TE, Lawson HW, Xia Z, Atrash HK. Surveillance for ectopic pregnancy—United States, 1970–1989. MMWR CDC Surveill Summ Morb Mortal Wkly Rep CDC Surveill Summ. 1993;42(6):73–85.
109. Centers for Disease Control. Current trends ectopic pregnancy: United States, 1990–1992. MMWR Wkly. 1995;44(3):46–8.
110. Chang J, Elam-Evans LD, Berg CJ, Herndon J, Flowers L, Seed KA, et al. Pregnancy-related mortality surveillance—United States, 1991–1999. MMWR Surveill Summ. 2003;52(2):1–8.
111. Grimes DA. Estimation of pregnancy-related mortality risk by pregnancy outcome, United States, 1991 to 1999. Am J Obstet Gynecol. 2006;194(1):92–4.

112. Creanga AA, Shapiro-Mendoza CK, Bish CL, Zane S, Berg CJ, Callaghan WM. Trends in ectopic pregnancy mortality in the United States: 1980–2007. Obstet Gynecol. 2011;117(4):837–43.
113. Tamai K, Koyama T, Saga T, Kido A, Kataoka M, Umeoka S, et al. MR features of physiologic and benign conditions of the ovary. Eur Radiol. 2006;16(12):2700–11.
114. Tamai K, Koyama T, Togashi K. MR features of ectopic pregnancy. Eur Radiol. 2007;17(12): 3236–46.
115. Si M-J, Gui S, Fan Q, Han H-X, Zhao Q-Q, Li Z-X, et al. Role of MRI in the early diagnosis of tubal ectopic pregnancy. Eur Radiol. 2016;26(7):1971–80.
116. Takahashi A, Takahama J, Marugami N, Takewa M, Itoh T, Kitano S, et al. Ectopic pregnancy: MRI findings and clinical utility. Abdom Imaging. 2013;38(4):844–50.
117. Yoshigi J, Yashiro N, Kinoshita T, O'uchi T, Kitagaki H. Diagnosis of ectopic pregnancy with MRI: efficacy of T2-weighted imaging. Magn Reson Med Sci. 2006;5(1):25–32.
118. Gamzu R, Almog B, Levin Y, Pauzner D, Lessing JB, Jaffa A, et al. The ultrasonographic appearance of tubal pregnancy in patients treated with methotrexate. Hum Reprod. 2002;17(10):2585–7.
119. Bouyer J, Coste J, Fernandez H, Pouly JL, Job-Spira N. Sites of ectopic pregnancy: a 10 year population-based study of 1800 cases. Hum Reprod. 2002;17(12):3224–30.
120. Filhastre M, Dechaud H, Lesnik A, Taourel P. Interstitial pregnancy: role of MRI. Eur Radiol. 2005;15(1):93–5.
121. Bourdel N, Roman H, Gallot D, Lenglet Y, Dieu V, Juillard D, et al. Interstitial pregnancy. Ultrasonographic diagnosis and contribution of MRI. A case report. Gynécologie Obstétrique Fertil. 2007;35(2):121.
122. Moawad NS, Mahajan ST, Moniz MH, Taylor SE, Hurd WW. Current diagnosis and treatment of interstitial pregnancy. Am J Obstet Gynecol. 2010;202(1):15–29.
123. Cohen J, Weinreb J, Lowe T, Brown CMR. imaging of a viable full-term abdominal pregnancy. Am J Roentgenol. 1985;145(2):407–8.
124. Wagner A, Burchardt A-JMR. Imaging in advanced abdominal pregnancy a case report of fetal death. Acta Radiol. 1995;36(2):193–5.
125. Malian V, Lee JE. MR imaging and MR angiography of an abdominal pregnancy with placental infarction. Am J Roentgenol. 2001;177(6):1305–6.
126. Ozdemir I, Demirci F, Yucel O, Alper M. Primary omental pregnancy presenting with hemorrhagic shock. Gynecol Obstet Invest. 2003;55(2):116–8.
127. Wong WC, Wong BPY, Kun KY, Ng TK, Kwok SY, Lee CK. Primary omental ectopic pregnancy. J Obstet Gynaecol Res. 2004;30(3):226–9.
128. Børlum K-G, Blom R. Primary hepatic pregnancy. Int J Gynecol Obstet. 1988;27(3):427–9.
129. Cormio G, Santamato S, Vimercati A, Selvaggi L. Primary splenic pregnancy. A case report. J Reprod Med. 2003;48(6):479–81.
130. Werber J, Prasadarao PR, Harris VJ. Cervical pregnancy diagnosed by ultrasound. Radiology. 1983;149(1):279–80.
131. Jung SE, Byun JY, Lee JM, Choi BG, Hahn ST, Characteristic MR findings of cervical pregnancy. J Magn Reson Imaging. 2001;13(6):918–22.
132. Gun M, Mavrogiorgis M. Cervical ectopic pregnancy: a case report and literature review. Ultrasound Obstet Gynecol. 2002;19(3):297–301.
133. Sherer DM, Gorelick C, Dalloul M, Sokolovski M, Kheyman M, Kakamanu S, et al. Three-dimensional sonographic findings of a cervical pregnancy. J Ultrasound Med. 2008;27(1):155–8.
134. Herbertsson G, Magnusson SS, Benediktsdottir K. Ovarian pregnancy and IUCD use in a defined complete population. Acta Obstet Gynecol Scand. 1987;66(7):607–10.
135. Ash A, Smith A, Maxwell D. Caesarean scar pregnancy. BJOG. 2007;114(3):253–63.
136. Rotas MA, Haberman S, Levgur M. Cesarean scar ectopic pregnancies: etiology, diagnosis, and management. Obstet Gynecol. 2006;107(6): 1373–81.
137. Timor-Tritsch IE, Monteagudo A. Unforeseen consequences of the increasing rate of cesarean deliveries: early placenta accreta and cesarean scar pregnancy. A review. Am J Obstet Gynecol. 2012;207(1):14–29.
138. Lipscomb GH, Bran D, McCord ML, Portera JC, Ling FW. Analysis of three hundred fifteen ectopic pregnancies treated with single-dose methotrexate. Am J Obstet Gynecol. 1998;178(6):1354–8.
139. Lipscomb GH, Stovall TG, Ling FW. Nonsurgical treatment of ectopic pregnancy. N Engl J Med. 2000;343(18):1325–9.
140. Lipscomb GH, McCord ML, Stovall TG, Huff G, Portera SG, Ling FW. Predictors of success of methotrexate treatment in women with tubal ectopic pregnancies. N Engl J Med. 1999;341(26):1974–8.
141. Tzafettas JM, Stephanatos A, Loufopoulos A, Anapliotis S, Mamopoulos M, Kalogeropoulos A. Single high dose of local methotrexate for the management of relatively advanced ectopic pregnancies. Fertil Steril. 1999;71(6):1010–3.
142. Romero R, Copel JA, Kadar N, Jeanty P, Decherney A, Hobbins JC. Value of culdocentesis in the diagnosis of ectopic pregnancy. Obstet Gynecol. 1985;65(4):519–22.
143. Vermesh M, Graczykowski JW, Sauer MV. Reevaluation of the role of culdocentesis in the management of ectopic pregnancy. Am J Obstet Gynecol. 1990;162(2):411–3.

Traumatic Abdominal Compartment Syndrome

12

Luigia Romano, Carlo Liguori, Ciro Acampora, Nicola Gagliardi, Antonio Pinto, Sonia Fulciniti, and Massimo Silva

Abstract

Traumatic abdominal compartment syndrome (ACS) can result from a blunt or penetrating trauma which involves abdominal and pelvic cavity. A direct injury to the abdomen or pelvis can cause vascular, tissue, and organ injuries which are frequently associated with ongoing hemorrhage. The severe bleeding causes hypoperfusion to organs and tissues, whereas the collection of blood within the abdominal and pelvic cavity can cause intra-abdominal hypertension (IAH). Both conditions can result in tissue and organ hypoxia. Traumatic ACS is diagnosed when the intra-abdominal pressure is greater than 20 mmHg, with the development of single- or multiple-organ dysfunction. In the acute setting of a severely injured patient, it is mandatory to control bleeding and restore coagulation function. Many patients need massive fluid resuscitation and are treated with abdominal packing. In presence of life-threatening hemorrhage, these treatments are necessary, but these same factors also increase the risk of developing ACS. Traumatic ACS is a clinical syndrome which may easily be misinterpreted, and can lead to worsening of patient outcome. It is essential to diagnose and manage ACS early, because without a rapid intervention the risk of death is high. It is considered a complication that is potentially reversible. Abdominal decompression of ACS rapidly improves cardiac, pulmonary, and renal functioning. With the use of multi-detector computed tomography (MDCT) for the assessment and follow-up of severe blunt and penetrating injuries, an unsuspected ACS can be diagnosed early, before the development of severe organ or multi-organ dysfunction. CT can provide evidence of some indicative features of increased intra-abdominal pressure in patients at risk for developing ACS, including large hematomas. The partnership between the radiologist and surgeon to utilize both clinical and CT findings to detect early ACS provides a more precise method for the detection and rapid treatment of this lethal but potentially reversible syndrome. Radiologists could be increasingly likely to evaluate patients with ACS in the presence of abdominal and/or pelvic hemorrhage and/or postsurgical application of packs. Correct early radiological diagnosis of ACS is based on the knowledge of the MDCT findings, as well as awareness of the pathophysiology of the syndrome.

Keywords

Traumatic abdominal compartment syndrome Intra-abdominal hypertension · Blunt or penetrating abdominal and pelvic trauma Traumatic space-occupying processes · Organ and tissue hypoperfusion · Single- or multiple-organ dysfunction · Bladder pressure measurement · Damage-control surgery

L. Romano (✉) • C. Liguori • C. Acampora
N. Gagliardi • A. Pinto • S. Fulciniti • M. Silva
Department of General and Emergency Radiology, A.O.R.N A. Cardarelli, Naples, Italy

M. Patlas et al. (eds.), *MDCT and MR Imaging of Acute Abdomen*,
https://doi.org/10.1007/978-3-319-70778-5_12

12.1 Introduction

Posttraumatic abdominal compartment syndrome (ACS) is diagnosed when there is ongoing intra-abdominal hypertension (IAH) greater than 20 mmHg, with the development of single- or multiple-organ dysfunction [1]. Patients generally have major intraperitoneal and/or retroperitoneal bleeding, typically due to blunt or penetrating abdominal and/or pelvic trauma. It is generally the effect of decreasing blood flow and increased abdominal cavity pressure on solid organs and vessels.

ACS is a silent process which can be easily overlooked or misinterpreted, so patient may be undiagnosed and the risk of death is therefore high, especially if massive fluid and blood product resuscitation are administered [2]. Rapid recognition and sudden treatment of ACS are mandatory [3]. Patients requiring post-injury damage-control surgery are also at high risk for developing ACS. Damage-control surgery is as a potentially lifesaving maneuver in severely blunt injured patients, who develop hypothermia, acidosis, and coagulopathy. It is based on placing of packs in the abdominal and/or pelvis cavity for obtaining hemostasis, and temporarily stabilizing vascular and solid organ injuries [4, 5].

Both experimental and clinical studies [6, 7] have shown that increasing intra-abdominal pressure reduces cardiac, pulmonary, and renal function, raising the possibility of developing multi-failure organ syndrome (MOF). In addition, ACS promotes mesenteric ischemia and bacterial translocation outside the intestinal lumen, through the bowel wall, contributing to the development of MOF [8].

Risk factors for development of ACS include massive fluid resuscitation, multiple transfusions, and hypothermia. High-volume fluid resuscitation sufficient to cause ACS has been defined as >3500 mL given in 24 h or less [9].

In the acute setting of a severely injured patient, it is mandatory to control bleeding and restore coagulation function for optimizing oxygen availability. Many patients need massive fluid resuscitation, develop mesenteric reperfusion bowel edema, and are treated with abdominal packing. In the presence of life-threatening hemorrhage, lifesaving treatment is needed, but these same factors also increase the risk of developing ACS [10].

There are three different types of ACS: primary, secondary, and tertiary.

Primary ACS is due to a principal intra-abdominal cause, particularly abdominal trauma and/or retroperitoneal hemorrhage [11] (Fig. 12.1). Secondary ACS is usually the result of massive bowel edema secondary to trauma, sepsis, burns, or other conditions which require massive fluid resuscitation [12]. It occurs most commonly after hemorrhagic shock or severe burn injuries. Tertiary ACS occurs after resolution of an earlier episode of either primary or secondary ACS. It is less frequent, and is sometimes due to abdominal surgical closure in an edematous patient.

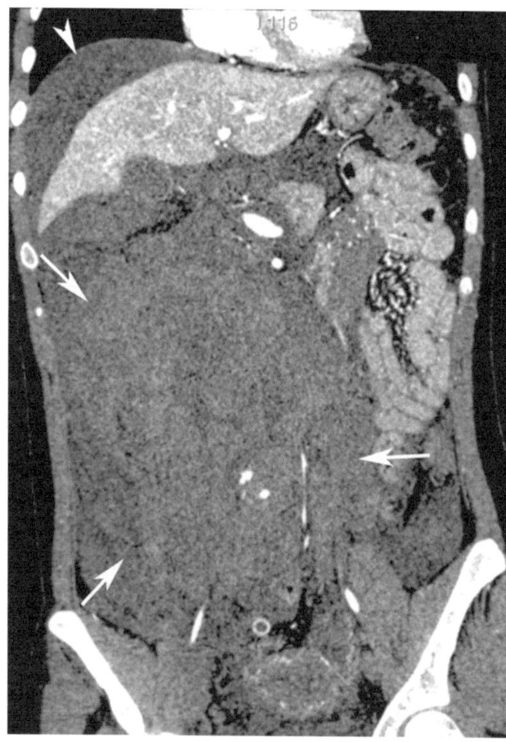

Fig. 12.1 A 37-year-old man was admitted for polytrauma from a motor vehicle collision. IV contrast-enhanced coronal abdominal CT image shows a large hemoretroperitoneum (*arrows*) associated with hemoperitoneum and elevation of right hemidiaphragm (*arrowhead*). CT findings suggested an abdominal compartment syndrome and the intravesical pressure was measured, confirming the diagnosis

Because the patient can die from the development of a multi-failure organ syndrome caused by ACS and not necessarily from the injuries themselves, it is important that the radiologist during the MDCT assessment of the severe trauma patient pays careful attention to ACS signs and alerts the surgeon before these impairments become irreversible. Early diagnosis of ACS is based on MDCT findings and knowledge of the causes of the syndrome.

12.2 Intra-abdominal Pressure

Normal values of intra-abdominal pressure (IAP) are considered to be close to atmospheric pressure, 0–5 mmHg. Consensus definitions propose IAH as an IAP greater than 12 mmHg [13]. However, there are differences of opinion in the literature regarding the value at which IAH becomes abnormal. Some authors [14] note that the range in which the abdominal decompression is needed is around 20–25 mmHg, because the highest incidence of mortality occurs with an IAP of >25 mmHg. Individual physiology and comorbidities can influence the patient's tolerance of IAH [15].

Intra-abdominal pressure can be measured by direct or indirect monitoring. Direct methods are based on the introduction of an intraperitoneal cannula for measuring intra-abdominal pressure, or a femoral venous line for measuring inferior vena cava pressure. There is a close correlation between IAP and inferior vena cava pressure [16]. Other indirect methods are based on intragastric and rectal pressure evaluation. With the use of an intragastric tube, water is instilled into the gastric lumen and the pressure within the abdominal compartment is measured within the stomach, by a manometer or pressure transducer. Rectal pressure measurement can be achieved with a tube which is introduced 10 cm above the anal edge [16]. The bladder pressure method is considered the reference standard [17] and is considered the most valid measurement of IAP via indirect measurement. 100 mL of water is instilled into the bladder, and pressure is measured by a manometer [17].

12.3 Pathophysiology of Abdominal Compartment Syndrome

ACS can involve any organ and system. Organ impairment typically starts subtly, and at varying intra-abdominal pressures, depending on the individual's abdominal conformity. In ACS, there is a decrease of the cellular blood supply which reduces the aerobic metabolism pushing the cells into an anaerobic state, leading to lactic acidosis [18]. The compression of the capillary network of organs and tissue interrupts transfer of the carbon dioxide. This further increases acidity at a cellular level, particularly in the intestines. Systemic acidosis develops, as more vascular impairment and organ dysfunction occur.

As the pressure increases within the abdominal cavity, it begins to compress the inferior vena cava (Fig. 12.2) with stagnation of the blood at periphery of the body, and consequent reduction in cardiac output and blood pressure. The elevation and compression of the diaphragm due to ACS increase intrathoracic pressure. As intrathoracic pressure increases, it further limits cardiac output and venous return, leading to pulmonary vascular resistance and impaired right ventricular activity [19]. Furthermore, the heart, compressed by the abdomi-

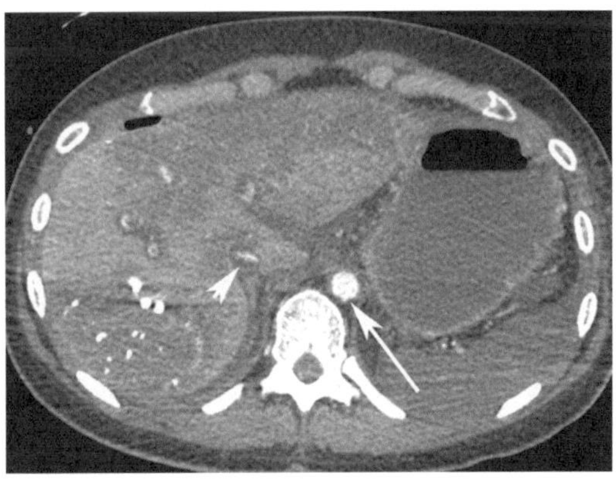

Fig. 12.2 A 45-year-old man after a fall from a high tree. IV contrast- enhanced axial CT scan depicts a large liver contusion, a small abdominal aorta (*white arrow*), a flattened inferior vena cava (*white arrowhead*) and extraluminal free air bubble anterior to the liver due to a small intestinal loop laceration. The patient has a large retroperitoneal hematoma associated with multiple pelvic and lumbar vertebral fractures

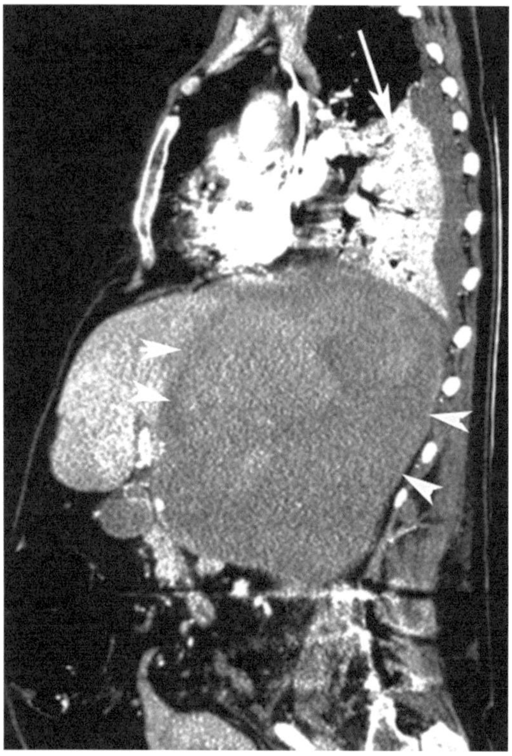

Fig. 12.3 A 32-year-old man involved in a motorcycle collision with an open-book pelvic fracture, was treated in another hospital with pelvic packing for large hematoma. After a few days, he was trasferred to our hospital for liver dysfunction and anuria. IV contrast- enhanced axial CT image shows bilateral renal infarctions (*arrows*) liver ischemia (*arrowheads*) and a splenic laceration. There were a small portal vein, a small aorta, a flattened inferior vena cava and a left pleural effusion do to left inferior ribs fractures. These CT findings were interpreted as post-packing abdominal compartment syndrome (ACS). After surgical removal of packing, only the liver function became progressively normal

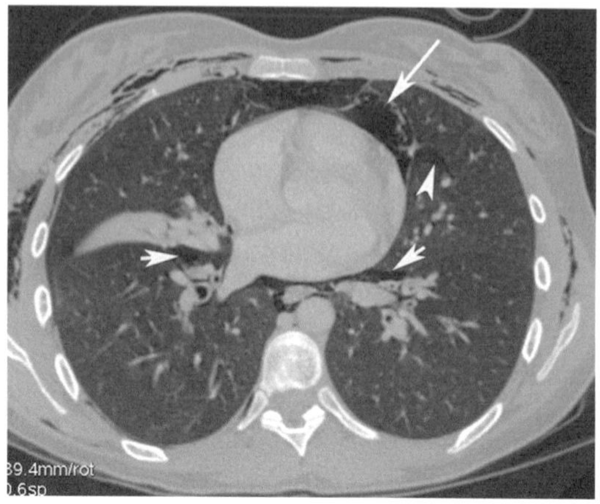

Fig. 12.4 A 48-year-old woman was admitted to the Intensive Care Unit for polytrauma in a motor vehicle collision. The patient had brain injury and hemoretroperitoneum from right renal lacerations; both were treated conservatively. The patient developed respiratory distress and axial CT image of the thorax shows multiple interstitial empysema due to barotrauma (*arrowheads*) associated with pneumomediastinum (*arrow*) and subcutaneous emphysema, due to high mechanical ventilator pressure

nal high pressure and diaphragm elevation, can contribute to increase in the elevated central venous pressure and pulmonary capillary pressure [20].

The reduction in cardiac output is an early clinical finding of ACS, and is caused by the attempt to compensate for the reduced stroke volume [20]. Hypotension is considered a late clinical finding [21]. Additionally, the high pressure on the abdominal aorta wall leads to a further reduction in cardiac output. Increased intra-abdominal pressure proceeds through the diaphragm, compressing the lower lungs (Fig. 12.3) with subsequent hypoxemia and hypercarbia. In order to correct hypoxemia and hypercarbia, the clinician frequently increases mechanical ventilator pressure, increasing the risk of barotrauma and development of interstitial emphysema, pneumomediastinum, and subcutaneous emphysema (Fig. 12.4) [22].

The rise in intrathoracic pressure limits venous flow from the cranial circulation. This causes a high intracerebral pressure, and impairs brain perfusion pressure [23, 24, 25]. When the IAP is more than 15 mmHg, the high pressure on the renal veins and parenchyma causes a decrease in renal perfusion, leading to oliguria (Fig. 12.5) [26].

Renal dysfunction from increased IAP is also due to cortical arteriolar compression, which leads to decreased glomerular filtration rate. This increases water and sodium retention due to the activation of the renin-angiotensin system, which can lead to acute tubular necrosis, and irreversible renal failure (Fig. 12.6) [27]. The effect of increased IAP on the kidney depends also on other factors. The urinary tract is compressed and antidiuretic hormone secretion increases; limited cardiac output reduces blood flow to the kidney, with a reduction in efferent flow, leading to compromised renal perfusion gradient [28].

Hepatic artery blood flow is impaired at a relatively low IAH; portal vein blood flow is also compromised by direct compression and by reduced cardiac output, leading to severe hepatic dysfunction. The impaired intestinal perfusion

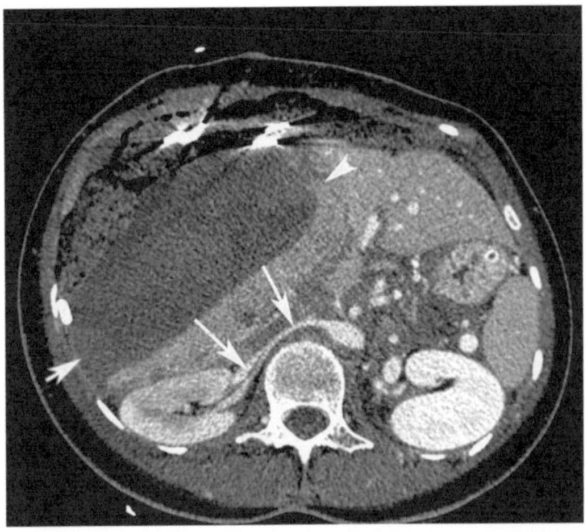

Fig. 12.5 A 25-year-old woman with a large subcapsular liver hematoma was treated at another hospital with perihepatic packing following a motor vehicle collision. After few days, she was transferred to our hospital for treatment of liver and renal dysfunction. IV contrast-enhanced axial CT scan shows a large subcapsular liver hematoma (*arrowhead* and *short arrow*), surrounded by packing, causing the compression of the liver, inferior vena cava, right renal artery and vein (*arrows*). The right renal parenchyma enhancement was less than the left kidney. The CT findings were interpreted as abdominal compartment syndrome, developing from perihepatic packing. Packs were promptly surgically removed, and liver and renal function returned to normal

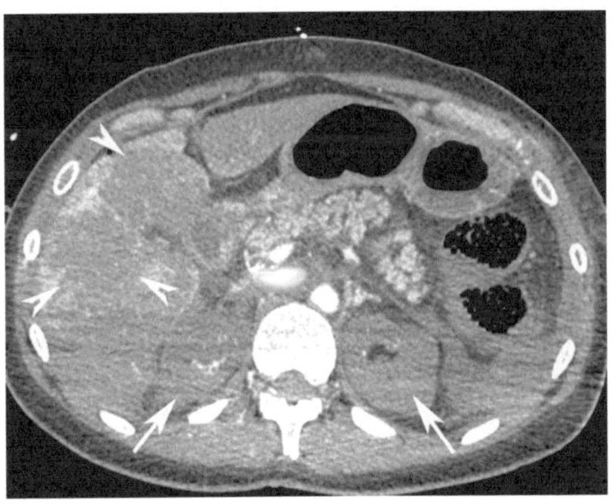

Fig. 12.6 A 32-year-old man involved in a motorcycle collision with an open-book pelvic fracture was treated in another hospital with pelvic packing for large hematoma. After a few days, he was transferred to our hospital for liver dysfunction and anuria. IV contrast-enhanced axial CT image shows bilateral renal infarctions (*arrows*) and liver ischemia (*arrowheads*) and a splenic laceration. There were a small portal vein, a small aorta, a flattened inferior vena cava and a left pleural effusion do to left inferior ribs fractures. There was a small portal vein and small aorta, and flattened inferior vena cava. These CT findings were interpreted as post-packing abdominal compartment syndrome (ACS). After surgical removal of packing, only the liver function became progressively normal

that results from IAH produces anaerobic cellular metabolism, acidosis, and free radical production in the blood. Gastrointestinal hypoperfusion also causes a reduction of the gastric and intestinal mucosa thickness, which contributes to the passage of microorganisms and toxins through the intestinal wall, from the bowel lumen to the systemic circulation [27]. Bacteria and toxins also move from the intestinal wall to the mesenteric lymph nodes, which are the initial site of sepsis, and the main source of the resultant systemic inflammatory response syndrome (SIRS) [29].

Trauma with hemorrhagic shock can lead to a capillary leak syndrome, resulting in the extravasation of fluid into bowel interstitium, with the development of massive bowel edema (Fig. 12.7).

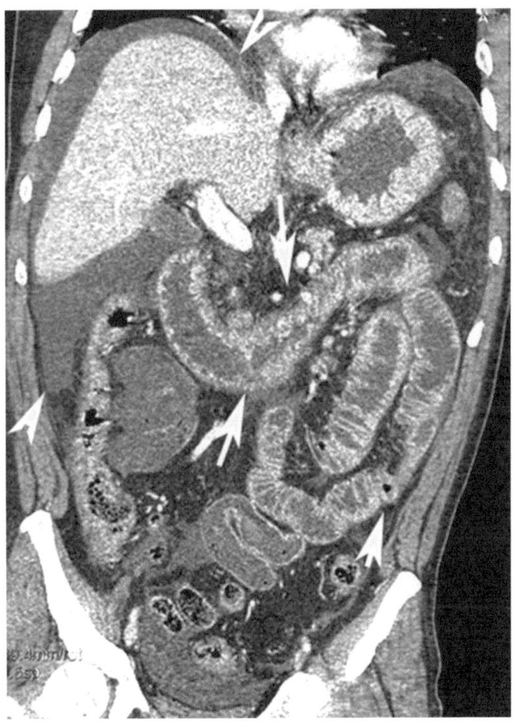

Fig. 12.7 A 25-year-old woman with a large subcapsular liver hematoma, was treated at another hospital with perihepatic packing following a motor vehicle collision. After few days, she was trasferred to our hospital for treatment of liver and renal dysfunction. IV contrast- enhanced axial CT scan shows a large subcapsular liver hematoma (*arrowhead*), surrounded by packing, causing the compression of the liver, inferior vena cava, right renal artery and vein (*arrows*). The right renal parenchyma enhancement was less than the left kidney. The CT findings were interpreted as abdominal compartment syndrome, developing from perihepatic packing. Packs were promptly surgically removed, and liver and renal function returned to normal

The intestinal wall has a great capacity to retain water, and can hold up to several liters of fluid. Intestinal wall edema increases pressure within the abdominal cavity, which can lead to decreased bowel perfusion [18]. Increased IAP also obstructs lymphatic efflux of fluid from the abdomen, worsening the process [29]. All of these factors can contribute to the increasing mesentery and intestinal wall edema, and IAP continues to increase (Fig. 12.7).

Furthermore, the trauma which leads to hemorrhagic shock may need massive fluid infusion. The initial traumatic event leads to direct blood loss from abdominal vascular leak. Whether the patient needs surgery to stop the bleeding or is managed conservatively, the patient generally has already lost a considerable quantity of blood, and needs blood transfusions and crystalloid fluid infusions to replace blood volume. Blood loss followed by fluid resuscitation or blood transfusion can result in an ischemia-reperfusion injury to the bowel, which can lead to an increased capillary permeability [29]. The result is progressively swollen bowel loops, and consequently ACS.

12.4 Main Causes of Traumatic Abdominal Compartment Syndrome

The traumatic bleeding can cause hypoperfusion to organs and tissues (Fig. 12.6). After active resuscitation, tissue reperfusion occurs and promotes interstitial edema. This is known as reperfusion syndrome and increases the volume and pressure inside the abdominal cavity, adding to the already rising IAP [30, 31].

A strategy to limit abdominal hemorrhage is to perform a damage-control laparotomy. This attempts to stop bleeding from organs or vessels by placing surgical packs in the patient's abdominal cavity, near the source of bleeding (Fig. 12.8). However, this potentially lifesaving procedure leaves patients at risk of developing primary ACS [2], because the packs are space occupying, and create increased abdominal pressure (Fig. 12.9). Also, the injured bowel loops can become edematous, worsening the IAH (Fig. 12.7) [32]. Furthermore, if the abdomen is

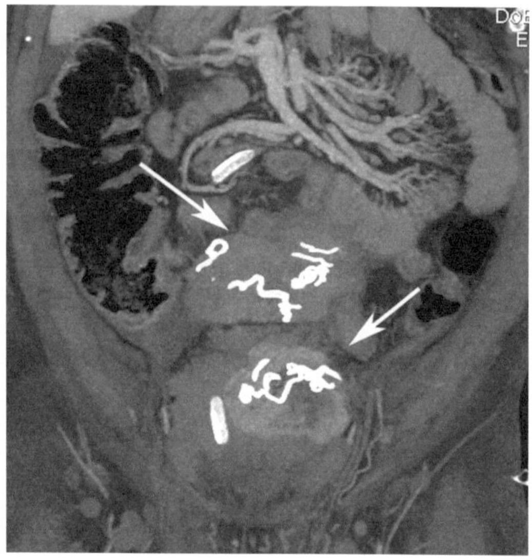

Fig. 12.8 A 64-year-old man with a pelvic hematoma following a fall from a height. IV contrast-enhanced coronal abdominal maximal intensity project image shows a pelvic packing (*arrows*) utilized for treating a pelvic hematoma due to a traumatic hypogastric vein laceration

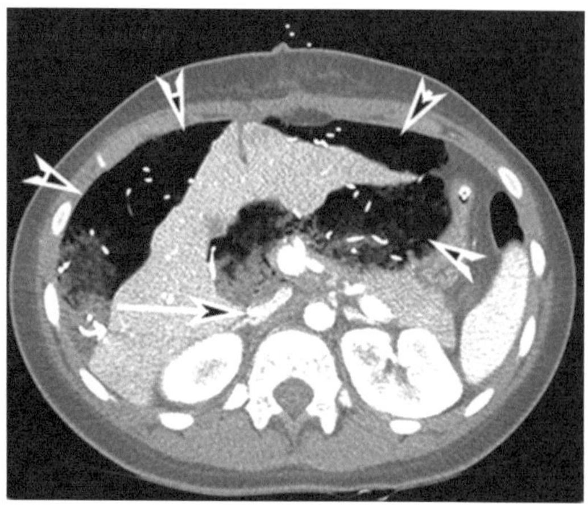

Fig. 12.9 A 57-year-old woman after fall from a window. She had a deep bleeding laceration of the liver dome which was treated with perihepatic packing (*arrowheads*). IV contrast-enhanced axial abdominal CT image shows the large perihepatic packing (*arrowheads*) compressing the liver parenchyma, and the inferior vena cava which has a flat appearance (*white-black arrow*), indicating ACS. After CT, the packing was removed

closed under tension, the risk of ACS is increased as the abdominal wall has little compliance. Since the introduction of damage-control laparotomy, more individuals are surviving extensive abdominal and pelvic trauma [33]. However, the risk of ACS could be increased. Usually the patient will return to the operating room for removal of the packs, once stabilized. If the patient's condition is complicated with ACS, the abdominal pressure needs to be reduced immediately to prevent severe consequences [34].

Secondary ACS can be seen in patients with severe shock (Fig. 12.10) and who have received massive fluid for hemorrhage, sepsis, or major burns. It is due to fluid shifts from the vascular space into the interstitial space, resulting in intestinal wall edema, and fluid accumulation in and around the abdomen [35]. These patients are at higher risk of not being recognized because of the absence of an abdominal wound [3].

Patients that have had a laparotomy, massive fluid infusion, pneumoperitoneum, hemoperitoneum, or other injuries should be evaluated with a high index of suspicion for IAH and ACS. Indications for IAP monitoring include trauma, posttraumatic abdominal surgery, and a distended abdomen with ACS signs and symptoms including oliguria, hypoxia, hypotension, unexplained acidosis, mesenteric ischemia, and/or elevated intracranial pressure.

Monitoring of IAP should be considered for patients who have had temporary closure with abdominal packs, and who have received large volumes of resuscitation fluids for septic or hypovolemic shock. There needs to be careful observation in assessment of the patient's IAP and organ function to optimize early recognition.

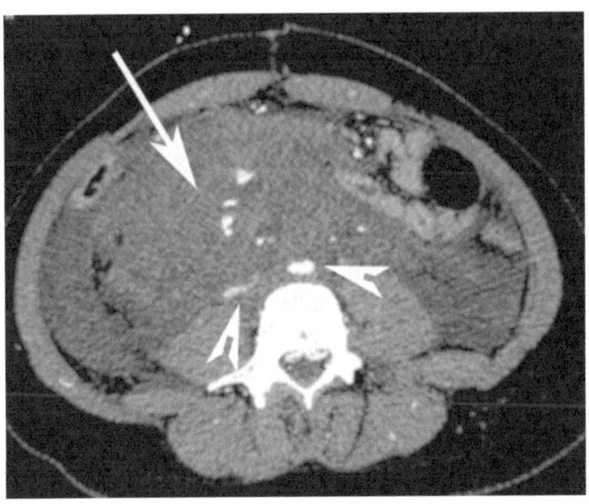

Fig. 12.10 A 28-year-old man with penetrating trauma (stabbing). IV contrast-enhanced axial abdominal CT image reveals a large amount of hemoperitoneum and hemoretroperitoneum, with extravasation of contrast (*arrow*) from a mesenteric artery injury, compressing the inferior vena cava and abdominal aorta (*arrowheads*), and causing ACS

12.5 MDCT Technique

CT is the main diagnostic imaging examination tool in patients with blunt and penetrating trauma. The MDCT protocol which is given here is designed for a 64-row CT scanner. Images are acquired at 0.625 collimation, with reconstruction axial slice of 2.5 mm, pitch of 0.984, and gantry rotation time of 0.5 s. The standard radiation dose is about 15 millisievert.

At our institution, preliminary non-enhanced chest and abdomen CT acquisitions can be obtained to depict blood collections and clots inside the thoracic cavity, peritoneum, retroperitoneum (Fig. 12.11), tissue, and organs.

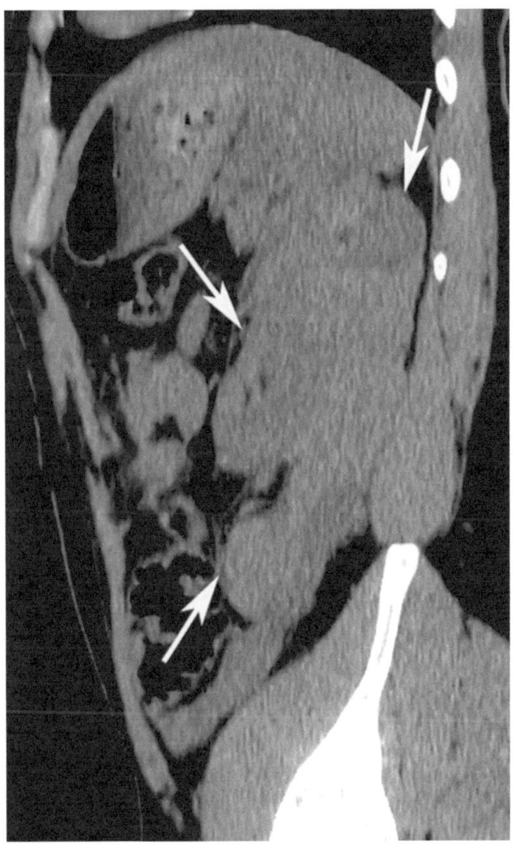

Fig. 12.11 A 55-year-old man with blunt back trauma. Patient is anticoagulated with history of cardiac surgery. Non-contrast sagittal abdominal CT image shows a retroperitoneal hematoma (*arrows*)

Intravenous administration of contrast is mandatory for evaluating organ and vessel injuries and ongoing hemorrhage. For superior enhancement of organs, tissues, and vessels, contrast agents with a higher concentration of iodine (400 mg/mL) and high injection rates (at least 3–4 mL/s) are preferred, and are followed by a 30–50 mL saline chaser, also injected at a rate of 3–4 mL/s. The arterial phase is used to detect arterial injuries, including pseudoaneurysms. The portal phase acquisition, obtained with a scan delay of 70 s, gives maximum enhancement of organs, intestinal wall, tissues, and venous structures.

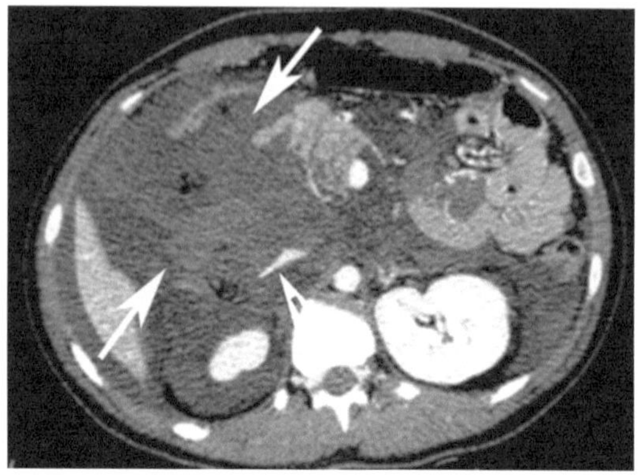

Fig. 12.12 A 23-year-old woman after fall from a balcony. IV contrast-enhanced axial abdominal CT image depicts a large amount of hemoretroperitoneum (*arrows*), associated with a flattened inferior vena cava (*arrowhead*). The small intestine is compressed and displaced to the left abdomen

12.6 CT Findings

The imaging diagnosis of abdominal compartment syndrome is based on color Doppler and CT of trauma patients, combined with the clinical information.

Sonography with color Doppler can demonstrate reduced diastolic flow in the portal, hepatic, and renal veins in patients with ACS.

The most important CT features are substantial hemoperitoneum associated with an elevated diaphragm (Fig. 12.7) and/or massive retroperitoneal hemorrhage with obvious mass effect (Fig. 12.12), with prominent involvement of the pararenal spaces and sometimes perirenal spaces. Another important CT finding is a rounded represented by the evidence of a rounded configuration of the abdominal wall. Significant abdominal distention has a more rounded appearance, with anteroposterior-to-lateral girth ratio >0.8 (without the inclusion of subcutaneous fat). This finding had been called the "round belly sign," and can be associated with the presence of bilateral epiploic or peritoneal fluid inguinal herniation [36].

Direct extrinsic compression of the inferior vena cava and renal veins results from large retroperitoneal and/or intraperitoneal hematomas. Flattened inferior vena cava and renal veins (Fig. 12.12) are frequently associated with an increased unilateral or bilateral renal volume with post-contrast enhancement reduction, due to function impairment [37]. The compression of the urinary tract due to the presence of perinephric fluid collection can be associated with unilateral or bilateral hydronephrosis [38, 39].

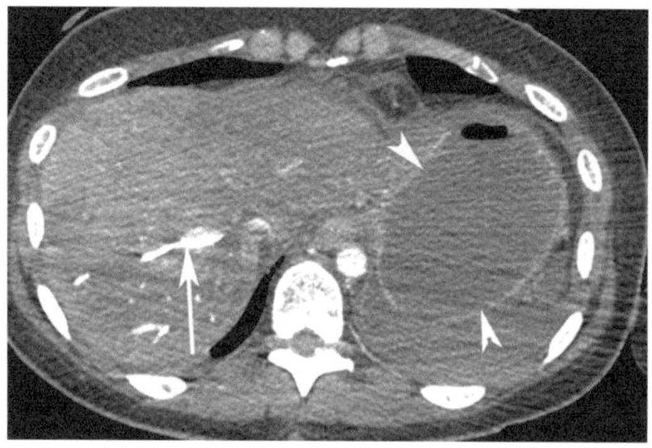

Fig. 12.13 A 48-year-old man with a stab wound. IV contrast-enhanced axial abdominal CT image demonstrates an exsanguinating liver laceration (*arrow*), hemoperitoneum, and increased gastric wall enhancement associated with gastric distension (*arrowheads*), in association with HAP

Another important CT finding is intestinal ischemia. This is manifested as increased bowel wall enhancement with edema and increased gastric wall enhancement associated with gastric lumen overdistension by fluid (Fig. 12.13) [40]. Mosaic liver perfusion and splenic ischemia or infarct are related to hypoperfusion of these organs.

Flattened inferior vena cava (Fig. 12.12) and increased bowel enhancement are not specific for

ACS, because they are also and more commonly present in patients with hypovolemic shock, but without ACS.

Elevated diaphragm (Figs. 12.3 and 12.7) is a sensitive finding, but is not specific for ACS.

However, when a combination of the described findings is present in the appropriate clinical setting, or if these findings worsen on follow-up CT of trauma patients, it is important to think about the potential development of ACS [41–43]

12.7 Management of Intra-abdominal Hypertension

Abdominal decompression of ACS rapidly improves cardiac, pulmonary, and renal function. So, for patients with primary ACS, it is necessary to perform an abdominal decompression as soon as possible. Minimally invasive options include percutaneous drainage of intra-abdominal and intrapelvic fluid collections, under CT or ultrasound guidance. Several studies have shown outcome benefits when these minimally invasive techniques are utilized [44, 45]. Decompressive laparotomy is the most effective treatment for ACS [45]. The abdominal muscle fascia is usually left open (Fig. 12.14), and alternative dressing closure such as polypropylene mesh is sutured to the abdominal fascia to give the visceral layer more expansion.

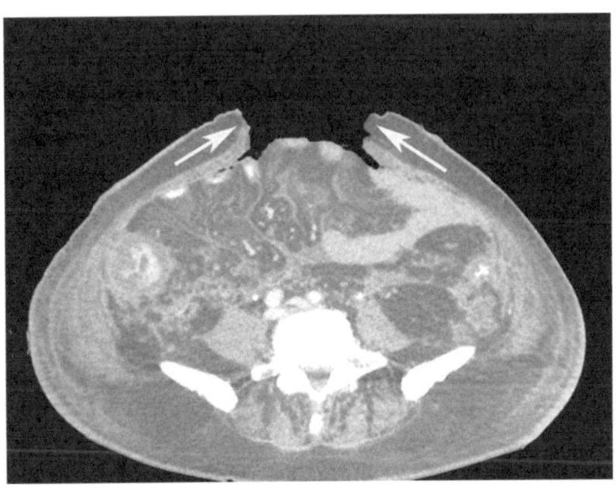

Fig. 12.14 A 55-year-old man developed ACS after a laceration of the pancreas, followed by pancreatitis with mesenteric and retroperitoneal fluid collections. The patient was treated surgically and the collections were drained. IV contrast-enhanced axial abdominal CT image shows an open abdominal wall and muscle fascia of the abdomen (*arrows*), performed for the decompression of ACS

Conclusion

Acute compartment syndrome occurs in a substantial number of severely injured abdominal trauma patients, and develops rapidly. It is a clinical syndrome that can easily be misinterpreted, and can lead to worsening outcome of trauma patients.

It is essential to diagnose and manage ACS early, because without a rapid intervention the risk of death is high [14, 46]. Most patients who develop ACS have had recent severe abdominal/pelvic trauma, which required staged laparotomy and packing to control hemorrhage secondary to coagulopathy. Abdominal packing combined with an abdominal closure is often employed in these patients, and increases the risk of developing ACS. This syndrome is a complication which develops over the course of the staged laparotomy approach; therefore, the timing of the decompression is particularly related to the management of these patients. Paradoxically, while increased IAP may be critical in stopping bleeding, excessive IAP may promote coagulopathy through cellular shock.

Soon after injury, the benefits of the compression provided by staged laparotomy are clear; however, later, as intra-abdominal pressure is greater than capillary perfusion pressure and the abdominal hypertension raises diaphragmatic pressure, the risk of ACS may cancel out benefits of the compression. ACS is a subtle and potentially life-threatening disease that requires good clinical expertise to diagnose and manage properly. With the use of MDCT for the assessment and follow-up of severe trauma patients, the early diagnosis of ACS can be facilitated, especially with the color Doppler ultrasound and bladder pressure measurement.

Radiologists are increasingly likely to evaluate patients with ACS following abdominal and/or pelvic traumatic hematomas, and then after application of packs. An awareness of the CT features of ACS is important, because this syndrome has to be managed with the immediate decompression of abdomen and/or pelvis and because lack of recognition may lead rapidly to multi-organ failure and death of the patient. Radiologists should be aware of ACS, and should be vigilant for CT features indicating possible increased intra-abdominal pressure in patients at risk for developing the syndrome. In the appropriate clinical setting, CT findings suggestive of the abdominal compartment syndrome should be communicated by the radiologist to the clinical staff without any delay.

References

1. Malbrain ML, Cheatham ML, Kirkpatrick A, et al. Results from the international conference of experts on intra-abdominal hypertension and abdominal compartment syndrome. I. Definitions. Intensive Care Med. 2006;32(11):1722–32.
2. Morken J, West M. Abdominal compartment syndrome in the intensive care unit. Curr Opin Crit Care. 2001;7:268–74.
3. Balogh Z, McKinley BA, Cox C, et al. Abdominal compartment syndrome: the cause or effect of post-injury multiple organ failure. Shock. 2003;20(16):483–92.
4. Moore EE, Burch JM, Franciose RJ, et al. Staged physiologic restoration and damage control surgery. World J Surg. 1998;22:1184–91.
5. Meldrum DR, Moore FA, Moore EE, et al. Prospective characterization and selective management of the abdominal compartment syndrome. Am J Surg. 1997;174:667–73.
6. Moore EE. Staged laparotomy for the hypothermia, acidosis and coagulopathy syndrome. Am J Surg. 1996;172:405–10.
7. Schein M, Wittmann DH, Aprahamian CC, et al. The abdominal compartment syndrome: the physiological and clinical consequences of elevated intra-abdominal pressure. J Am Coll Surg. 1995;180:745–53.
8. Magnotti LJ, Upperman JS, DZ X, et al. Gut-derived mesenteric lymph but not portal blood increases endothelial cell permeability and promotes lung injury after haemorrhagic shock. Ann Surg. 1998;228:518–27.
9. Malbrain ML, Chiumello D, Pelosi P, et al. Incidence and prognosis of intra-abdominal hypertension in a mixed population of critically ill patients: a multiple-center epidemiological study. Crit Care Med. 2005;33:315–22.
10. Meldrum DR, Moore FA, Moore EE, et al. Cardiopulmonary hazards of perihepatic packing for major liver injuries. Am J Surg. 1995;170:537–42.
11. Leppaniemi A, Kirkpatrick AW, Salazar A, et al. Miscellaneus conditions and abdominal compartment syndrome. In: Ivatury R, Cheatham M, Malbrain M, et al., editors. Abdominal compartment syndrome. Austin, TX: Landes Bioscience; 2006. p. 195–214.
12. Balogh Z, McKinley BA, Cocanour CS, et al. Secondary abdominal compartment syndrome in an elusive early complication of traumatic shock resuscitation. Am J Surg. 2002;184:538–43.
13. Malbrain M. Is it wise not to think about intra-abdominal hypertension in the ICU? Curr Opin Crit Care. 2004;10:132–45.
14. Cheatham M, White M, Sagraves S, et al. Abdominal perfusion pressure: a superior parameter in the assessment of intra-abdominal hypertension. J Trauma. 2000;49:621–6.
15. Cheatham M, Malbrain M, Kirkpatrick A, et al. Results from the international conference of experts on intra-abdominal hypertension and abdominal compartment syndrome. II. Recommendations. Intern Care Med. 2007;33:951–62.
16. Kimball EJ, Kim W, Cheaham ML, et al. Clinical awareness of intra-abdominal hypertension and abdominal compartment syndrome in 2007. Acta Clin Belg. 2007;62:66–73.
17. Joynt GM, Gomersall CD. Intra-abdominal hypertension-an intensive care perspective. Crit Care Shock. 2003;6(3):131–8.
18. Ivatury RR, Sugerman HJ, Peitzman AB. Abdominal compartment syndrome: recognition and management. Adv Surg. 2001;35:251–69.
19. Malbrain M, Van Miegham N, Verbrugghe W. PICCO derived parameters versus filling pressures in intrabdominal hypertension. Intensive Care Med. 2003;29(suppl. 1):S123–45.
20. Been Saleem T, Ahmed I. Recent advances in the management of abdominal compartment syndrome. J Coll Physicians Surg Pak. 2004;14(6):382–5.
21. Nebelkopf H. Abdominal compartment syndrome. Am J Nurs. 1999;99(11):53–9.
22. Malbrain M, Nieuwendijk R, Verbrugghe W. Effect of intrabdominal pressure on pleural and filling pressures. Intensive Care Med. 2003;29(suppl 1):564–78.
23. Joseph DK, Dutton RP, Aarabi B, et al. Decompressive laparotomy to treat intractable intracranial hypertension after traumatic brain injury. J Trauma. 2004;57(4):687–93.
24. Saggi BH, Bloomfield GL, Sugerman HJ, et al. Treatment of intracranial hypertension using non-surgical abdominal decompression. J Trauma. 1999;46(4):646–51.
25. Deeren DH, Dits H, Malbrain ML. Correlation between intrabdominal and intracranial pressure in non traumatic brain injury. Intensive Care Med. 2005;31(11):1577–81.
26. Malbrain M. Abdominal pressure in the critically III. Curr Opin Crit Care. 2000;6:17–29.
27. Walker J, Criddle L. Pathophysiology and management of abdominal compartment syndrome. Am J Crit Care. 2003;12(4):367–71.

28. Sugrue M, Jones F, Deane SA, et al. Intra-abdominal hypertension is an independent cause of postoperative renal impairment. Arch Surg. 1999;134(10):1082–5.
29. Shah SK, Jimenez F, Letourneau PA, et al. Strategies for modulating the inflammatory response after decompression from abdominal compartment syndrome. Scand J Trauma Resusc Emerg Med. 2012;20:25–36.
30. Balogh Z, Moore FA. Intraabdominal hypertension: not just a surgical critical care curiosity. Crit Care Med. 2005;33(2):447–9.
31. Gallagher J. How to recognize and manage abdominal compartment syndrome. Crit Care Choices. 2004;34(suppl. May):36–42.
32. Lozen Y. Intra-abdominal hypertension and abdominal compartment syndrome in trauma: pathophysiology and interventions. Am Assoc Crit Care Nurses. 1999;10(1):104–12.
33. Sutton E, Bochicchio G, Bochicchio K, et al. Long term impact of damage control surgery: a preliminary prospective study. J Trauma Inj Infect. Crit Care. 2006;61(4):831–6.
34. Zacharias S, Offner P, Moore E, et al. Damage control surgery. AACN Clin Issues. 1999;10(1):95–103.
35. Moore FA, McKinley BA, Moore E. The next generation in shock resuscitation. Lancet. 2004;363:1988–96.
36. Laffargue G, Taourel P, Saguintaah M, et al. CT diagnosis of abdominal compartment syndrome. AJR. 2002;178:771–2.
37. Doty JM, Saggi BH, Blocker CR, et al. Effects of increased renal parenchymal pressure on renal function. J Trauma. 2000;48:874–7.
38. Harman PK, Kron IL, McLachlan HD, et al. Elevated intra-abdominal pressure and renal function. Ann Surg. 1982;196:594–7.
39. Waschberg RH, Sebastiano LLS, Levine CD. Narrowing of the upper abdominal inferior vena cava in patients with elevated intraabdominal pressure. Abdom Imaging. 1998;23:99–102.
40. Patel A, Lall CG, Jennings SG, et al. Abdominal compartment syndrome. AJR. 2007;189:1037–43.
41. Maxwell RA, Fabian TC, Ma C, et al. Secondary abdominal compartment syndrome: an underappreciated manifestation of severe hemorrhagic shock. J Trauma. 1999;47:995–9.
42. Pickhardt PJ, Shimony JS, Heiken JP, et al. The abdominal compartment syndrome: CT findings. AJR. 1999;173:575–9.
43. Epelman M, Soudack M, Engel A, et al. Abdominal compartment syndrome in children: CT findings. Pediatr Radiol. 2002;32:319–22.
44. Watson RA, Howdieshell TR. Abdominal compartment syndrome. South Med J. 1998;91:326–32.
45. Burch J. New concepts in trauma. Am J Surg. 1997;173(1):44–6.
46. Mailbrain ML, Cheatham ML, Kirkpatrick A, et al. Results from the international conference of experts on intra-abdominal hypertension and abdominal compartment syndrome. I. Definitions. Intensive Care Med. 2006;32(11):1722–32.

13 Imaging of the Acute Abdomen in the Pediatric Patients

Grazia Loretta Buquicchio, Margherita Trinci, Riccardo Ferrari, Stefania Ianniello, Michele Galluzzo, and Vittorio Miele

Abstract

The acute abdomen and pelvis is a serious clinical condition which may require urgent surgery. The potential causes of the acute abdomen and pelvis in pediatric patients are numerous, as in adults, and diagnosis is often delayed due to misleading signs and symptoms. Clinical signs and symptoms are often nonspecific; abdominal and pelvic pain and abdominal distention are common in a wide variety of disorders. Other signs and symptoms can include bilious vomiting, other signs of intestinal obstruction, urinary tract signs, fever, and weakness. Although in adult patients with an acute abdomen/pelvis, computed tomography (CT) is the mainstay of diagnosis and for discriminating conditions requiring surgery from those which can be treated conservatively, the use of CT in pediatric patients in recent years has decreased due to the potential risks of radiation exposure. The role of ultrasound (US) has become increasingly important. US does not use ionizing radiation, is usually readily available in emergency departments, is inexpensive, is portable, and does not require patient sedation. Furthermore, US allows assessment of intestinal peristalsis, and allows compression of the bowel. Magnetic resonance imaging (MRI) also does not use ionizing radiation, and can be used to diagnose a wide variety of pediatric acute abdominal and pelvic conditions, but MRI is more expansive, is not always available in emergency departments, and often requires sedation of pediatric patients to obtain good-quality images. Despite this, in line with radioprotection criteria, MRI should be considered as an alternative to CT, for its excellent ability to depict the causes of acute abdominal and pelvic disease, to provide valuable assistance in differential diagnosis, and for evaluation of any complications.

Keywords

Emergency radiology · Pediatric acute abdomen
Nontraumatic pediatric abdominal emergencies
Computed tomography · Ultrasound · Magnetic resonance imaging

G. L. Buquicchio, M.D. • M. Trinci, M.D.
R. Ferrari, M.D. • S. Ianniello, M.D.
M. Galluzzo, M.D.
Department of Emergency Radiology, S. Camillo Hospital, Rome, Italy

V. Miele, M.D. (✉)
Department of Radiology, Careggi University Hospital, Florence, Italy
e-mail: vmiele@sirm.org

M. Patlas et al. (eds.), *MDCT and MR Imaging of Acute Abdomen*,
https://doi.org/10.1007/978-3-319-70778-5_13

13.1 Introduction

Abdominal and pelvic pain is one of the most frequent reasons why pediatric patients are evaluated in pediatric emergency departments. The role of the pediatric emergency physician is to verify the existence of an emergency condition, and to differentiate between medical and surgical emergencies. Abdominal and pelvic pain in the pediatric population is a challenging condition. Approximately 15% of children will go to the doctor during the first 15 years of life for abdominal pain, but only one-third will need hospitalization or surgery [1].

In all age groups, the most common cause of abdominal pain is gaseous colic and/or constipation. The pediatrician must be able to distinguish serious illness from benign causes. Clinical signs are often nonspecific; abdominal pain and abdominal distention are common in different diseases. Other symptoms can include bilious vomiting, other signs of intestinal obstruction, urinary tract signs, fever, and weakness. Early clinical manifestations are often nonspecific, and can be confused with medically treated conditions including flu and gastroenteritis, resulting in delays in diagnosis. The need for adequate clinical observation in acute abdominal pain is particularly recommended in the first 3–4 years of life, when both manifestations and clinical assessment are often nonspecific.

Abdominal pain can be a single acute event, acute but recurrent, or chronic. Differential diagnosis is difficult, and varies in relation to age. Although some situations are present throughout pediatrics (including constipation and gastroenteritis), some occur only at certain ages (for example, intussusception in infants). The clinical history and physical examination are therefore essential for a proper diagnostic framework. Laboratory examinations and imaging are fundamental for diagnosis. In approximately 55% of children with acute abdominal pain, a specific medical diagnosis is established, while in 35% no specific cause is found [1].

Although in adult patients with acute abdominal and pelvic pain computed tomography (CT) is the mainstay of diagnosis and for discriminating conditions requiring surgery from those which can be treated conservatively, the use of CT in pediatric patients in recent years has decreased due to the potential risks of ionizing radiation exposure [2]. To avoid radiation exposure in pediatric patients, in recent years US has become increasingly important. Multiple clinical studies have demonstrated that in the pediatric emergency department, US should be used as the first-line imaging technique [3], and only if the findings are negative or equivocal CT can be used as a subsequent method [4, 5]. Since US has multiple advantages, it is the ideal method and it should almost always be used for initial evaluation in the pediatric population, although it does have some limitations. US does not use ionizing radiation, is always available in emergency departments, is relatively inexpensive, and does not require patient sedation. Furthermore, US allows assessment of intestinal peristalsis, and permits compression of the bowel [3].

Magnetic resonance imaging (MRI), which also does not use ionizing radiation, can be used to diagnose the pediatric acute abdomen, but MRI is more expensive, is not always available in emergency departments, and often requires sedation of pediatric patients to obtain good-quality images. Despite this, in line with radioprotection criteria, MRI should be considered as an alternative to CT, for its excellent ability to depict the causes of abdominal and pelvic disease, to assist in differential diagnosis, and for evaluation of any complications. Currently, the use of fast MR sequences substantially reduces the examination time, and in some patients avoids the need for sedation; with wider MR gantries or "open" MR equipment, it is easier to monitor pediatric patients. Also, IV contrast is not always necessary for the evaluation of some clinical situations of the acute abdomen and pelvis.

13.2 Clinical Management

Evaluation of acute abdominal pain is a frequent problem in the pediatric emergency department, and the assessing health-care practitioners need to discriminate amongst multiple potential etiologies.

13.2.1 Distribution by Age

The variability and complexity of diseases associated with abdominal and pelvic pain at different ages of pediatric patients explain the nonspecificity and potential for diagnostic error. The causes of the acute abdomen in pediatric population are numerous but can be divided into two main groups, inflammatory causes and occlusive causes. The most frequent inflammatory causes are acute appendicitis, which are often due to occlusion of the appendicular lumen by appendicolith; the most frequent occlusive causes are internal hernia, intussusception, and adhesions, caused by either previous surgical intervention or congenital nonsurgical adhesions.

With respect to the age of clinical onset, the acute abdomen can be categorized into three major groups: the acute abdomen in newborns/infants, the 2–6-year-old child, and the child over 6 years old. In the first months of life, the main cause of abdominal pain is colic. The main pathologic causes are necrotizing enterocolitis, intestinal malrotation, volvulus, and intestinal stenosis, i.e., hypertrophic pyloric stenosis (HPS) and bowel atresia. Before of the age of 2, the main causes of acute abdominal pain are gastroenteritis, intestinal obstruction, congenital megacolon, intussusception, and incarcerated inguinal hernia. From 2 to 6 years, the most frequent causes are gastroenteritis, constipation, appendicitis, urinary tract infection, trauma, basilar pneumonia, and mesenteric adenitis. Less frequent causes include Henoch-Schonlein purpura, nephrolithiasis, and various neoplasms (neuroblastoma and Wilms tumor). After 6 years, other causes include gastroenteritis, constipation, trauma, urinary tract infection, mesenteric adenitis, appendicitis, and other intestinal disorders.

Genitourinary emergencies can present both in the neonate and in the older infant or child, with acute abdominal pain, fever, and an abdominal mass. These include hydronephrosis, in particular, which is the most common cause of a neonatal abdominal mass, neonatal adrenal hemorrhage, nephro-urolithiasis, pyelonephritis, an acute scrotum, hydrometrocolpos, and ovarian torsion.

13.2.2 Location of Pain: Onset of Pain

In pediatric patients, unlike in adults, pain localization does not have precise diagnostic value, since pediatric patients, especially under 3 years of age, are often uncooperative, and pain is frequently reported in the periumbilical area. Therefore, it is very difficult to identify the point of greatest pain on palpation. However, the topography of acute abdominal pain can be useful for initial differential diagnosis.

Even when the pain is related to a specific abdominal quadrant, it can be indicative of more than one disease. Pain in the upper right quadrant may indicate retrocecal appendicitis, pyelonephritis, basilar pneumonia, acute hepatitis, or cholecystitis. In the upper left quadrant, the most common causes include pyelonephritis and basilar pneumonia. In the right and left lower quadrants, causes of acute pain include acute appendicitis, nephrolithiasis, incarcerated inguinal hernia, ovarian torsion, and ectopic pregnancy. Periumbilical pain may indicate peritonitis, acute pancreatitis, intestinal obstruction, constipation, or bowel colic.

When diagnosing abdominal and pelvic pain in pediatric patients, the chronology of the onset of pain is fundamental. It is not always possible to get this information because the patient may be too young to explain the symptoms, or was not with the parents when the pain started. However, when possible, the time of onset of pain, localization of pain, characteristics of pain, degree of activity of the child, presence of gastrointestinal symptoms (including anorexia and nausea, vomiting, diarrhea, and constipation), presence of any other systemic symptoms, and family history should all be evaluated.

Since some patients with acute abdominal and pelvic pain require urgent surgery, delayed diagnosis may result in increased morbidity, and, in some pediatric patients, death. Surgical diagnoses represent less than 10% of the causes of acute abdominal and pelvic pain in the infants and young children [1], but if not diagnosed they can lead to severe complications. The role of imaging is to help distinguish amongst the causes of abdominal and pelvic pain which require surgical intervention, from those which can be treated conservatively.

As the discussion of this chapter specifically focuses on the acute abdomen in children, the following are the main causes in this age group. In the toddler and older child, and in the adolescent, the most common causes which require surgery are acute appendicitis and Meckel diverticulum. In this chapter we discuss disorders which generally require surgery: ileocolonic intussusception, appendicitis, and Meckel diverticulum. We also discuss the differential diagnosis, and the potential complications. Mesenteric adenitis is often found in children with abdominal pain, and is briefly covered. We do not discuss other specific diseases of newborns and small infants (2–3 months old).

13.3 Intussusception

Intussusception is a relatively common surgical emergency in children. The reported incidence is variable, between 0.66 and 4 per 1000 births, with a male/female ratio of 3:1 [6]. Intussusception affects mainly children in the first 3 years of life, with two peaks of incidence. The first peak is at 3–9 months, and the cause of the intussusception is generally idiopathic or related to reactive infectious right lower quadrant adenopathy. In the second group, children older than 2 years, a pathologic leading point is usually present [7]. Approximately 95% of pediatric patients with intussusception do not have a fixed pathologic leading point. The cause is lymphatic tissue hyperplasia, usually resulting from viral infections as noted (e.g., adenovirus, rotavirus, and herpesvirus) [8].

Intussusception occurs when one portion of the intestinal tract is drawn into the adjacent bowel. The intestine also carries the mesentery with lymph nodes and vessels, which are then stretched. In addition to an occlusive event, given by the intestine intussuscepted, there is also an ischemic component. The most common site in pediatric patients is the terminal ileum and cecum (80–95%), with the ileocecal valve as the receiving loop and the ileum as the donor loop. Isolated small bowel intussusception is much less frequent in pediatric patients and usually spontaneously reduces and does not require further treatment. However, it may be due to underlying celiac disease.

There are various hypotheses as to why intussusception is more frequent at the ileocecal valve, including greater disproportion between the size of the ileum and the ileocecal valve in younger children than those of older age, or increased intestinal peristalsis and relaxation of the ileocecal valve due to increased nitric oxide production caused by inflammatory reactions which usually precedes intestinal intussusception [7].

In 1–6% of pediatric patients, intussusception occurs in children older than 5 years. In this age group, there is a much higher likelihood that the invagination is due to a pathologic leading point. In these patients, it is important to look for underlying conditions including appendicitis, Meckel diverticulum, and a gastrointestinal duplication cyst.

Intussusception presents with a palpable mass, irritability, intermittent crying, abdominal colic, bilious vomiting, and “currant jelly” or bloody stools. Children are initially irritable, and then, if the intussusception does not resolve spontaneously, there may be alternating of drowsiness and abdominal pain episodes. The simultaneous presence of intermittent abdominal pain, vomiting, and a palpable mass in the right upper abdominal quadrant has a positive predictive value of intussusception of approximately 93%; if rectal bleeding is added to these, this positive predictive value increases to 100% [9–11].

13.3.1 Diagnostic Imaging and Nonoperative Treatment

The clinical diagnosis of intussusception is confirmed by imaging. The diagnosis of intussusception is made with fluoroscopic enema, currently performed primarily using air, or with a hydrosoluble contrast agent mixed into a water solution. Air or liquid enema is still used today in many hospitals worldwide as the standard examination for the diagnosis of intussusception in children [10]. During the examination, the contrast medium reaches the intussuscepted segment, demonstrating the point of obstruction (Fig. 13.1). The intussuscepted segment appears as a "coiled spring" endoluminal filling defect, with a convex upper profile (Fig. 13.2).

Currently, in accordance with radioprotection criteria, it is preferable to initially diagnose intestinal intussusception using US. US is performed to confirm the diagnosis, because of its high sensitivity (97.9%) and specificity (97.8%), combined with its noninvasiveness and absence of ionizing radiation [12, 13]. US also reveals the presence of other diagnoses, as well as predisposing conditions. US is performed in infants and younger children using a high-frequency linear array transducer (5–12 MHz), while in the older child the convex probe (3.5 MHz) is used which allows for greater panoramic views. Most intussusceptions are ileocolic, and should be looked for in the right upper quadrant, in the subhepatic region, in particular. There are direct and indirect US signs of intussusception.

US images are quite specific; in the transverse view, the intussusception has a "target" or "doughnut" sign, due to the alternating concentric layers of the receiving loop and the intussuscepted loop, with the addition of mesenteric fat, vascular structures, and lymph nodes (Fig. 13.3). In these axial images, there is an outer hyperechoic ring (the intussuscepted loop) and an inner hypoechoic ring (the intussuscipiens loop), which mimic the presence of a large, rounded mass. In longitudinal US, a "pseudo-kidney" appearance

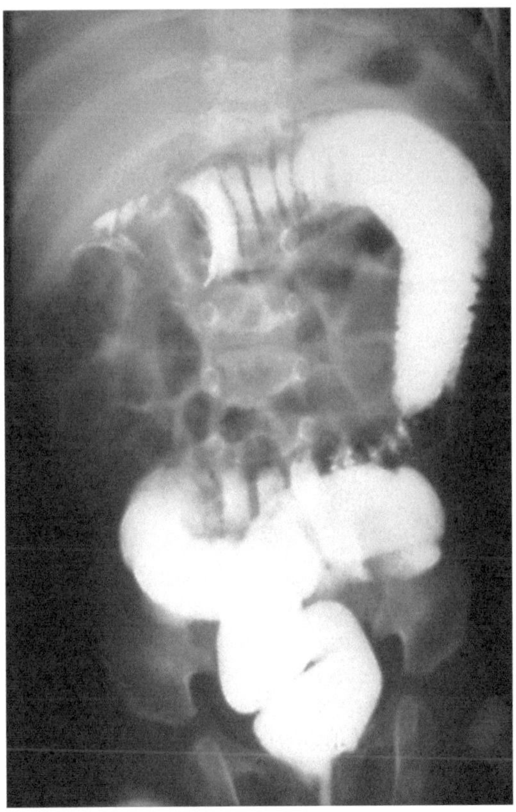

Fig. 13.1 Twenty-eight-month-old previously healthy boy with sudden onset of abdominal pain. Barium enema image shows an intestinal intussusception, with the typical filling defect with a convex upper profile. This figure is shown only for historical/demonstration purposes and does not reflect current techniques used

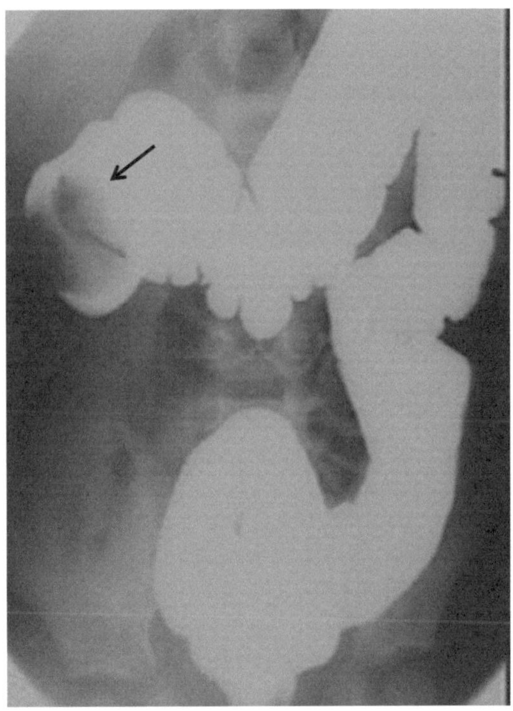

Fig. 13.2 Intestinal intussusception, barium image: detail of the intussusception, with the typical filling defect with a convex upper profile due to the intussuscepted loop (*arrow*)

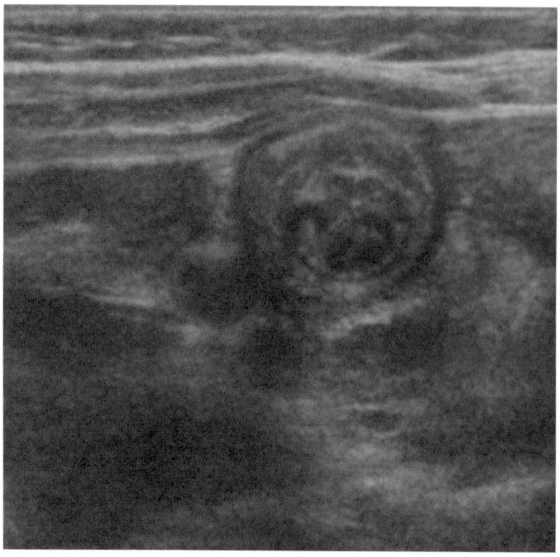

Fig. 13.3 Three-year-old boy presenting with acute abdominal colicky pain, without fever, who was diagnosed with intussusception. Transverse US image shows the "target" or "doughnut" sign, due to the alternating concentric layers of the receiving loop and the intussuscepted loop with the addition of mesenteric fat, and lymph nodes

is the characteristic finding, resulting from the entrance of the intussuscepted loop, mesenteric fat, vascular structures, and sometimes lymph nodes, which are dragged into the intussuscipiens loop (i.e., the receiving loop) (Fig. 13.4). Often, it is possible to find both the appendix and the ileum invaginated into this process; in the older toddler or child, appendicitis can be the cause of the invagination (Fig. 13.5) [10]. The incorporation of mesenteric vascular structures into the intussuscipiens loop can cause venous congestion with consequent wall edema and, if not resolved promptly, subsequent necrosis and perforation.

The typical appearance at color Doppler US is a double-ring appearance due to the vascularization of the two sections of the intestinal loops. The absence of vascularization at color Doppler within the invagination is a sign of bowel necrosis and irreducibility without surgery [14]. The presence of free fluid in the abdomen or between bowel loops is also associated with a high risk of necrosis, and with a much lower reduction rate. Indirect signs of intussusception at US include free fluid in the abdomen or between bowel loops, associated with signs of intestinal occlusion. Also, numerous enlarged lymph nodes in the right iliac fossa are often present.

To date, the abdominal radiography is indicated for identifying complications, including peritonitis and/or intestinal perforation with pneumoperitoneum (sensitivity 45%) [15].

If not recognized and not adequately treated, intussusception exposes patients to a high risk of severe complications, including intestinal perforation, peritonitis, and shock; the intervention must therefore be as timely as possible.

Spontaneous reduction of invagination occurs in about 17% of all pediatric intussusceptions. Conservative treatment can be carried out by a US-guided hydrostatic contrast enema, or a fluoroscopic enema. In these patients, successful reduction occurs most of the time (80–92%). The absolute contraindications for conservative treatment (nonsurgical reduction of intussusception) are peritonitis and perforation [16].

The purpose of nonsurgical imaging treatment is to reduce the intussusception by exerting pressure to push the intussuscepted loop out of its position, and to bring it back to its original position. Fluoroscopic guidance with enema or a water-soluble contrast agent can also be performed. Fluoroscopic guidance can be performed with a solution of 100 mL of iodinated contrast agent diluted to 10% with warm water. The iodinated contrast medium is used to show, at the end of the procedure, the positive or negative outcome. The solution is made by diluting the iodinated contrast medium with water, and is placed inside a bag positioned approximately 1 m (3 ft) above the patient's position. Through a Foley or similar catheter positioned in the rectum, the iodinated solution extends by gravity, and the water distends bowel and reaches the point of invagination, where it penetrates between the intestinal rings, and if successful produces a progressive relaxation of the intussuscepted loop.

Abdominal radiography is possible to see the degree of distention of the intestine. If the loop appears too distended and the water cannot overcome the point of invagination (Fig. 13.6), the

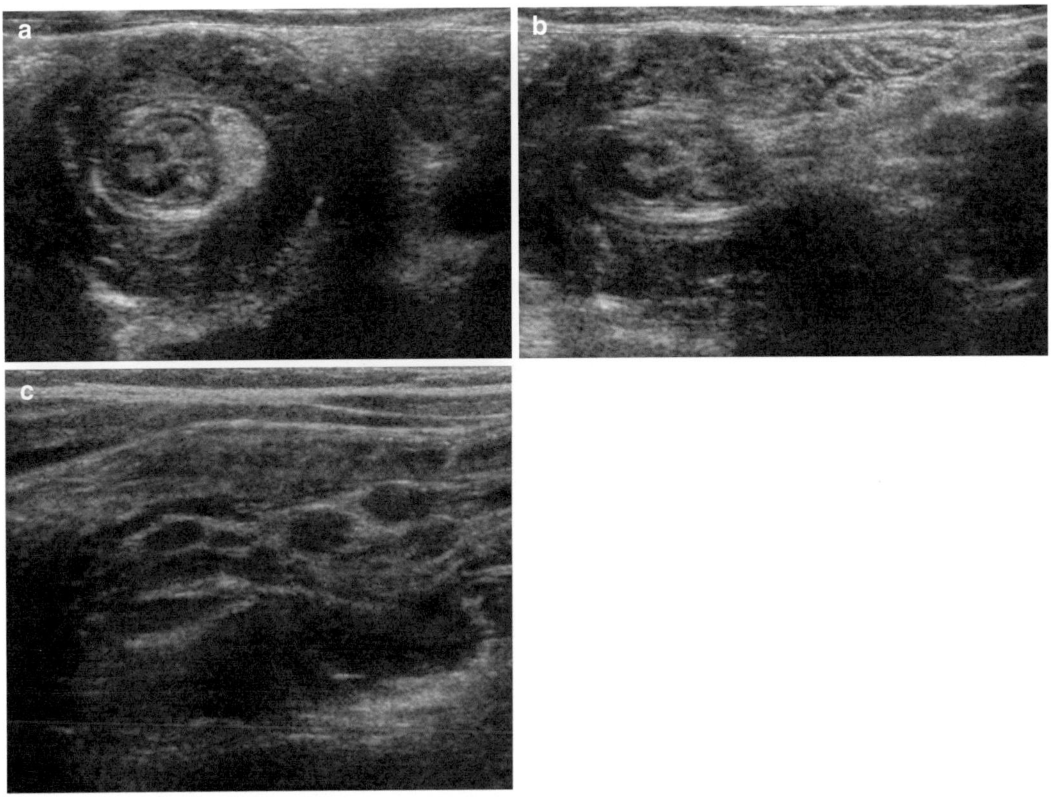

Fig. 13.4 Two-year-old boy presenting with acute abdominal pain, due to enteritis starting a few days earlier, and then intussusception. US transverse (**a**) and longitudinal (**b**, **c**) images with the typical transverse target sign and the longitudinal "pseudo-kidney" appearance. This morphology is due to the entrance of the intussuscepted loop, mesenteric fat, vascular structures, and sometimes lymph nodes, which are dragged into the receiving loop

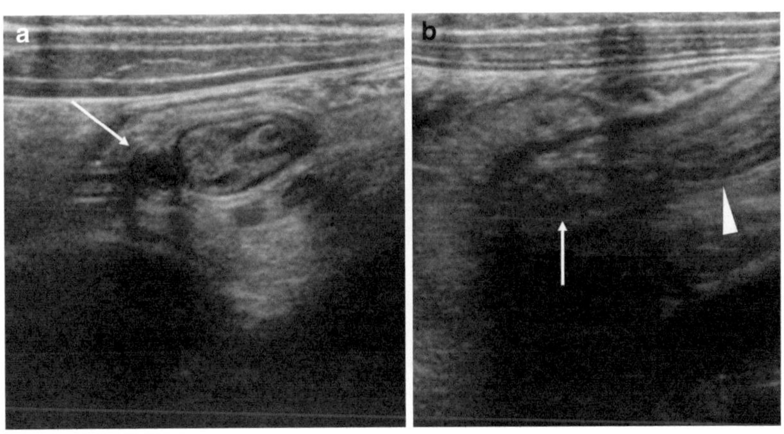

Fig. 13.5 Five-year-old boy presenting with acute abdominal pain, fever, and intussusception. Axial (**a**) and longitudinal (**b**) US images show the typical target aspect of an intussuscepted bowel loop. Note that both the appendix (white arrow) and the ileum (arrowhead) are intussuscepted

catheter must be removed; the water will flow out of the colon, and another attempt can be made (Fig. 13.7). Usually there are no more than three attempts. If bloody fluid emerges from the rectum, the examination must be stopped immediately, because there is danger of perforation [17]. In North America, also air enema under fluoroscopic guidance is commonly used; this method is quick and clean, and has a high reduction rate (73–95%) [18].

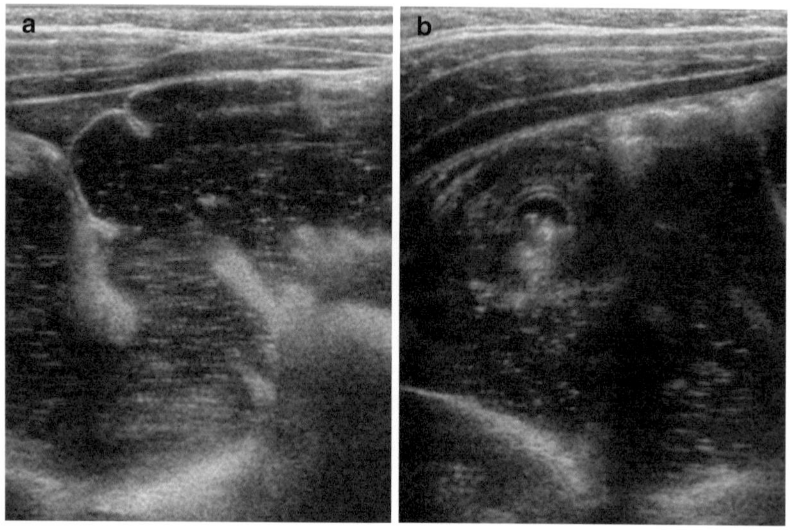

Fig. 13.6 (**a**, **b**) 4-year-old previously healthy boy presenting with acute abdominal pain. Intestinal intussusception. US enema shows the water solution which dilates the loop, and reaches the intussuscepted loop, but the water stops close to the intussuscepted segment. The procedure has failed and intussusception was not reduced. In this patient, surgical reduction was needed

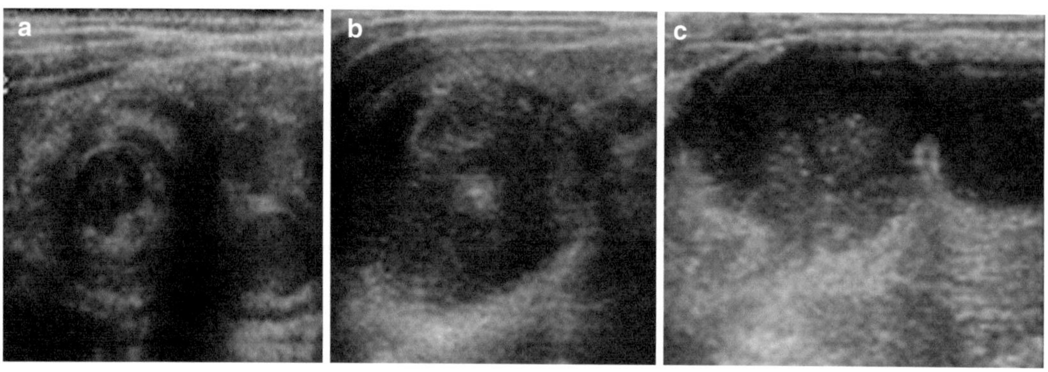

Fig. 13.7 (**a**–**c**) Three-year-old boy presenting with acute abdominal pain, without fever, with intussusception. Hydrostatic US-guided reduction shows an intussuscepted loop (**a**, **b**). The water solution dilated the loop, reached the intussusception, reduced it, and completely cleared the lumen of the colon (**c**)

When the procedure is successful, the intestinal loops are progressively stretched and the invagination morphology changes gradually. At the end of the procedure, a radiograph of the abdomen demonstrates complete filling of the cecum, and passage of contrast into the lumen of the small bowel (Fig. 13.8). An abdominal radiographic examination should also be performed if there is failure, to demonstrate the invagination point, and that no complications, particularly perforation, have occurred during the procedure.

Several studies have reported a high percentage of successful reduction with few complications [19]. The rate of recurrence in surgically reduced intestinal invagination is ≤5%. The rate of recurrence of intestinal invagination after nonsurgical US-guided reduction with water, saline, or gas enema varies from 5 to 20%. In 50% of patients with recurrence, this occurs within 48 h [16]. One should not attempt a US-hydrostatic procedure of reduction of the invagination if the invagination is not recent, if at the US there are signs of occlusion with possible ischemia such as fluid between the loops and/or lack of peristalsis, if the patient is very young, or if the patient is much older. Differential diagnosis

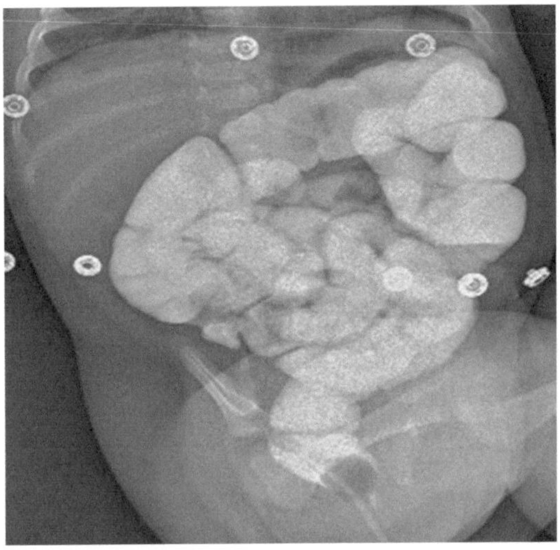

Fig. 13.8 Same patient as shown in Fig. 13.6. Radiograph at the end of US enema demonstrates that the procedure was successful

includes appendicitis, lymphoma, Meckel diverticulum, mesenteric adenitis, and gastrointestinal duplication cyst.

13.4 Acute Appendicitis

Acute appendicitis is the most common abdominal emergency in pediatric patients, and clinical diagnosis today is still relatively difficult [20–24].The incidence of acute appendicitis is an estimated 4 per 1000 cases per year in school-age children. It has a higher incidence in children between 5 and 15 years of age, and is rare under 2 years. In approximately one-third of school-age children, the onset is classic, characterized by periumbilical pain which migrates to the right lower quadrant (McBurney's point), followed by anorexia and vomiting, leukocytosis, and low-grade fever [8]. In children under 5 years of age, the clinical presentation of acute appendicitis is generally subtle, frequently resulting in a delayed diagnosis and potential complications, ranging from perforation, abscess formation, and rarely death. Furthermore, younger children often are unable to localize pain, or to clearly describe their symptoms. Early diagnosis is fundamental to reduce morbidity. Moreover, the risk of progression to diffuse peritonitis and perforation in children is higher than in adults, ranging from 20 to 50% [25]. Appendicitis is often confused clinically with gastroenteritis, due to diarrhea and vomiting occurring in 33–41%; in acute appendicitis, abdominal pain usually precedes vomiting, contrary to what happens in gastroenteritis [26]. Appendicitis is usually the result of the obstruction of its lumen, which becomes distended. The first event is obstruction caused by a fecalith(s), lymphoid hyperplasia, foreign bodies, and rarely parasites or tumor. Once the obstruction has occurred, the continuous mucus secretion inside the lumen causes increase in pressure, resulting in overdistention of the lumen. As the internal pressure exceeds capillary perfusion, venous engorgement leads to progressive ischemia. Since the mucous barrier is compromised by ischemia, bacterial proliferation occurs with the passage through the appendix wall, and consequent transparietal inflammation. Continued tissue ischemia results in appendiceal infarction and perforation.

13.4.1 Imaging

US is currently the initial imaging examination in the evaluation of children with suspected acute appendicitis. US is performed using a linear array transducer (5–12 MHz). The sensitivity and specificity of US alone in the diagnosis of appendicitis in children are estimated at 88 and 94%, respectively [27]. The anatomical references in the right lower quadrant to look for the appendix are the cecum, iliac vessels, and psoas muscle. The gradual pressure applied with the probe to bowel loops helps to differentiate normally collapsible bowel from the appendix, which is not compressible in appendicitis [28]. The appendix arises from the posteromedial wall of the cecum, a few centimeters below the ileocecal valve, although its distal tip may have a variable location. When imaging the appendix with US, it is important to try to visualize all of it, lumen up to the tip, but this is not always possible because both the length of the appendix and the site of the tip are very variable [29]. A normal appendix has an outer wall diameter of 6 mm or less, its lumen is compressible at the pressure of the probe, and it does not have substantial flow on color flow Doppler imaging [4]. The outer wall diameter is measured in the transverse plane of the appendix.

The maximal mural thickness (MMT) is also measured, which is an important morphologic criteria used to identify a normal or abnormal appendix on US. It is defined as the distance from the hyperechoic luminal interface to the outer hyperechoic line. Normal MMT in the young children, older children, and adolescent are 1.9 mm ± 0.4, 2.0 mm ± 0.5, and 2.1 mm ± 0.5, respectively. Other US findings of appendicitis include distention of the lumen, an outer wall diameter greater than 6 mm, non-compressibility of the lumen, and one or more appendicoliths (Fig. 13.9). On longitudinal images, the lumen of the appendix is distended by fluid, and often one or more appendicoliths can be found (Fig. 13.10). Increased vascularity of the appendicular wall at color Doppler is visible due to the inflammation, while decreased vascularity is appreciable in perforation/gangrenous changes (Fig. 13.11) [30].

The appearance of appendicular wall changes in advanced appendicitis. Thickened wall stratification is maintained in catarrhal forms, while stratification is lost in phlegmonous and gangrenous appendicitis; in those patients, there is a high risk of perforation (Fig. 13.12).

Perforation is generally associated with a diagnostic delay of more than 36 h. In tip appendicitis the rest of the appendix is normal (Fig. 13.13). Indirect signs of acute appendicitis on US include inflamed periappendiceal fat hyperechogenicity, enlarged lymph nodes, and free fluid. In secondary peritonitis, bowel loops are distended, there may be absent peristalsis, there is fluid between the bowel loops, there is hyperechogenicity of the pericecal fat, there is loss of the echogenic submucosal layer, and there may be abscess formation.

In the more complex or equivocal patients, CT with iodinated intravenous contrast can be

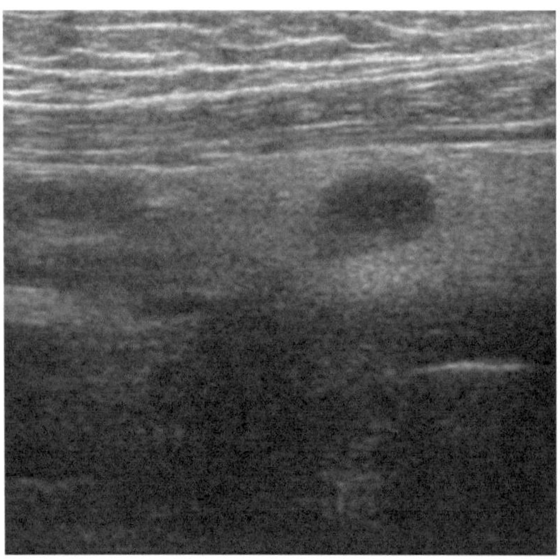

Fig. 13.9 Seven-year-old girl presenting with acute recurrent abdominal pain and fever which started 2 days earlier, as well as diarrhea, with appendicitis. US transverse image shows the distended lumen of the appendix, surrounded by hyperechoic mesenteric fat

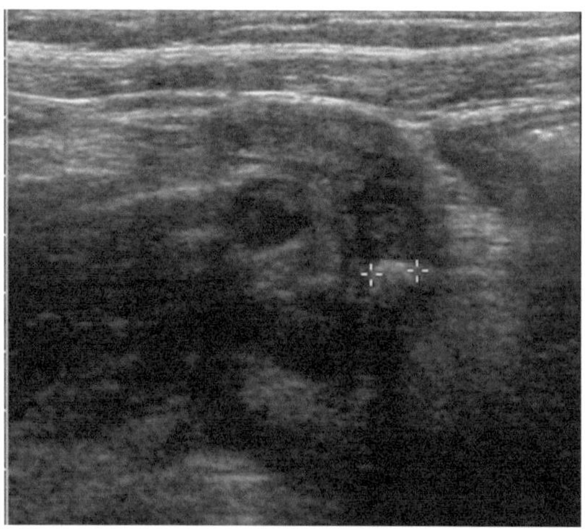

Fig. 13.10 Appendicitis. Nine-years-old boy presenting with severe abdominal pain; no fever. US longitudinal image shows thickening of the appendiceal wall, fluid distending the appendicular lumen, and an appendicolith (calipers)

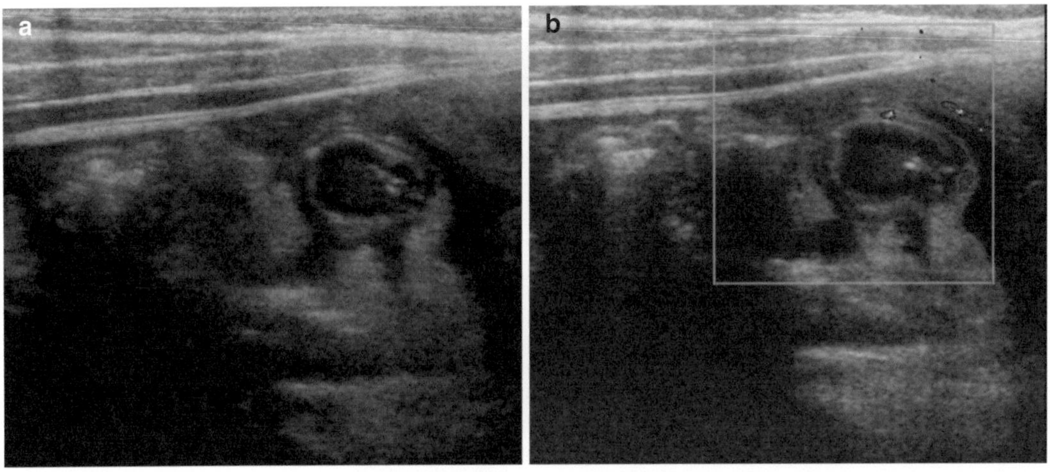

Fig. 13.11 (**a**, **b**) Ten-year-old boy presenting with fever and abdominal pain for 5 days, with appendicitis. US transverse image scan (**a**) shows the appendicular lumen distended with fluid, and an appendicolith. The appendix is surrounded by free fluid and hyperechoic mesenteric fat. The wall stratification is maintained; color Doppler shows parietal flow (**b**)

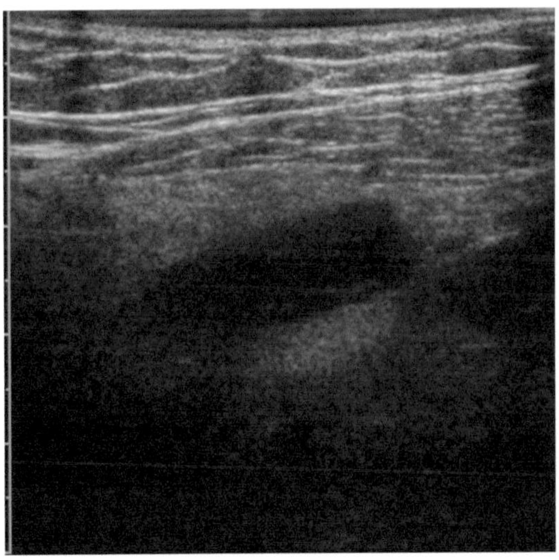

Fig. 13.12 Appendicitis. Ten-years-old boy with abdominal pain, abdominal distention, fever, diarrhea. US longitudinal image shows the appendiceal lumen distended by fluid, as well as loss of wall stratification. The appendix is surrounded by hyperechoic mesenteric fat

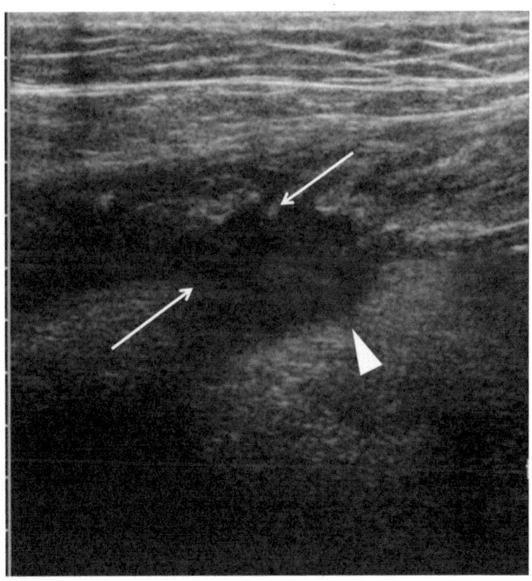

Fig. 13.13 Thirteen-year-old girl presenting with recent onset of pain in the lower abdominal quadrants. Tip appendicitis. US longitudinal image shows the tip of the appendix distended by fluid (arrows). Note loss of wall stratification and irregularity of the wall, whose profile blends into the surrounding mesenteric fat (arrowhead)

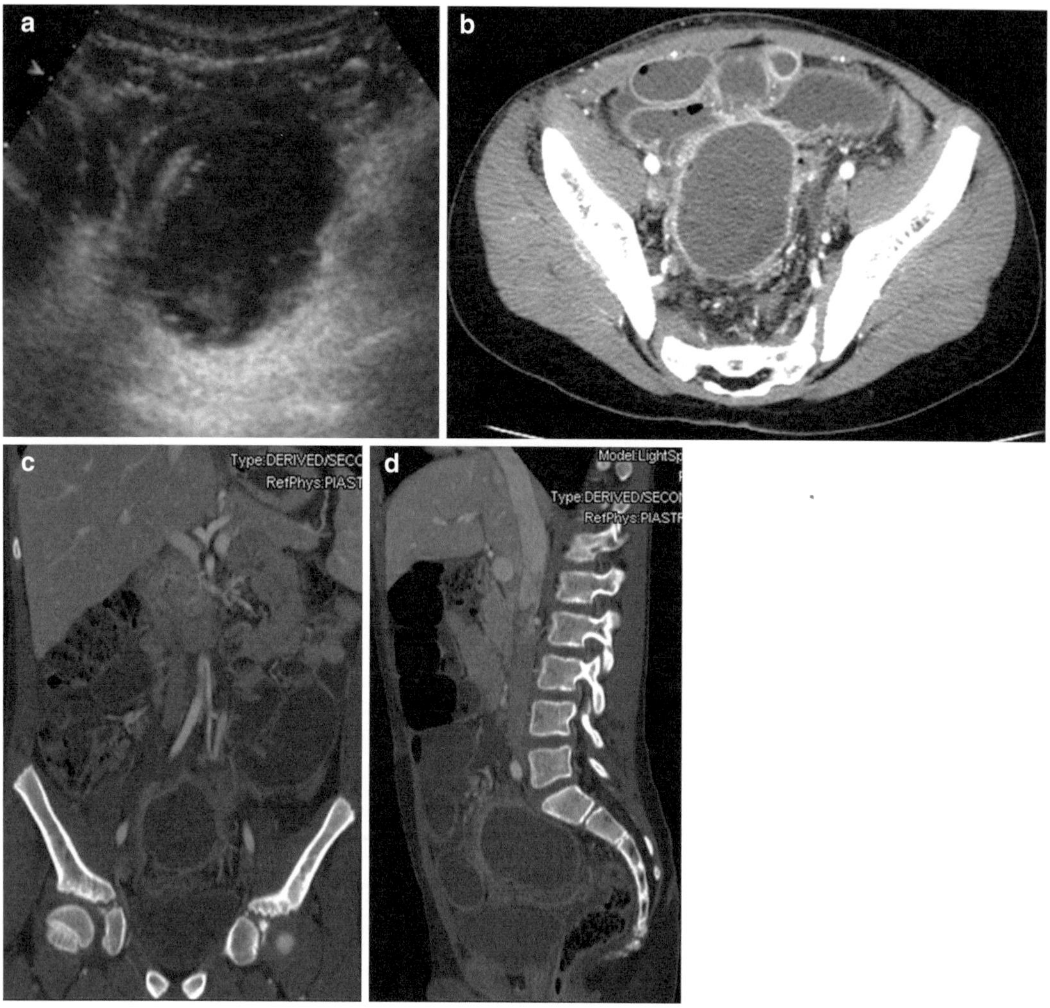

Fig. 13.14 (**a**–**d**) Nine-year-old boy presenting with abdominal pain and fever, and an appendiceal abscess. US transverse image with convex probe (**a**) shows a complex pelvic mass. Axial CT image (**b**) and multi-planar reconstructions (**c**, **d**) show a pelvic abscess surrounded by distended intestinal loops and free fluid, due to generalized peritonitis

performed (Fig. 13.14). In peritonitis, the infected fluid can extend from the pelvis to the scrotum (Fig. 13.15). Generalized bowel wall thickening may be found in the right lower quadrant [31]. In some patients, the clinical and laboratory diagnosis of appendicitis remains equivocal, even after US is performed [32]. In this scenario, the use of CT is becoming more frequent with the utilization of modern dosage reduction techniques. The radiologist, however, must not forget the ALARA principle and minimization of the radiation dose, and the responsibility for choosing the most accurate and appropriate imaging examination [33].

For these reasons, in the last few years, in patients with equivocal appendicitis, magnetic resonance imaging (MRI) is being increasingly used after US. The absence of ionizing radiation and the use of fast sequences make MR optimal [34]. Sequences usually include T2 half Fourier multi-planar images with and without fat saturation and T1-GRE images (Figs. 13.16 and 13.17). MRI also provides differential diagnoses, including Crohn disease, Meckel diverticulitis, mesenteric adenitis, ovarian torsion, and ovarian hemorrhagic cyst (Figs. 13.18 and 13.19).

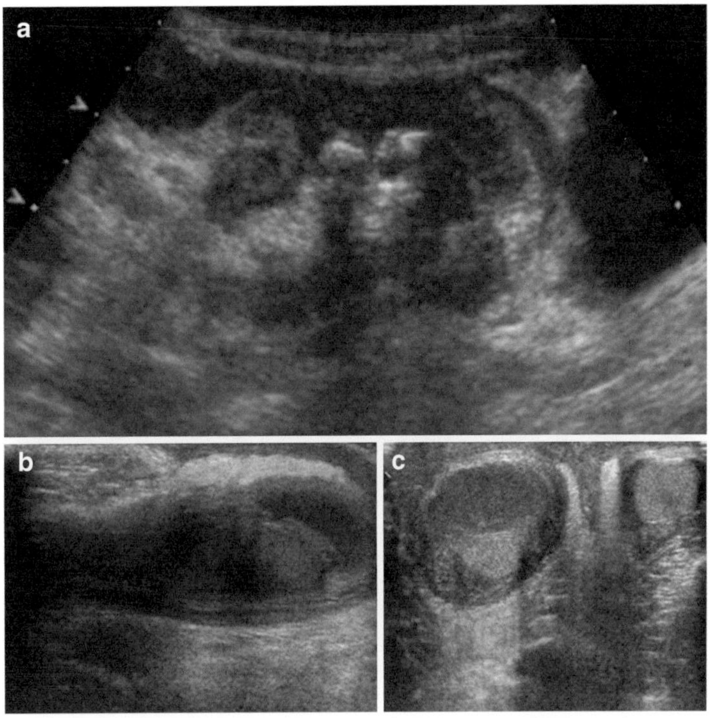

Fig. 13.15 (**a**–**c**) Ten-year-old boy, with 10 days of abdominal pain, and an appendiceal abscess. US transverse image with convex probe (**a**) shows a complex mass in right lower abdominal quadrant. US longitudinal and transverse images using a linear probe (**b**, **c**) show fluid, most noticeable in the right scrotum. Note the thickening and inhomogeneity of the scrotum wall due to the extension of the abscess through the inguinal canal

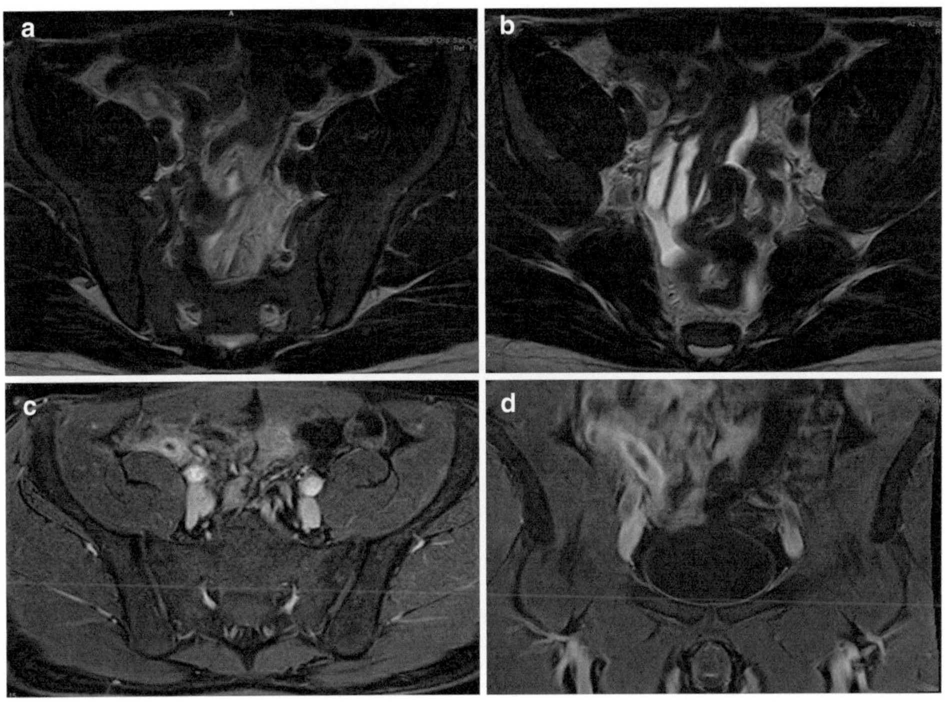

Fig. 13.16 (**a**–**d**) Seven-year-old girl with a positive US examination for appendicitis (not shown) but a nonspecific clinical presentation. T2-weighted axial images (**a**, **b**) show thickening of the appendiceal wall and of the mesenteric fat; (**c**, **d**) IV contrast-enhanced GRE T1-weighted MR images show enhancement of appendicular wall and of the adjacent mesenteric fat

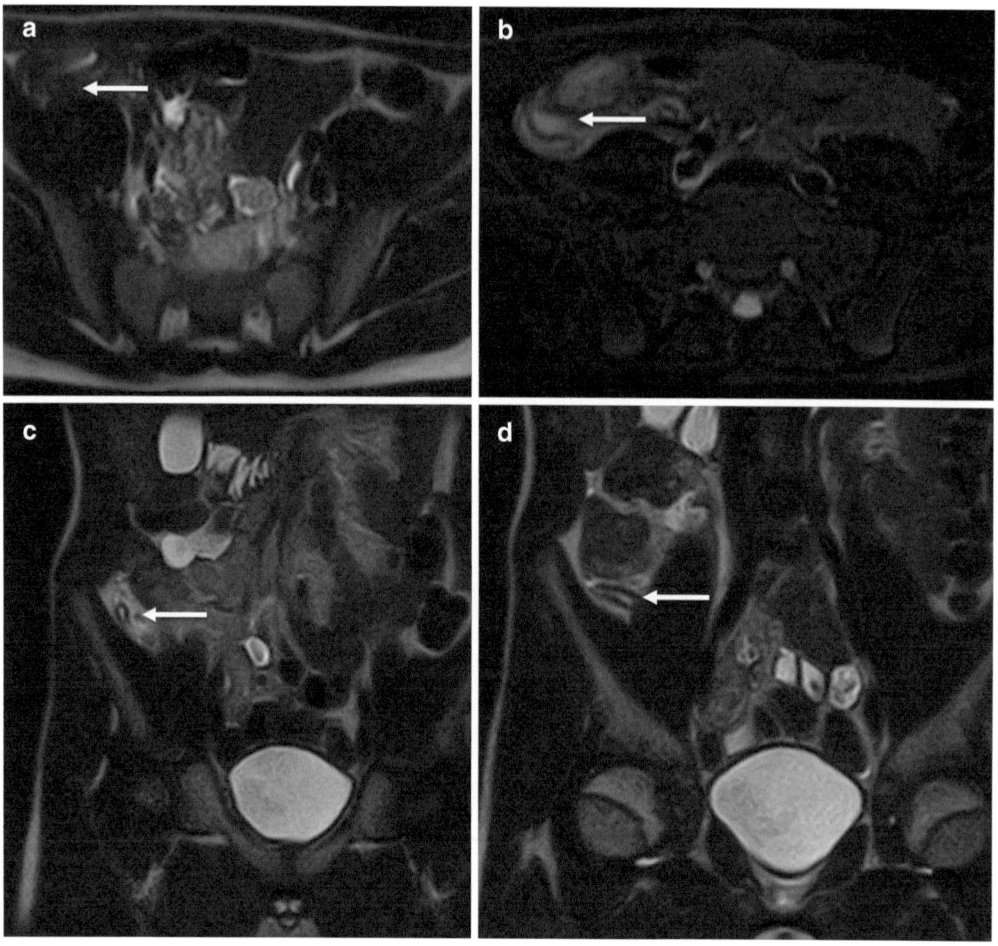

Fig. 13.17 (**a–d**) Ten-year-old girl with a positive US examination but with a nonspecific clinical presentation. T2-weighted axial MR image (**a**) shows a distended appendix (arrow), with a slightly thickened wall. T2-weighted fat-saturation MR axial image (**b**) demonstrates periappendicular edema (arrow). On T2-weighted coronal MR images (**c**, **d**), it is possible to follow the entire course of the appendix

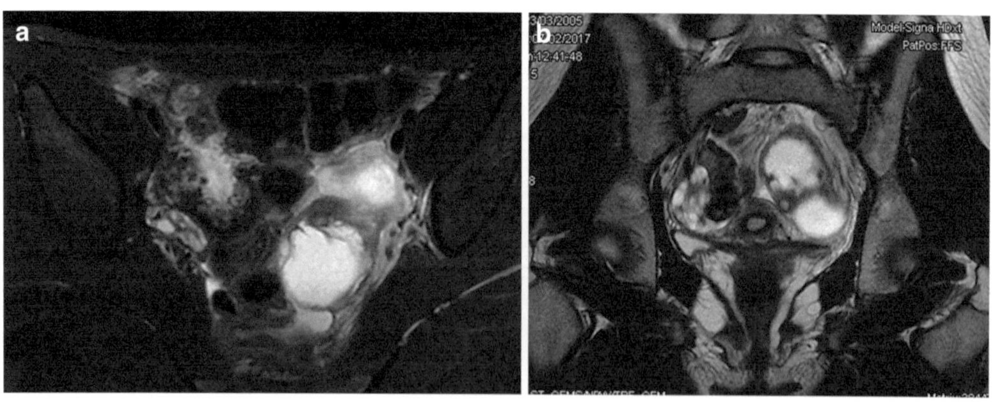

Fig. 13.18 (**a**, **b**) Thirteen-year-old girl with pain in the right lower quadrant, no fever, and normal serum white blood cell counts. T2-weighted axial (**a**) and coronal (**b**) MR images demonstrate a left ovarian cyst. There are also findings of torsion, with cyst wall thickening and a periovarian fluid collection. All these findings were proven at surgery

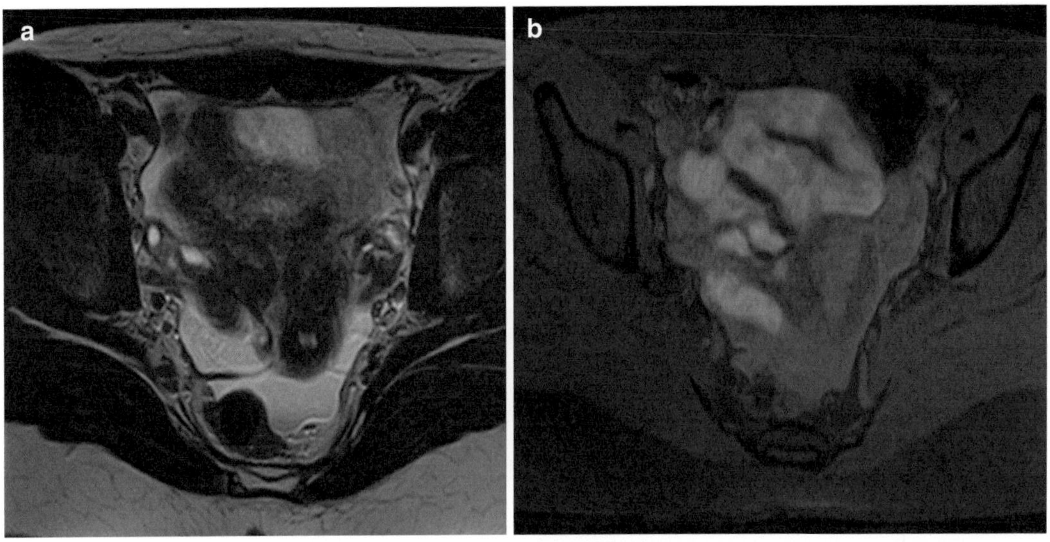

Fig. 13.19 (**a**, **b**) Twelve-year-old girl with pain in the lower abdominal quadrants, without fever. T2-weighted axial MR image (**a**) shows a complex ovarian mass and a large fluid collection in the pelvis. A T1-weighted 3D fat-saturation axial MR image (**b**) reveals high signal of the fluid, typical of hemorrhage

13.5 Meckel Diverticulitis

Meckel diverticulum is one of the most common congenital anomalies affecting the gastrointestinal tract, with a prevalence of 2%. It affects about 2% of the population, with slight male predominance [35]. Acute Meckel diverticulitis usually manifests with abdominal pain, fever, and vomiting. The clinical presentation cannot be distinguished from acute appendicitis. The differential diagnoses include appendicitis, inflammatory bowel disease, and pelvic inflammatory disease in female patients. Meckel diverticulum is a true diverticulum, due to an obliteration failure of the omphalomesenteric (vitelline) duct, which normally occurs at 7–8 weeks of gestation. It involves all layers of the ileal wall, and is lined by normal small bowel mucosa. It frequently contains heterotopic mucosa, usually of the gastric type. The ectopic tissue can also be pancreatic. It is located on the antimesenteric border of the intestine, at 80–85 cm above the ileocecal valve, and in 90% measures between 1 and 10 cm in length.

Most individuals are asymptomatic, and the Meckel diverticulum remains undiscovered. Many Meckel diverticula are discovered incidentally. Complications occur in around 15–30%, commonly before 2 years of age; Meckel diverticulum is the most common cause of intestinal hemorrhage in infants and children. Hemorrhage is usually due to erosion of adjacent ileal mucosa by acid produced by the ectopic gastric mucosa. Other complications include obstruction due to volvulus about the diverticulum, or intussusception, with the diverticulum as the leading point. Inflammation, or perforation, is another potential complication [36].

The clinical diagnosis of Meckel diverticulum is difficult, and usually the diagnosis is made by a radiologist or at surgery [37]. US is the imaging method which may reveal a Meckel diverticulum. It shows a right lower quadrant tubular blind-ending structure, which is connected to the small bowel, but not the cecum. The structure is noncompressible, with a thick and irregular hyperechoic internal wall (mucosa and submucosa), and a hypoechoic external wall (muscularis propria). The diverticulum may contain an air-fluid level, a fluid level suggestive of recent hemorrhage, simple fluid, or fecal-like material. When obstructed, the diverticulum is overdistended with fluid (Fig. 13.20) [38]. Other US features of Meckel diverticulitis include wall thickening, increased wall vascularization, fat stranding, and adjacent fluid collections. US and CT can demonstrate complications, including intestinal obstruction and intussusception (Fig. 13.21). The most frequent complication is enteric hemorrhage from peptic ulceration of ectopic gastric mucosa; this is usually painless. It can be massive, manifesting as red blood in the stool, with a texture comparable to "currant jelly" [40].

Technetium-99m pertechnetate scintigraphy is the imaging modality of choice for evaluating pediatric patients with gastrointestinal hemorrhage from a suspected Meckel diverticulum. Since mucous cells in the gastric epithelium uptake pertechnetate, after intravenous injection of Tc-99m pertechnetate, a Meckel diverticulum containing gastric-type epithelium will appear at scintigraphy as a small, rounded area of increased activity [40]. CT should be used in suspected complications including volvulus or intestinal occlusion, or if further evaluating for an intestinal bleeding site [41, 42].

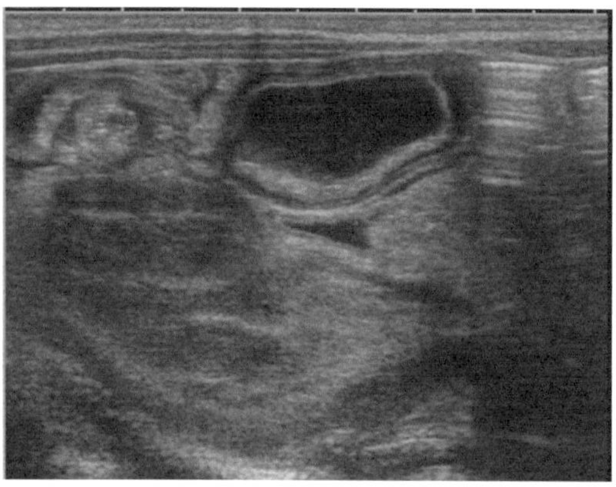

Fig. 13.20 Thirty-month-old boy, presenting with anemia. Meckel diverticulitis. US axial image shows a fluid-distended Meckel diverticulum, with a thickened wall. Note that the complex fluid content is consistent with recent hemorrhage

13.6 Henoch-Schonlein Purpura

Henoch-Schonlein purpura (HSP) is the most common childhood vasculitis. It can affect anyone, but is most common in children between 2 and 6 years, and more frequently involves boys. It is characterized by palpable purpura, arthritis or arthralgia, colicky abdominal pain, and nephritis. It is generally an acute self-limited vasculitis involving the small vessels of the skin, gastrointestinal tract, kidneys, joints, and rarely lungs and central nervous system. The most striking feature of HSP is a purplish palpable rash, typically on the lower legs and buttocks. It is a multisystemic small vessel vasculitis which involves the gastrointestinal tract, causing diffuse abdominal pain due to submucosal bowel hemorrhage and edema.

Henoch-Schonlein purpura is generally benign and has a good prognosis, responding to

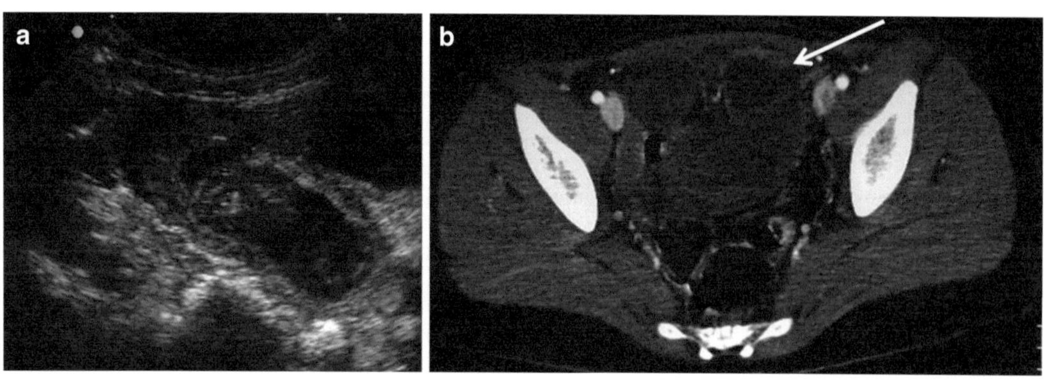

Fig. 13.21 (**a**, **b**) Three-year-old boy, presenting with an acute abdomen. US (**a**) shows a Meckel diverticulum intussuscepted within an intestinal loop, causing obstruction. IV contrast-enhanced abdominal CT (**b**) confirms the Meckel diverticulum and the intussusception (arrow) and associated intestinal obstruction

corticosteroid therapy in most patients. However, severe complications including intussusception, massive gastrointestinal bleeding, and intestinal perforation can occur.

HSP can be confused clinically with appendicitis, intussusception, and other disorders. Gastrointestinal symptoms include abdominal pain, melena, bloody diarrhea, hematemesis, duodenal ulcers, and massive hemorrhage. No specific diagnostic laboratory test is available to assess for HSP. Treatment remains primarily supportive in most patients, and surgery may also be considered in specific circumstances including severe bowel ischemia.

Early detection of intestinal ischemia is crucial. Delayed diagnosis can result in intestinal perforation and peritonitis, which are severe and potentially life-threatening complications.

If a fluoroscopic examination is performed, irregular caliber loops of jejunum and ileum with hypertonic, contracted loops alternating with dilated ones may be seen. The margins of the contracted, hypertonic loops are very irregular, with loss of mucosal architecture in some areas. The irregular mucosal outline is suggestive of ulceration. US findings include thickening of the bowel wall, which appears hyperechoic, or hypoechoic if there is substantial edema of the wall, dilatation of the lumen, and prominence of the valvulae. Often, free fluid is present (Fig. 13.22). This condition can be complicated by ileoileal intussusception, as noted [43, 44].

13.7 Mesenteric Adenitis

Mesenteric lymphadenitis is one of the most common diagnoses identified at US (or CT) performed for abdominal pain in pediatric patients. Mesenteric lymphadenitis is due to an inflammatory process which occurs most frequently in the right lower quadrant. However, it may also be secondary to appendicitis, intussusception, and intestinal occlusion [45]. Mesenteric lymphadenitis often mimics appendicitis clinically. Lymph node enlargement can be found in approximately 40% of patients with appendicitis, but the absence of a blind-ending tubular structure in the right lower quadrant suggests the diagnosis of mesenteric lymphadenitis, if no other reason is found [9, 28, 45]. US shows multiple, enlarged, rounded, and hypoechoic mesenteric clustered lymph nodes, which may be painful when graded compression is applied with the US

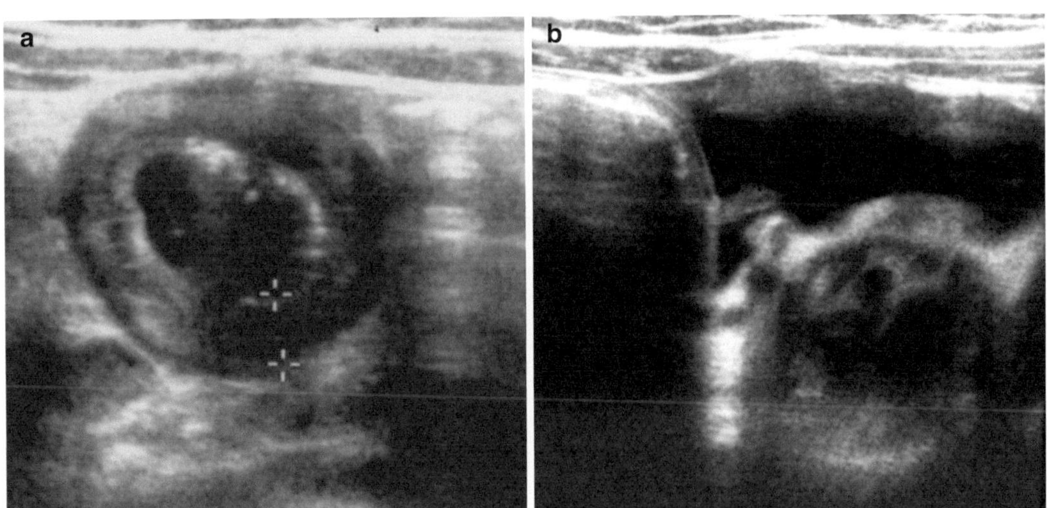

Fig. 13.22 (**a**, **b**) Ten-year-old boy, presenting with acute abdominal pain and palpable purpura on the body, due to Henoch-Schonlein purpura. US shows thickening of hypoechoic bowel wall (calipers). The lumen is distended by fluid (**a**), and free fluid is also present (**b**)

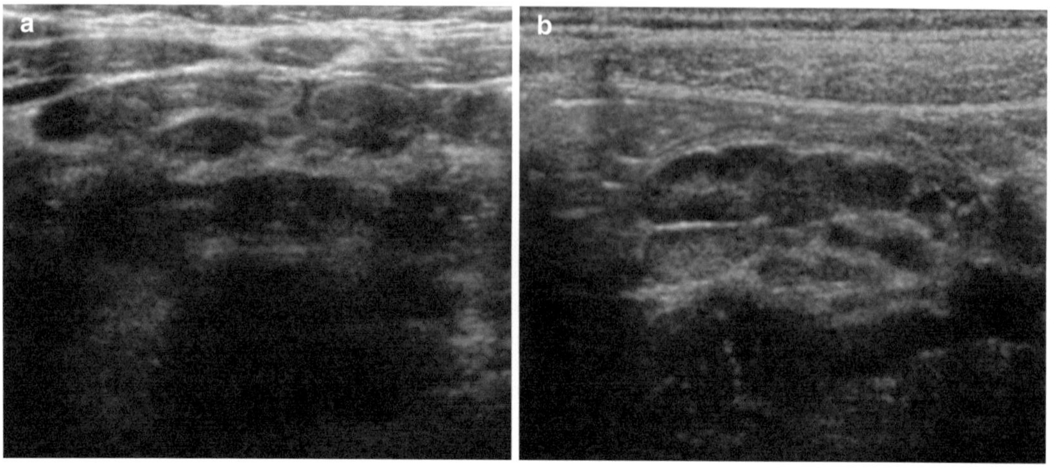

Fig. 13.23 Mesenteric adenitis. Axial (**a**) and longitudinal (**b**) US images show multiple enlarged lymph nodes in the mesenteric fat, which is hyperechoic

probe (Fig. 13.23). Enlarged lymph nodes are often associated with thickening of the adjacent bowel wall.

Conclusion

Abdominal pain is one of the most frequent reasons for a visit to the pediatric emergency department, whose main task is to identify or exclude an emergency condition, and particularly a surgical emergency (acute appendicitis and intussusception, in particular).

After 2 years of age, the most common cause of acute abdominal pain usually requiring surgery is acute appendicitis, whose evolution is often rapid and progressive. Clinical observation and imaging of acute abdominal and pelvic pain especially with ultrasound are particularly recommended in the first 3–4 years of life, when clinical findings are often nonspecific and these young patients cannot provide a reliable history.

References

1. Cardoni G, Fabiani E, Vignini M. Il dolore addominale acuto. Rivista di emergenza ed urgenza pediatrica. 2009;3(1):5–17.
2. Hernanz-Schulman M. CT and US in the diagnosis of appendicitis: an argument for CT. Radiology. 2010;255:3–7.
3. Brenner DJ, Hall EJ. Computed tomography: an increasing source of radiation exposure. N Engl J Med. 2007;357:2277–84.
4. Cogley JR, O'Connor SC, Houshyar R, et al. Emergent pediatric US: what every radiologist should know. Radiographics. 2012;32:651–65.
5. Hryhorczuk AL, Mannix RC, Taylor GA. Pediatric abdominal pain: use of imaging in the emergency department in the United States from 1999 to 2007. Radiology. 2012;263:778–85.
6. Lochead A, Jamjoom R, Ratnapalan S. Intussusception in children presenting to the emergency department. Clin Pediatr (Phila). 2013;52:1029–33.
7. Galluzzo M, Gaudino F, Palliola R, et al. Intestinal intussusception. In: Miele V, Trinci M, editors. Imaging non-traumatic abdominal emergencies in pediatric patients. Switzerland: Springer International Publisher; 2016. p. 133–47.
8. Strouse PJ. Sonographic evaluation of the child with lower abdominal or pelvic pain. Radiol Clin North Am. 2006;44(6):911–23.
9. Di Giacomo V, Trinci M, Van der Byl G, et al. Ultrasound in newborns and children suffering from non-traumatic acute abdominal pain: imaging with clinical and surgical correlation. J Ultrasound. 2014;18:385–93.
10. del-Pozo G, Albillos JC, Tejedor D, et al. Intussusception in children: current concepts in diagnosis and enema reduction. Radiographics. 1999;19:299–319.
11. John SD. The value of ultrasound in children with suspected intussusception. Emerg Radiol. 1998;5:297–305.
12. Hryhorczuk AL, Strouse PJ. Validation of US as a first-line diagnostic test for assessment of pediatric ileocolic intussusception. Pediatr Radiol. 2009;39:1075–9.

13. Ko HS, Schenk JP, Tröger J, et al. Current radiological management of intussusception in children. Eur Radiol. 2007;17:2411–21.
14. Lim HK, Bae SH, Lee KH, et al. Assessment of reducibility of ileocolic intussusception in children: usefulness of color Doppler sonography. Radiology. 1994;191:781–5.
15. Sargent MA, Babyn P, Alton DJ. Plain abdominal radiography in suspected intussusception: a reassessment. Pediatr Radiol. 1994;24:17–20.
16. Niramis R, Watanatittan S, Kruatrachue A, et al. Management of recurrent intussusception: nonoperative or operative reduction? J Pediatr Surg. 2010;45:2175–80.
17. Flaum V, Schneider A, Ferreira CG, et al. Twenty years' experience for reduction of ileocolic intussusception by saline enema under sonography control. J Pediatr Surg. 2015;51:179–82.
18. Stein M, Alton DJ, Daneman A. Pneumatic reduction of intussusception: 5-years experience. Radiology. 1992;183:681–4.
19. Grosfeld JL. Intussusception then and now: a historical vignette. J Am Coll Surg. 2005;201:830–3.
20. Kaiser S, Frenckner B, Jorulf HK. Suspected appendicitis in children: US and CT—a prospective randomized study. Radiology. 2002;223:633–8.
21. Kosloske AM, Love CL, Rohrer JE, et al. The diagnosis of appendicitis in children: outcomes of a strategy based on pediatric surgical evaluation. Pediatrics. 2004;113:29–34.
22. Rabah R. Pathology of the appendix in children: an institutional experience and review of the literature. Pediatr Radiol. 2007;37:15–20.
23. Sivit CJ, Siegel MJ, Applegate KE, et al. When appendicitis is suspected in children. Radiographics. 2001;21:247–62.
24. Wiersma F, Toorenvliet BR, Bloem JL, et al. US examination of the appendix in children with suspected appendicitis: the additional value of secondary signs. Eur Radiol. 2009;19:455–61.
25. Klein MD. Clinical approach to a child with abdominal pain who might have appendicitis. Pediatr Radiol. 2007;37:11–4.
26. van Breda Vriesman AC, Puylaert JB. Mimics of appendicitis: alternative nonsurgical diagnoses with sonography and CT. Am J Roentgenol. 2006;186(4):1103–12.
27. Doria AS, Moineddin R, Kellenberger CJ, et al. US or CT for diagnosis of appendicitis in children and adults? A meta-analysis. Radiology. 2006;241:83–94.
28. Puylaert JB. Acute appendicitis: US evaluation using graded compression. Radiology. 1986;158:355–60.
29. Birnbaum BA, Wilson SR. Appendicitis at the millennium. Radiology. 2000;215:337–48.
30. Buquicchio GL, Cuneo G, Giannecchini S, et al. Acute appendicitis. In: Miele V, Trinci M, editors. Imaging non-traumatic abdominal emergencies in pediatric patients. Switzerland: Springer International Publisher; 2016. p. 149–70.
31. Kessler N, Cyteval C, Gallix B, et al. Appendicitis: evaluation of sensitivity, specificity, and predictive values of US, Doppler US, and laboratory findings. Radiology. 2004;230:472–8.
32. Papes D, Medancic SS, Antabak A, et al. What is the acceptable rate of negative appendicectomy? Comment of the prospective evaluation of the added value of imaging within the Dutch National diagnostic appendicitis guideline—do we forget our clinical eye? Dig Surg. 2015;32:181–2.
33. Singh S, Kaira MK, Shenoy-Bhangle AS, et al. Radiation dose reduction with hybrid iterative reconstruction for pediatric CT. Radiology. 2012;263:537–46.
34. Imler D, Keller C, Sivasankar S, et al. Magnetic resonance imaging versus ultrasound as the initial imaging modality for pediatric and young adult patients with suspected appendicitis. Acad Emerg Med. 2017;24:569–77.
35. Moore MM, Kulaylat AN, Hollenbeak CS, et al. Magnetic resonance imaging in pediatric appendicitis: a systematic review. Pediatr Radiol. 2016;46:928–39.
36. Cullen JJ, Kelly KA, Moir CR, et al. Surgical management of Meckel's diverticulum: an epidemiologic, population-based study. Ann Surg. 1994;220:564–8.
37. Pantongrag-Brown L, Levine MS, Buetow PC, et al. Meckel's enteroliths: clinical, radiologic, and pathologic findings. Am J Roentgenol. 1996;167:1447–50.
38. Maglinte DD, Elmore MF, Isenberg M, et al. Meckel diverticulum: radiologic demonstration by enteroclysis. Am J Roentgenol. 1980;134:925–32.
39. Daneman A, Lobo E, Alton DJ, et al. The value of sonography, CT and air enema for detection of complicated Meckel diverticulum in children with nonspecific clinical presentation. Pediatr Radiol. 1998;28:928–32.
40. Levy AD, Hobbs CM. From the archives of the AFIP. Meckel diverticulum: radiologic features with pathologic correlation. Radiographics. 2004;24:565–87.
41. Blumhardt R, Growcock GW, Hartshorne MF, et al. Patterns of intestinal activity with Meckel's scintigraphy. Gastrointest Radiol. 1984;9:353–6.
42. Miele V, De Cicco ML, Andreoli C, Buffa V, Adami L, David V. US and CT findings in complicated Meckel diverticulum. Radiol Med. 2001;101:230–4.
43. Esposito JJ. Small intestinal abnormalities in anaphylactoid purpura: report of two cases. Radiology. 1950;55:548–52.
44. Miller JH, Kemberling CR. Ultrasound scanning of the gastrointestinal tract in children: subject review. Radiology. 1984;152:671–7.
45. Quillin SP, Siegel MJ. Color Doppler US of children with acute lower abdominal pain. Radiographics. 1993;13:1281–93.

MIX
Papier aus verantwortungsvollen Quellen
Paper from responsible sources
FSC® C105338

If you have any concerns about our products,
you can contact us on
ProductSafety@springernature.com

In case Publisher is established outside the EU,
the EU authorized representative is:
Springer Nature Customer Service Center GmbH
Europaplatz 3, 69115 Heidelberg, Germany

Printed by Libri Plureos GmbH
in Hamburg, Germany